More Advance Praise fo

"Patients and family members often
but increasingly burdensome admini........... ... .
it challenging for care providers to spend enough time with their patients. To cope,
clinicians may refer patients to other sources of information, use asynchronous
forms of communication, or rely on sophisticated diagnostic tests or medical procedures to answer questions that may not have been needed if only they had more
time to spend with their patients.

"Communication between clinician and patient is the cornerstone of accurate
and timely diagnosis, and critically important for establishing the therapeutic alli-
ance and empowering the patient and family to be active participants. But if we
can't undo the pressures of today on the practice of medicine, what can we do? How
can care providers stay true to the Hippocratic Oath and 'remember that there is art
to medicine as well as science, and that warmth, sympathy, and understanding may
outweigh the surgeon's knife or the chemist's drug' and that clinicians 'do not treat
a fever chart, a cancerous growth, but a sick human being' (http://en.wikipedia.org/
wiki/Hippocratic_Oath)?

"The answer may be found in 'How Many More Questions?' Techniques for
Clinical Interviews of Young Medically Ill Children. Drs. Caplan and Bursch, both
very experienced and renowned clinicians, provide the necessary tools to make the
most efficient use of clinical interviews, and in particular interviews with medically
ill children.

"With sensitivity and compassion for young children, and a focus on pragmatic
and feasible solutions, the authors stress the importance of approaching clinical
interviews in the contexts of the developmental stage of the child's communication skills, the impact of the specific illness on those skills, and the emotional and
behavioral issues that so often arise from physical and psychological suffering, at
times overshadowing the underlying illness, as may occur with epilepsy. Further
compounding the barriers to effective communication, and also addressed by the
authors, are the stresses and uncertainties of an acute and serious illness and the
bewildering complexity of the medical establishment.

"Clinicians who learn and adopt the techniques described in this unique and
essential book will quickly see benefits in their understanding of their patients' conditions and in addition will feel more enriched by the time they spend with patients,
happily remembering why they dedicated their lives to caring for patients."
—*Steven C. Schachter, MD,* Beth Israel Deaconess Medical Center, Boston, MA

"Caplan and Bursch have teamed up to write a textbook that addresses the topic of
the clinical assessment of the young medically ill child. This book fills a unique spot
in the scientific literature. Condensing years of clinical wisdom, the authors outline twelve essential developmental guidelines that should be considered in interviews of all children. These guidelines are accompanied by detailed, real life case
vignettes that illustrate specific interviewing approaches and, equally important,
which words and questions to avoid. These principles come to life in the second section of the book where they are used to show how careful, developmentally appropriate interviewing techniques form the cornerstone of the diagnostic assessment.

The reader of this book will gain a practical and detailed knowledge of ways to assist the young child in explaining their psychological reactions to physical illness.

"One of the unexpected pleasures in reading this book is that it provides a concise yet remarkably comprehensive review of the psychological issues in children with epilepsy. Using the developmental guidelines outlined earlier in the book, Caplan and Bursch emphasize the presence and significance of comorbid psychiatric illness with a series of detailed case vignettes. This topic is expanded in the thorough review of cognitive and language difficulties in pediatric epilepsy and the impact of these issues on the child's family. The topics of pediatric pain, medical trauma, and terminal illness receive a similarly thoughtful analysis. Throughout, the text is supplemented with summaries and numerous informative tables that help consolidate the reader's learning. This book will appeal not only to new trainees in the field but also serves as a valuable resource for seasoned practitioners. It is undoubtedly destined to become one of the core texts for professionals who work with young medically ill children."

—*Richard J. Shaw, MD,* Professor of Psychiatry and Pediatrics,
Department of Psychiatry and Behavior Sciences,
Stanford University School of Medicine, Palo Alto, CA

"In this important and innovative book, Caplan and Bursch utilize a developmentally sensitive framework to provide professionals from a variety of disciplines with the interviewing skills necessary to conduct challenging clinical interviews with young children who have medical, psychiatric, and/or neurological illnesses. They proffer developmental guidelines for how to obtain accurate clinical information from young children. The authors also present engaging and excellent clinical vignettes throughout the volume that illustrate the principles of developmentally sensitive interviewing with a variety of high-risk youngsters. I enthusiastically recommend this book. It is a major addition to the literature. It will be of great benefit to a wide range of professionals who work with young children with medical illnesses."

—*Dante Cicchetti, PhD,* McKnight Presidential Chair,
William Harris Professor, and Professor of Child Psychology and Psychiatry,
Institute of Child Development, University of Minnesota, Minneapolis, MN

"Caplan and Bursch understand how to talk to, and how to listen to, children. They also understand how to talk to adults who are struggling to do the same. In this remarkably successful book they provide us with a clear understanding of the child's world view, and with example after example, they show how what we think we are saying as adults can be heard differently. The range of this exploration is significant, moving from common anxieties about common medical procedures to the more rare expressions of psychosis. With confidence borne from experience, they deal skillfully with the variety and richness of material and allow one to practice and explore our own habits. They have achieved something rare with this volume. It is scholarly and authoritative, but accessible and practical."

—*Christopher Eccleston, PhD,* Centre for Pain Research,
The University of Bath, UK

"*'How Many More Questions?' Techniques for Clinical Interviews of Young Medically Ill Children* by Rochelle Caplan and Brenda Bursch is an essential, practical, developmentally sensitive guide for clinicians learning to elicit useful and accurate information from young children including those with language deficits or other mild cognitive impairments. They perceptively cover a broad range of challenging topics from talking with children who have epilepsy and its concomitant psychiatric, cognitive, linguistic, and psychosocial comorbidities to talking with children who have experienced medical trauma or are dying of a terminal illness. In the same conversational manner they might use with a child, the authors patiently and systematically walk the reader through how to sort out the nuances between whether psychological symptoms arise from a disease, from the treatment of the disease, from the impact of other complex psychosocial factors or from the onset of a pre-existing psychiatric syndrome. They provide step-by-step ways to approach talking about psychological symptoms and discuss how these can come together to develop into specific disorders such as major depression or separation anxiety disorder. Through the use of actual cases that emphasize how children are essential informants in their care, we also see how children, parents and interviewers can mislead or misinterpret one another when the interview is not led in a thoughtful and intentional manner. As the authors suggest, children can detect the genuinely caring and interested interviewer and appreciate when the interviewer helps them express themselves. The gentle wisdom and accumulated knowledge of Caplan and Bursch comes shining through as they take our hand and walk us through the many questions we have to ask children to understand their cognitive and emotional experiences of medical care. Just as children often ask, 'Are we there yet?', Caplan and Bursch take us on a learning journey and expertly help us arrive at our destination of how to communicate clearly with children."

—*Maryland Pao, MD,* Bethesda, Maryland

"Thanks to Caplan and Bursch for providing an excellent reference for all practitioners who interact with young children as they sort out differential diagnoses involving physical, emotional and cognitive symptoms. The book contains many sample interviews that illustrate effective techniques along with examples of well-intended questions that can shut down a child's communication leading to misdiagnosis or inappropriate treatments. The authors give practical guidelines so that clinicians can become the child's 'communication assistant' or 'coach' partnering with the child and family to find the best possible solutions for their presenting issues. I particularly appreciate the section that focuses on two of the most common somatic complaints, headaches and stomach aches, providing a laundry list of potential causes. The chapter discussing terminal illness is another invaluable component. This book is like having the Child Psychiatric Consult/Liaison team in your pocket."

—*Beatrice Yorker, RN, MS, JD,* Dean and Professor of Nursing, College of Health and Human Services, California State University, Los Angeles

"History is without question the most important diagnostic tool in the armamentarium of anyone who provides healthcare to children, and yet it is often the most challenging thing to obtain. Critical portions of the history can only be obtained from the child him or herself. Parents cannot feel the quality or intensity of a child's pain, describe what they see or feel prior to the onset of a seizure or a headache, nor why they feel angry, sad, or afraid. Recognizing the need for this information, however, does not tell the provider how to effectively elicit it. That is why this wonderful book by Rochelle Caplan and Brenda Bursch is such a gift to any healthcare professional who needs to communicate effectively with kids, be it pediatricians, pediatric subspecialists such as neurologists or psychiatrists, nurses, psychologists, or social workers. By providing clear and concise information on developmental differences in how children understand and use language and translating this into practical guidelines in how to most effectively communicate with children of different ages, this book provides an essential reference for pediatric healthcare professionals."

—*Amy Brooks-Kayal, MD,* Chief and Ponzio Family Chair in Pediatric Neurology, Children's Hospital Colorado, Professor of Pediatrics, Neurology, and Pharmaceutical Sciences, University of Colorado, Denver, CO

"At last—a book that teaches the keys to clinical practice with children! This book is long overdue in numerous fields of work with medically ill children. How can we help children if we don't know how to talk with them and to help them talk with us? This book is a goldmine of information; it provides an excellent review of symptoms of a number of childhood disorders associated with medical conditions. The choice of epilepsy as a disorder for in-depth examination is appropriate because it is a chronic medical disease with a number of psychosocial, behavioral, cognitive, and psychiatric co-morbidities. The principles of interviewing demonstrated for use with a variety of conditions experienced by children with epilepsy can easily be transferred to other disorders.

"The authors present an excellent review of symptoms of a number of emotional and behavioral disorders associated with medical and psychiatric conditions. The concise literature reviews provide a comprehensive basis for conceptualizing the conditions and the concrete examples of questions provide the starting point for gaining rapport and conducting effective interviews. The provision of sample interviews illustrating the rights and wrongs of asking children about their symptoms and opinions are invaluable. These vignettes also illustrate how to bring the parents into the picture by obtaining the permission and establishing the readiness of the child.

"The clear guidelines and concrete tools for interviewing can be used by a wide variety of clinicians ranging from beginners to seasoned professionals. This book will be invaluable for trainees in a variety of mental health, counseling, and medical programs, and for more advanced practitioners to enhance their skills. I will certainly be using this book in my teaching and to enrich my own practice."

—*Mary Lou Smith, PhD, CPsych,* Department of Psychology, University of Toronto; and Neuropsychologist and Associate Senior Scientist, Neurosciences and Mental Health Program, The Hospital for Sick Children, Toronto, Ontario, Canada

"How Many More Questions?"

"How Many More Questions?"

Techniques for Clinical Interviews of Young Medically Ill Children

ROCHELLE CAPLAN, MD

PROFESSOR EMERITUS

DEPARTMENT OF PSYCHIATRY & BIOBEHAVIORAL SCIENCES

DAVID GEFFEN SCHOOL OF MEDICINE

UNIVERSITY OF CALIFORNIA, LOS ANGELES

LOS ANGELES, CA

BRENDA BURSCH, PhD

PROFESSOR

DEPARTMENT OF PSYCHIATRY & BIOBEHAVIORAL SCIENCES

DEPARTMENT OF PEDIATRICS

DAVID GEFFEN SCHOOL OF MEDICINE

UNIVERSITY OF CALIFORNIA, LOS ANGELES

LOS ANGELES, CA

ILLUSTRATED BY AMARA LEIPZIG

OXFORD
UNIVERSITY PRESS

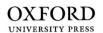

UNIVERSITY PRESS

Oxford University Press is a department of the University of Oxford. It furthers the University's
objective of excellence in research, scholarship, and education by publishing worldwide.

Oxford   New York
Auckland   Cape Town   Dar es Salaam   Hong Kong   Karachi
Kuala Lumpur   Madrid   Melbourne   Mexico City   Nairobi
New Delhi   Shanghai   Taipei   Toronto

With offices in
Argentina   Austria   Brazil   Chile   Czech   Republic   France   Greece
Guatemala   Hungary   Italy   Japan   Poland   Portugal   Singapore
South Korea   Switzerland   Thailand   Turkey   Ukraine   Vietnam

Oxford is a registered trademark of Oxford University Press in the UK and certain other countries.

Published in the United States of America by
Oxford University Press
198 Madison Avenue, New York, NY 10016

© Oxford University Press 2013

Library of Congress Cataloging-in-Publication Data
Caplan, Rochelle.
  "How many more questions?" : techniques for clinical interviews of young
  medically ill children/Rochelle Caplan, Brenda Bursch.
     p. ; cm.
  Includes bibliographical references.
  ISBN 978-0-19-984382-4 (pbk)
  I. Bursch, Brenda. II. Title.
  [DNLM: 1. Medical History Taking—methods. 2. Child Psychology.
  3. Child. 4. Interview, Psychological—methods. 5. Mental Disorders—diagnosis.
  WB 290]
  LC Classification not assigned
  618.92'8914—dc23
  2012006848

Printed in the United States of America on acid-free paper

I dedicate this book to my four master clinician mentors. Alexander Fallik, MD, and Lydia Peket, MD, taught me the importance of talking with each and every patient in the patient's language (whatever it might be, including a psychotic language) and establishing rapport through genuine interest in the patient's life, humor, and empathy. From Avraham G. Szekely, MD, and Aliza Blum, MD, I learned how to talk to toddlers and older children, respecting them as essential informants about their lives.

This book is the product of knowledge gained from applying these clinical principles and my developmental psycholinguistic clinical studies. And most importantly, it represents what the children I have treated have taught me about how to ask them questions while making sure they do not ask me, "How many more questions?" My thanks go to my pediatric neurology, psychiatry, and other multidisciplinary colleagues for referring me all these children.

Last but not least, none of this would have happened without the love and support of my husband, Dick, and daughters, Leah and Sarit Platkin, and the joy of working together with my amazing co-author and colleague, Brenda Bursch, PhD.

—Rochelle Caplan

During my college years, I worked in a café at a marina. One summer day, a houseboat exploded at the gas dock. The houseboat was filled with disabled children and several adults. I was trained as an emergency medic, but was still surprised that I could improve the vital signs of the burn victims by my verbal and nonverbal communication. This experience revealed to me that there was a need to teach the psychological side of medicine and that communication skills can impact health outcomes. This has become the theme of my career. Needless to say, it was an honor to be asked by Rochelle Caplan to join her in writing this book. She had the vision for the book as well as the generosity to allow me to be a true partner in writing it.

I dedicate this book to my parents, Jack Bursch and Charlene Jetter, for their emotional and financial support that has allowed me to achieve my educational goals; to David Beck, MD, and Margi Stuber, MD, for recognizing me as one of their people before I even had sufficient knowledge or training to function as one; and to Jim for being Jim, especially on Saturdays.

—Brenda Bursch

CONTENTS

PART V Brief Review and Next Steps

ACKNOWLEDGMENTS

We wish to express our gratitude to Craig Panner at Oxford University Press for his longstanding interest in our book and encouragement to tackle this project. We thank Craig, as well as Kathryn Winder and Karen Kwak, also at Oxford University Press, for their helpful, patient, and prompt responses to our many questions and requests.

We thank several family members for their assistance. Jim Bursch put in hours of time to review earlier drafts of our chapters and to figure out how to tell us when our writing was incomprehensible. Despite their time constraints, Dick, Leah, and Sarit Platkin gave us very helpful comments and critiques.

A number of our colleagues also reviewed our work and provided us with much appreciated feedback, including Miya Asato, MD, Assistant Professor, Pediatrics and Psychiatry, University of Pittsburgh School of Medicine; Sue Yudovin, RN, MN, CPNP, Associate Clinical Professor, UCLA School of Nursing; and Jessica Joseph Bernacki, MS, Pediatric Consultation-Liaison Psychology Intern, UCLA Semel Institute for Neuroscience and Human Behavior. Thank you very much for making time in your busy schedules to support us in this way.

Also enthusiastically contributing to our book were three children who drew pictures for us with the support of their family members. Cassandra Martinez, Lacresha Collins, and Aaron Watson are three brave children with the hospital experience to be considered experts on this subject. Their drawings were made after they heard a description of the book and were asked if they wished to draw something about being sick, being in a health-care setting, or communicating with an adult. Thank you for your excellent work and for teaching us so much, Good job!

We were extremely grateful for our illustrator, Amara Leipzig, who listened to our ideas, read our book, and produced visual images that neither one of us can even imagine having the talent to create. She then patiently listened to our detailed feedback as we shared our perfectionistic tendencies with her … *Are they sitting too close? Does she look too young? Is that psychosis or delirium?* Bottom line, your artwork is amazing. Thank you so much, Amara!

We wish to thank our longtime friends and supportive colleagues from the UCLA Division of Pediatric Neurology, the Department of Psychiatry & Biobehavioral Sciences, and the Department of Pediatrics. We have been privileged to work within many multidisciplinary teams and to participate in the training of scores of exceptional young professionals.

Finally, we wish to thank our many young patients and their families who have touched our hearts and inspired us to try to do better for them. You have truly been our best teachers. Thank you.

WHO SHOULD READ THIS BOOK, AND WHY?

This book is intended for the wide range of professionals who work with medically ill children including pediatricians, neurologists, psychiatrists, psychologists, neuropsychologists, social workers, nurses, child life specialists, and others, as well as trainees for these professions. It aims to provide skills needed to conduct the most complex and challenging clinical interviews, those of young medically ill children, aged 5–10 years. To do this, it presents a comprehensive and developmentally sensitive framework to familiarize professionals with how young children understand questions about their emotions, behavior, and illness, and how they use language to formulate and communicate their thoughts and feelings to the listener. Acquisition of developmentally sensitive interviewing skills will enable professionals to transition from novice to expert competency in clinical interviewing.

Although young medically ill children are the focus of this book, many of the techniques can be used to interview older children and adults who have communication challenges involving language, cognition, and/or emotions. Other interested professionals (such as teachers or lawyers) and parents may find this book useful.

WHAT READERS WILL LEARN FROM THE BOOK

Part I of this book introduces the reader to twelve developmental guidelines to adopt when interviewing young children and encouraging them to talk about themselves. Part II describes techniques to obtain clinical information from children about common emotional and behavioral symptoms that often occur with pediatric disorders. These techniques are reviewed in the following chapters: Mood, Anger, and Irritability; Fears and Anxiety; Attention; Aggression; Impaired Insight, Judgment, and Reality Testing; Somatization (physical complaints in response to stress); and Symptoms Associated with Autistic Spectrum.

Part III of this book applies the developmental guidelines and techniques described in part II to the interview of young children with epilepsy. Pediatric epilepsy serves as a model for demonstrating how to apply the developmental guidelines to comprehensively assess the emotions and behavior of young chronically ill children using a biopsychosocial approach. Epilepsy, like many other pediatric chronic illnesses, is associated with daily illness-related stressors, acute medical events (seizures), and social stigma. Additionally, epilepsy has the added challenge of being a chronic disorder that involves the brain and related functions, such as behavior, emotions, cognition, language, and social skills. Identification of the complex biopsychosocial factors that impact children with epilepsy and their families is essential for the comprehensive assessment and treatment of children with this disorder. Individuals who master the

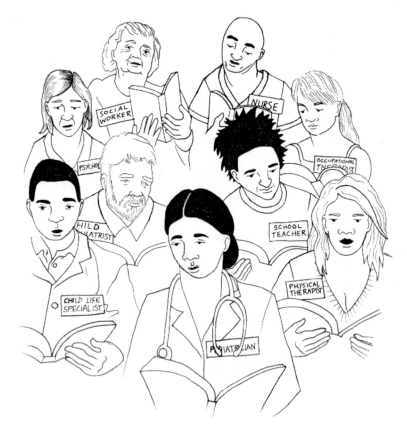

skills required for such complex clinical interviewing will easily be able to apply their knowledge and skills to other patient populations.

Part IV of this book applies the developmental guidelines and techniques described in parts I and II to interviews of young children with pain, iatrogenic trauma symptoms (trauma symptoms due to frightening medical experiences), and a terminal illness. These topics are included in the book because seriously medically ill children struggle with these problems and they pose specific challenges to the interviewer.

Examples of interviews are presented throughout the book. These fictional clinical examples include useful techniques for encouraging children to talk about themselves and illustrate how to make sense of what young children mean when they respond to questions about their feelings and behavior. They also highlight that young children are essential informants about their behavior, emotions, and response to illness.

WHY IS THIS IMPORTANT?

Most professionals who work with children receive minimal formal training on the developmental aspects of children's communication skills other than learning about the milestones of the acquisition of language during the toddler period. They are rarely trained to use interview techniques that help young children talk about topics they might not want to talk about, such as fears regarding their illness, their emotions, and their behavior. Similarly, they are not taught how to make sense of children's communication about these topics. Finally, there is a dearth of literature on specific techniques for the comprehensive biopsychosocial assessment of young ill children with epilepsy, pain, treatment-related traumatic symptoms, or terminal illness.

Professionals do the best they can when they interview young children about the topics presented in this book, both in terms of how they ask the questions and how they understand the child's responses. Well-intentioned professionals often incorrectly believe that children have qualitatively similar but quantitatively less skill than their older counterparts in cognitive, linguistic, and social behavioral domains. This faulty assumption can limit the yield of valuable information elicited during an interview and cause the interviewer to misunderstand the information that is gathered. Consequently, it is essential for those working with young children to understand how they use language to formulate and communicate their thoughts to the listener, how best to elicit information from them about difficult topics and how to understand the essence of what they are communicating.

Acquisition of developmentally sensitive and practical information on effective interviewing techniques will help professionals working with children feel more confident as competent interviewers. Those who master the ability to interview and correctly interpret the communication of young medically ill children will also be well equipped to apply these skills to other challenging interviews, such as with children who have language impairment and intellectual disabilities, as well as older individuals with cognitive limitations. Ultimately, those who will benefit the most will be the young children with medical, neurological, and/or psychiatric illness from whom we have learned so much and to whom we dedicate this book.

"How Many More Questions?"

PART I

Interview Basics

Developmental Guidelines for Interviewing Young Children

The twelve guidelines described in this chapter (Table 1–1) provide interviewers with a framework for understanding young children's communication. They focus primarily on how to communicate with the young child during an interview, a formal situation in which an adult professional with whom the child might have some or no familiarity asks the child questions. Although children are usually told not to talk with strangers, in this situation the "helpful" professional (pediatrician, psychologist, psychiatrist, social worker, nurse, physical therapist, and the like) encourages the child to talk on private topics related to emotions, behavior, and illness. To achieve this goal, the interviewer should act as the child's communication assistant. Knowledge of these developmental guidelines is the first step toward becoming a competent interviewer aware of the need to help young children provide the required information.

The first guideline sets the stage by correcting the common misperception among adults that children are little adults. Guidelines 2–4 describe features that differentiate children's communication from that of adults. Two of these guidelines involve the form of speech: spontaneous speech and elaborate speech; and two relate to cognitive function: concrete thinking and perception of time or chronology. Guidelines 5–6 involve children's behavior when communicating with unfamiliar, "helpful" professional adults. Guidelines 7–12 provide techniques adults should use when speaking to children to create an ambience that encourages children to talk with an unfamiliar adult about topics that might not be easy to talk about. They also provide techniques to formulate questions that children understand and can respond to with valid information. The last guideline emphasizes the adult interviewer's responsibility to make sense of what the child says based on the child's developmental level, fund of knowledge, and expressive linguistic skills.

DEVELOPMENTAL GUIDELINES

1. Children Are Not Little Adults

This guideline is probably the most difficult to understand because adults automatically assume that a speaking child understands speech and is competent at

Table 1–1. DEVELOPMENTAL GUIDELINES FOR INTERVIEWING CHILDREN

Topic	Guideline
Basic developmental concept	Children are not little adults
CHILDREN	
Speech	Children do not initiate spontaneous speech with strangers
	Children do not elaborate on a topic of conversation (nondiscursive speech)
Cognition	Children have poor perception of chronology and time
	Children use concrete language
Behavior	Children like to please adults
	Children figure out what the interviewer wants to hear
INTERVIEWER	
Ambience of interview	Children talk if they feel comfortable
Types of questions	Use "What" or "How" questions, not "Why" questions
	"Yes/No" questions are inefficient
Question structure	Use short, focused sentences without clauses
Behavior	Work on understanding

formulating and expressing thoughts and ideas, albeit at a simple level. Some adults might use less complex language in terms of sentence structure, abstract words, and concepts when speaking with young children whereas others do not.

Children aged 5–10 years do not understand language as adults do. Children might make different inferences when adults use abstract language while talking to children. For example, most adults would understand that the question, "How did the story end?" implies a need for a description of events that lead to the end of the story. A child's answer "With a period," demonstrates that the child inferred something quite different from this question. This child focused on the mechanics of writing a story rather than on the narrative. This example underscores the need to be aware that children and adults might have different assumptions about the meaning of words and sentences. A young child might not understand the over-arching idea an adult is trying to communicate to the child.

When we speak to people from a different country, we are cognizant of gaps in the knowledge we share about our native language, as well as in our culture and life experiences. Therefore, we usually adapt and/or modify how we speak with them accordingly. A similar approach should be used with children whose language and communication skills differ in both quality and quantity (e.g., less complex, fewer words, simple ideas) from those of adults.

Adults sometimes try to engage children in conversation by modifying physical differences and using techniques to establish rapport with their young conversation partners. Thus, they might bend down toward the child to minimize differences in stature, change the prosody of their speech to the more singsong quality characteristic of young children's speech, or decrease the volume of speech when

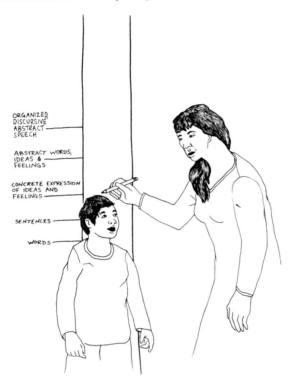

speaking to children. A common technique is use of terms of endearment such as "honey" and "sweetie." Although heart warming and well meaning, these physical modifications and techniques do not address the qualitative differences in the language skill of adults and children and do not bridge the developmental communication gap.

Aware that one needs good rapport to successfully engage young children in conversation, an adult might try to overcome this emotional hurdle through play. The impact of this helpful approach, however, falls flat if the adult then proceeds to speak with the child using abstract and difficult to follow language or misunderstands what the child is actually trying to communicate.

Understanding the underlying reason for quantitative and qualitative differences in the expressive and receptive communication skills of children and adults can help dispel these misconceptions. Communication involves integrated use of language, cognition, and social skill. The onset of speech during the toddler period is regarded as an important milestone in the development of children's communication and language. Although adults are aware that children's cognitive skills develop through adolescence, they usually do not know that language development continues from the toddler period through childhood and only reaches maturity at the end of adolescence (see review in Caplan 1996). This protracted course reflects the prolonged development of language-related regions in the brain (Sowell et al. 2003; Gogtay et al. 2004).

Mature language skills reflecting the integration of language and cognition enable youth to coherently express their thoughts and ideas both orally and through writing using well-constructed sentences within organized paragraphs. As a result, the listener or reader can follow who and what they are talking about and the flow of ideas. Parallel development throughout childhood of the social skills involved in communication (pragmatics) that allow turn-taking, understanding gestures, use of nonverbal communication, as well as online monitoring and repair of communication breakdown (e.g., clarification of the spoken message when the listener does not appear to follow what the speaker says) are essential for competent communication. Thus, children aged 5–10 years have a long way to go before these complex and integrated skills reach adult levels.

With the overarching understanding that children are not little adults, the additional eleven guidelines described below alert the reader to some of the qualitative differences in how children and adults communicate. Understanding these principles is imperative to successfully conducting interviews of young children about their illness and response to illness. These developmental principals are also applicable to conversations with children about other topics and when interviewing older children, adolescents, and adults who have subtle communication challenges involving language, cognition, and/or emotions.

Summary
- Children are not little adults.
- Being able to speak does not mean that a child is a competent communicator with mature linguistic, cognitive, and pragmatic skills.
- Children understand and use speech differently than adults.

2. Young Children Do Not Initiate Speech with Strangers

Young children rarely engage in spontaneous speech with strange adults, including professionals. It is up to the professional to elicit from the child information needed to help assess symptoms, diagnose the child's illness, and/or assess treatment effects. The statement, "the child said nothing about these symptoms," is meaningless and does not confirm whether the child is or is not experiencing the symptoms. The chapters of this book and their clinical examples will guide the reader and provide techniques on how to encourage young children to speak and become the child's communication assistant.

Summary
- Young children do not initiate speech with adult professionals.
- Using techniques that encourage young children to speak, interviewers need to act as the communication assistant of their young patients.

3. Children Do Not Elaborate on Conversation Topics

While adults elaborate on topics of conversation, children speak in one or two sentences (nondiscursive speech) (Caplan et al. 1989). Children also rarely engage in spontaneous speech in the interview situation. Therefore, the burden is on the adult interviewer (the child's communication assistant) to both encourage children to speak and provide the needed information. If a child's response of one or two sentences yields insufficient detail, the interviewer should help the child elaborate on

Table 1–2. NONDISCURSIVE SPEECH: INTERVIEWER PROMPTS

Interviewer Questions and Prompts	Child Responses
Question What brings you to the hospital?	My head
Prompt: "What" question What's not feeling good in your head?	It hurts
Prompt: Empathy Sorry to hear that. What makes it better?	My medicine
Prompt: Repeat child's statement So your head is hurting you bad.	It doesn't go away. Every day the same thing.
Prompt: Open ended sentence And when it hurts every day …	My mom says stay home from school
Prompt: "How" question How does that help?	I can rest
Prompt: Open-ended question And then … ?	I feel better
Prompt: Positive feedback Thank you. This really helps me understand what these headaches are doing to you.	You can also ask my mom. She'll tell you how bad they are.

the conversation topic using the prompts found in Table 1–2. These include using "What" and "How" questions (described below), expressing empathy, repeating a statement the child made followed by a pause, making an open-ended statement, asking an open-ended question, and giving the child positive feedback on the information the child provides.

Parents of children in this age group often complain that their child does not provide them with information about school or their friends when they come home from school and the parents ask them how their day went. Rather than resistance or an unwillingness to speak about these topics, this usually reflects the nondiscursive nature of young children's speech together with limited initiation of spontaneous speech with adults. Parents of young children, similar to professionals, can also use the techniques provided in Table 1–2 to encourage more speech in their children as demonstrated in the following examples.

Mary, aged 6 years, comes to see Dr. Simpson because of vomiting and diarrhea that began during the night.

Nondiscursive Speech

DR. SIMPSON: *Mary, are you sick?*
MARY: *Yes.*
DR. SIMPSON: *What part of you doesn't feel good?*
MARY: *I don't know.*
DR. SIMPSON: *How about you point to where it doesn't feel good?*
Mary sits and stares at Dr. Simpson.
DR. SIMPSON: *I see you really don't feel good. Should I ask you mother?*
Mary nods yes.

This is an example of a child's nondiscursive speech. When asked a "Yes/No" question, "Are you sick?" Mary answers, "Yes" without further elaboration. Her answer, "I don't know" to Dr. Simpson's question, "What part of your doesn't feel good?" could mean that she does not know, feels bad all over and cannot localize the source, or feels so bad that she has no energy to speak. Rather than regarding her as an uncooperative child, Dr. Simpson then clarifies if it would be easier for Mary to point to which part of her does not feel good or feels real bad. Since Mary does not respond, Dr. Simpson acknowledges that Mary might be feeling too ill to talk, and obtains her permission to ask if her mother would be able to help answer the question. The girl listlessly nods her head in agreement suggesting that she has no energy to talk.

SUMMARY

- Nondiscursive speech (one- to two-sentence responses) is age appropriate in young children.
- It does not reflect an unwillingness to speak.
- Interviewers have to use developmentally appropriate techniques to encourage children to speak.

4. Children Are Concrete Thinkers

This guideline relates to how children process and comprehend communication. Concrete thinking refers to thoughts about actions, objects, events, and people rather than thoughts about ideas and concepts. Children with concrete thinking also tend to understand and use the literal rather than the figurative meaning of words, phrases, or idioms. The ability for abstraction gradually develops from age seven through adolescence and involves both language and cognition.

Adults are often unaware of the abstract nature of how they speak, as well as young children's lack of or limited abstract thinking and their difficulty understanding abstract language. This is particularly evident when medical and para-medical professionals mix professional jargon and abstract concepts in the language they use with child patients. How we use speech is an automatic rather than a controlled process (Hahne et al. 2004). Therefore, it takes a considerable effort by adults to monitor how they word their sentences and avoid using abstractions when talking to young children. In fact, this process is somewhat akin to the effort needed when speaking in a foreign language. Thus, when speaking to young children, adults should rethink and rephrase their abstract language into concrete language. In essence, this means reformulating concepts expressed through abstract words into action-based language by using verbs. For example, rather than asking a child, "Are you arrogant (conceited, proud etc)?" one might say, "Do other kids say you show off?" Likewise, instead of asking a child "What physical symptoms do you have when you are separated from your parents?" one might ask, "What parts of your body don't feel good when you are not together with your parents?"

Similarly, the interviewer should also be aware that young children express their thoughts and ideas concretely. The dialogue below between Dr. Eastman and Jack presents three examples (in bold) of concrete thinking in this 8-year-old child. Dr. Eastman is seeing Jack because of problems with attention, aggressive outbursts, and insomnia. Although he is in a regular class at school, his teachers have threatened to make him repeat the current grade in the next school year.

Concrete Thinking

DR. EASTMAN: *What can I do for you today, Jack?*
JACK: *Give me medicine.*
DR. EASTMAN: *What for?*
JACK: *Sleep.*
DR. EASTMAN: *How do you sleep at night?*
JACK: **In my bed.**
DR. EASTMAN: *Is it easy or difficult for you to fall asleep?*
JACK: *I can't sleep.*
DR. EASTMAN: *The whole night?*
JACK: *Yes.*
DR. EASTMAN: *Then what happens in the morning when you have to go to school?*
JACK: **I catch the bus.**
DR. EASTMAN: *So what grade are you in now at school?*
JACK: *Third.*
DR. EASTMAN: *What's your teacher like?*
JACK: **She likes us to be quiet.**

In response to Dr. Eastman's question, "How do you sleep at night?" Jack concretely answered that he sleeps in his bed. When Dr. Eastman asked how he goes to school after a night of no sleep, the child concretely answered that he catches a bus. Dr. Eastman's subsequent question on what his teacher is like led to his response that the teacher likes the children to be quiet. In addition to concrete thinking, Jack's responses to these latter two questions demonstrate that young children might not share the same inferences as adults during a conversation. Although Dr. Eastman thought the child inferred that she was asking about his level of tiredness when going to school in the morning, Jack concretely understood that she meant how he physically gets to school. Similarly, rather than describing the teacher's attributes, the child focused on how she likes her students to behave.

Lack of knowledge about young children's concrete thinking, together with differences in the frame of reference and inferential skills between adults and children are a potential source of communication breakdown during a conversation. The potential for communication breakdown is illustrated in the following two examples. The first example clearly demonstrates that the child and interviewer did not share the same frame of reference. The second example shows what the interviewer does when she does not understand a young child's use of concrete language.

Emma, aged 9 years, has come for her annual anemia checkup with Dr. King, and is accompanied by her grandmother.

Differences in Frame of Reference

DR. KING: *Emma, we are going to have to do a blood test again to see if everything is okay with your blood.*
EMMA: *I'm 9 now. I'm not scared of shots.*
DR. KING: *You really are a big girl now.*
EMMA: *I'm already in fourth grade.*

DR. KING: *Is school going well, could be better, or not so good for you?*

EMMA: *Not so good.*

DR. KING: *What's making it not so good?*

EMMA: *The girls, they're mean.*

DR. KING: *All of them?*

EMMA: *Only one.*

DR. KING: *What does she do?*

EMMA: *Who does she think she is? Britney or someone?*

DR. KING: *Oh, so her name is Britney?*

EMMA: *No one in my class has that name.*

DR. KING: *So is Britney in another class?*

EMMA: *Don't you know Britney?*

DR. KING: *I am not sure.*

EMMA (smiling quite disdainfully): *Britney Spears, who else?*

DR. KING: *Oh, how stupid of me not to think of her.*

Diego, aged 6 years, is seeing Dr. Frost for a sore throat, fever, and coughing. Several months ago, his mother brought him to Dr. Frost because he had stomachaches while at school.

Action-based Concrete Thinking

DR. FROST: *Diego, let me check your throat; I see you have a high temperature.*

DIEGO: *Will it hurt?*

DR. FROST: *It will not hurt if you don't move while I put this in your mouth to check why your throat hurts.*

Diego nods yes and opens his mouth wide.

DR. FROST: *Good job not moving. Now how is your tummy feeling these days at school?*

DIEGO: *Okay.*

DR. FROST: *What do you like to do at school?*

DIEGO: *My teacher is weird*

DR. FROST: *What's weird about her?*

DIEGO: *She doesn't know how to talk.*

DR. FROST: *Does she talk like she is from another country?*

DIEGO: *No, she just doesn't know how to talk.*

DR. FROST: *Where do you sit in class?*

DIEGO: *In the front.*

DR. FROST: *Oh, so is it easy or difficult to hear her?*

DIEGO: *I can hear her, she talks loud, and a lot. But she just can't talk.*

DR. FROST: *Is it hard to understand the work she is teaching?*

DIEGO (angry): *I already said she doesn't know how to talk. She talks and talks, and I don't know what she is talking about.*

This example demonstrates how an interviewer can try to make sense of what the child meant in his statement that the teacher "doesn't know how to talk." Dr. Frost presented the child with different options expressed in action-based concrete terms to clarify what message the child was trying to get across to Dr. Frost. By asking Diego if the teacher speaks with an accent, if he does not hear the teacher (if he sits in the back of the class), or if he has difficulty understanding the work, Dr. Frost discovered that Diego has difficulty understanding the schoolwork.

Summary

- Interviewers of young children should monitor their own speech to ensure that they avoid using abstract language.
- They should use concrete action-based words (verbs) when talking with young children.
- Learning how to interpret children's concrete use of language is key to understanding the message they are conveying.
- When it is difficult to comprehend what a child is actually trying to communicate, an interviewer should present the child with action-based concrete options to help clarify what the child means.

5. Children Have Poor Perception of Chronology and Time

Children are poor historians regarding the onset, duration, frequency, and recurrence of their symptoms. Given this developmental limitation, interviewers should refrain from asking children to tell them "When," "How long," and "How often," they have symptoms. Interviewers should direct these questions to parents who are usually aware of the chronology of their children's physical condition and acting out (externalizing) behaviors (fidgeting, hyperactivity, distractibility, impulsivity, argumentativeness, irritability, physical or verbal aggression). Nevertheless, parents frequently are not cognizant of their children's internalizing symptoms (sadness, worrying, anxiety, fears, hurt feelings, unusual perceptions, such as hallucinations and illusions, thoughts about death and dying, suicidal thoughts, suicidal plans, delusions).

Young children are, therefore, the essential source of information to determine if they experience internalizing symptoms and of what intensity. Chapters 3–5 and 7–8 inform the reader how to ask young children questions about internalizing symptoms and how to assess their severity in the absence of information on chronology and time.

Given the emphasis of the DSM-IV and V on frequency and duration of symptoms to meet diagnostic criteria of psychiatric disorders, child mental health interviewers tend to ask "When," "How long," and "How often" questions when interviewing young children. In addition to the lack of validity of young children's answers to these questions, they often lead to the child asking, "How many more questions?" or "When are we done?" These questions herald the beginning of the end or the "kiss of death" of the interview, as evident from the following clinical example.

Eva is a 7-year-old girl who was brought to the emergency room because of stomach pain and severe constipation. While her parents were on an overseas trip, Eva had been staying with a neighbor, Mrs. Nelson, who brought her to the emergency room. After talking to Mrs. Nelson, who knew little about the child's medical history and bowel movement patterns, a new intern had the following conversation with Eva:

Chronology Questions
INTERN: *What seems to be the trouble?*
EVA: *My tummy hurts*

INTERN: *When did this start?*

EVA: *I don't know.*

INTERN: *Has it been a few days, a week, or a month?*

EVA: *Yes.*

INTERN: *For which option are you saying yes?*

EVA: *I don't know.*

INTERN: *Let's try again, has your tummy been hurting for a few days, a week, a month, or longer?*

EVA: *Longer.*

INTERN: *So this has been a chronic problem. How often does it hurt you?*

EVA: *I don't know.*

INTERN: *Is it once, twice, or more times a day?*

EVA: *More times.*

INTERN: *When did the constipation start?*

Eva shrugs her shoulders.

INTERN: *You do have constipation, right?*

EVA: *No.*

INTERN: *When did you have your last bowel movement?*

Eva looks befuddled.

INTERN: *Do you know what I mean? When did you last go pooh?*

EVA: *It hurts.*

INTERN: *I understand but when was the last time you had a pooh?*

EVA: *My tummy hurts when I go to the bathroom.*

INTERN: *How long has that been going on for? A week?*

EVA: *Yes.*

INTERN: *Has it been more than a week?*

EVA: *When are we going to be done?*

INTERN: *Please answer. Have you not gone pooh for more or less than a week?*

EVA: *Less.*

EVA (turning to Mrs. Nelson): *I want to go home.*

INTERN TO MRS. NELSON: *I still would like to get more information from Eva before I examine her.*

MRS. NELSON: *Eva, the doctor wants to help you. We will be done soon, and go home, okay.*

EVA NODS.

INTERN: *Okay, so let me summarize, you have had tummy aches for more than a month and constipation for less than a week, is that correct?*

EVA: *I guess.*

INTERN: *Do you have diarrhea?*

EVA: *Yes.*

INTERN: *How often?*

EVA: *Often.*

INTERN: *Is that once a day, twice a day, or more?*

EVA: *More.*

INTERN: *About how many times?*

EVA: *I am tired.*

INTERN: *When did the diarrhea start?*

EVA: *I don't know.*
INTERN: *Last week, yesterday, a month ago?*
EVA: *A month ago.*
EVA (turning to Mrs. Nelson): *I want to go home.*

The intern examines Eva and then tells Eva and Mrs. Nelson that he will return with Dr. Lowe to complete the examination. He tells Dr. Lowe that he has had a lot of difficulty taking a history because the neighbor has no information on the child's medical history and the child has been uncooperative. He reported that Eva says she has stomach pains probably for more than a month that occur many times a day, constipation for less than a week, and diarrhea more than twice a day that has gone on for about a month. The physical exam revealed a soft abdomen, some tenderness in the umbilical area, borborygmi (increased sounds of movement of the intestinal muscles), and no other findings. They then both go back to see Eva.

Developmentally Oriented Questions

DR. LOWE: *Hi, Eva. You must be getting tired being here in the ER for so long.*
EVA NODS YES.
DR. LOWE: *Please point to where your tummy hurts the most.*
Eva points to umbilical area.
DR. LOWE: *I understand that your parents went on a trip and that you are staying with your neighbor, Mrs. Nelson.*
Eva nods yes and appears quite sad.
DR. LOWE: *Is this the first time they have gone out of town without you?*
Eva nods yes, holding back tears.
DR. LOWE: *That must be hard for you.*
Eva nods with tears in her eyes.
DR. LOWE: *Is this also the first time you are sleeping over at Mrs. Nelson's house?*
EVA: *Yes.*
DR. LOWE: *Some kids find it difficult to go pooh in the bathroom of someone else's house. How about you?*
Eva nods yes.
DR. LOWE: *So while you have been at Mrs. Nelson's house, has it been difficult to go pooh?*
Eva nods yes.
DR. LOWE: *Before your parents went out of town, was it easy or difficult for you to go pooh?*
EVA: *Easy.*
DR. LOWE: *How about your tummy aches? Did you have them before mom and dad went on the trip?*
EVA: *No.*
DR. LOWE: *So they started for the first time at Mrs. Nelson's house.*
EVA: *Yes.*
DR. LOWE: *You are doing a great job telling me about all this.*
Eva smiles.
DR. LOWE: *Do you have diarrhea every time you go to the bathroom?*

EVA: *No.*

DR. LOWE: *Let's check if this is diarrhea. When you try go pooh, does it come out like water or something very soft?*

EVA: *Yes.*

DR. LOWE: *Does it also happen when you are not in the bathroom?*

Eva (nods with tears in her eyes): *It just comes out by itself.*

DR. LOWE: *That's embarrassing for you.*

EVA CRIES.

DR. LOWE: *Eva, you have been very helpful explaining this all to me. Let me examine you and figure out how we will get rid of these tummy aches and the trouble you have had going to the bathroom.*

The intern's focused questions on chronology did not yield the information needed to diagnose Eva. Young children do not provide valid answers when faced with "When" and "How often" questions. The intern's efforts to get answers to these questions by breaking down the onset (a week, a month, longer) and frequency (once a day, twice a day, more) of Eva's stomach pain, constipation, and diarrhea were unsuccessful. In fact, Eva consistently confirmed the last of the onset and frequency options because they are the easiest to remember. This common response occurs when young children are presented with question options that they do not understand and/or lack the knowledge base to answer. The child's "I don't know" and "I guess" answers indicated her mounting frustration which lead to "When are we going to be done?" "I want to go home," and "I am tired."

As evident from Dr. Lowe's interview with the child, the intern reached erroneous conclusions about Eva's symptoms based on Eva's invalid answers to his chronology questions. Using a developmental approach, Dr. Lowe obtained valid information that allowed her to diagnose the constipation, its cause, and severity of the associated abdominal pain and overflow diarrhea.

SUMMARY

- Young children have a poor sense of chronology and time.
- Although health-care professionals are trained to find out when symptoms start, their frequency, and duration, they should avoid asking young children these questions.
- Parents are usually better informants on the chronology, evolution, and duration of physical and externalizing behavior symptoms but not of internalizing symptoms.

6. Children Try to Please Adults

Young children typically want to make a good impression on adults. During an interview, they achieve this by answering the adult interviewer's questions. As a result, they feel competent and are willing to answer additional questions. It is essential that interviewers understand this principle, because it is the interviewer's obligation to ensure that the child is motivated to go on with the interview.

If the child perceives that he/she is not providing the interviewer with the requested answers, tension increases between the child (who wants to please the interviewer) and the interviewer. The resulting strained atmosphere detracts from the rapport between the child and the interviewer, and might lead to the child asking, "How many more questions?" or "When will we be done?"

In the clinical example above, Eva responded to the intern's chronology questions with any answer (not necessarily the correct answers) rather than tell the interviewer that she does not know when her symptoms started and how frequently they occur now and in the past. Similarly, in lieu of acknowledging difficulty understanding an interviewer's question, a young child might reply with "Yes," "No," "A little," "Maybe " or "When can I go home?"

The interviewer should be sensitive to red flags that suggest the young child might be having difficulty with the interviewer's questions. These include repeated "Yes," "No," "A little," "Maybe," "Because," "Not sure," or "I guess" answers. A child might also consistently respond to the last option the interviewer mentions in a question as in the following example. In response to the doctor's question "Is the pain in your tummy like a knife, something pressing on your tummy, or just on the skin of your tummy?" a young child answers, "On the skin."

In addition to questions on chronology, children have difficulty with questions that challenge their analytical skills, such as "Why" questions. Questions that include run-on sentences demand attention and good working memory and tax children's ability to understand the interviewer's main question. They also are not forthcoming in answering questions that focus on a sensitive topic. Since children like to please adults, they do not tell the interviewer they are having a problem answering a question. Instead, they respond with red flag answers.

When young children appear to be uncooperative or resistant to answering questions in an interview, the interviewer should determine what aspects of the interview have made the child feel she/he cannot or does not know how to answer the questions. Once the interviewer has figured out what has made the interview difficult for the child, it is important to then modify the interview approach accordingly.

Addressing the child's sense of competence by noting that it is difficult for most children to answer these questions or acknowledging that the child might find it hard to speak about a specific topic are helpful approaches that decrease the child's tension and resistance to speak. However, if the interviewer does not use age-appropriate language and the question formats described in the guidelines below, these expressions of empathy alone do not help the child provide valid information and feel that he/she is pleasing the interviewer.

Summary
- Children like to please adults.
- Children try to please an interviewer by answering the interviewer's questions (even incorrectly).
- Inability to answer questions makes children tense and resistant to additional interview questions.
- Red flags that suggest a child is having difficulty answering questions include repeated "Yes/No," "Maybe," "I guess," "A little," "Because," and "Not sure" responses, as well as confirming the last option in a series that the interview presents in questions to a child.

- Interviewers should structure their questions so that young children can successfully provide them with the needed information.

7. Children Figure Out What the Interviewer Wants to Hear

This guideline is relevant to questions about behavior, emotions, and school. In their quest to identify pathology, interviewers tend to word their questions in a leading manner. For example, an interviewer might inquire, "Are you a sad kid?" rather than providing the child with a choice as in, "Are you a happy, sad, or in-between kid?" Similarly, an interviewer might ask, "So are you having trouble at school?" in lieu of "What do you like about school and what don't you like?" or "What are you good at school and what is more difficult?" An additional frequently asked leading question is "Do you have lots of friends?" to which most children will answer "Yes" even if they have no friends.

Related to the previous guideline "Children try to please adults," if a child wants the interviewer to think he is well behaved, he will answer "No" if asked "Do you get mad and lose it?" But, if he realizes that the interviewer wants to hear "Yes," particularly when the interviewer repeats the question several times, he might answer in the affirmative. To avoid this pitfall, the interviewer should ask the child for examples to validate if the child, in fact, is experiencing anger. The interviewer should ask the child what different things make him angry. The interviewer should follow up the child's examples by asking what he does when he gets angry. The child's answers to these validation questions will help the interviewer determine if, in fact, the child gets angry. Alternatively, when an interviewer tries to minimize pathology, as in "So you don't lose your temper," the child will respond with a "No" and confirm what the interviewer seems to want to hear.

Interviewers should be cognizant that a child with a clear pattern of "Yes" or "No" responses to multiple questions might simply be giving the interviewer the information he wants. Repeat "Yes" or "No" answers might also represent the child's effort to tell the interviewer to get the interview over with as fast as possible. Therefore, the interviewer must evaluate the internal consistency of the child's responses to clarify inconsistencies and/or to identify inaccurate responses.

SUMMARY
- Young children figure out what the interviewer wants to hear.
- They respond to leading questions that either maximize or minimize pathology with the information the interviewer seems to want to hear.
- Young children might assume that the interviewer wants to hear that they are well behaved.

8. Children Talk If They Feel Comfortable

Establishing good rapport during an interview helps an interviewer obtain information from young children. Table 1–3 summarizes the "Dos" and "Don'ts" to make young children feel comfortable during an interview.

Table 1–3. DOS AND DON'TS FOR CHILDREN TO FEEL COMFORTABLE IN AN INTERVIEW

Do	Don't
Use developmentally appropriate language	Start interview with the most sensitive topic
Allow the child to engage in non-distracting yet calming activities	Demand that the child concentrate
Provide positive feedback at different points during the interview	Emphasize that you are asking questions
Reformulate unanswered questions	Repeat unanswered questions
Economize time spent with the child by carefully structuring questions	Spend more than 60 minutes on an interview Ask "Yes/No" questions
Use "What" or "How" questions	Use "When," "How often," "How long," and "Why" questions
Express empathy	Criticize the child's answer
When possible "normalize" and emphasize that symptoms are treatable	

Young children generally do not like being asked questions, particularly if they are asked by strangers. Medical professionals often introduce themselves to a child and then say that they are going to ask the child questions. Rather than emphasizing the need to ask the child questions, the interviewer might tell the child he wants to chat with the child in order to get to know the child and understand what brought the child to the professional in the first place. Throughout the interview, the interviewer should refrain from emphasizing and reminding the child that the interviewer is asking questions and expects answers to questions.

Providing positive feedback and saying the child is a good talker encourages the child to talk more. Expressing empathy for the information obtained from the child also encourages speech. For example, if the child describes a stomachache each morning before school, the interviewer should express sympathy and understanding that it is not a fun way to start the day.

Parents sometimes bring activities (games, drawings, books), snacks, or drinks for the child while waiting to be seen by the interviewer. The interviewer should let the child continue with these activities during the interview, unless they distract the child from speaking. Allowing activities decreases the child's anxiety, makes the child less aware of answering questions, and creates an atmosphere conducive to a successful interview. The interviewer's compliments on how well the child is doing the interview and the activity are additional rapport boosters.

Interviewers should not repeat questions, even if the child does not answer the question or provides an inadequate answer, because it communicates the interviewer's dissatisfaction with the answer and indirectly with the child. Repeating questions can make the child perceive the interviewer as a "nag." As a result, tension during the interview increases for both the child and the interviewer, and the child becomes resistant to speaking. However, the interviewer should clarify whether the child is having difficulty understanding what the interviewer said or does not know the answer.

If the interviewer needs to pursue the topic of an unanswered question, it is best to reformulate the question. For example, if the child acknowledges stomach pains, but in response to the question "What makes your tummy hurt bad?" says "Nothing," the interviewer can say "For some kids, their tummy hurts when they have to go to the bathroom, for others when they eat certain things, and for some when they wake up in the morning; how does it work for you?" If the child says none of these options apply, the interviewer should provide other concrete examples of possible causes of pediatric abdominal pain. In this way, rather than perceiving the interviewer as a badger, the child appreciates the efforts and interest in finding out what causing abdominal pain.

Alternatively, the interviewer can change the topic of conversation and revisit the questions when the child appears to be feeling more comfortable and talkative. When doing this, the interviewer should tell the child that, although he already asked the child this question, he is not sure if he really understood the child's answer. Asking the child to help the interviewer revisit a question and better understand what the child is saying makes the child feel respected and helpful. It also emphasizes that the interviewer values what the child is telling the interviewer. Since most young children are not used to adults talking to them with this level of respect and taking what they say seriously, this approach helps improve rapport.

An interview of a young child should last no longer than 50–60 minutes. To carefully budget time during the interview, the interviewer should plan and prioritize questions to elicit the information needed to rule in or rule out the diagnoses at hand. The interviewer should not start an interview with what appears to be the child's main problem if this might be an emotionally laden or difficult topic for the child to discuss. The interviewer should only approach a sensitive topic once the child appears comfortable enough to talk about it, and this might only occur toward the end of the interview.

Three techniques increase the amount of time the child will tolerate the interviewer. The first technique involves refraining from questions on chronology ("When," "How often," "How long") and causality ("Why"). The second technique avoids "Yes/No" questions. The third technique employs the interviewer's continued efforts to strengthen rapport with the child. To do this, the interviewer should respond to the information the child presents with appropriate empathy and understanding of the difficulties the child faces. The interviewer should also decrease the child's concern or embarrassment about symptoms/problems by telling the child that other children have similar problems. This normalizes the symptoms/problems for the child and decreases the child's resistance to talk about what he/she is experiencing. Being told that the interviewer has treated other children with similar difficulties—children who are now well—increases the child's trust in the interviewer.

Summary
- Young children speak during an interview if they feel comfortable.
- To achieve this, the interviewer should:
  - Use developmentally appropriate language.
  - Allow the child to continue an activity while talking.
  - Introduce sensitive topic(s) only once rapport is well established

- Reformulate unanswered questions.
- Ask "What" and "How" questions.
- Empathize with the child.
- "Normalize" symptoms/problems that might make the child embarrassed.
- Give positive feedback.
- Provide hope for treatment.
- To avoid making the child uncomfortable, the interviewer should not:
  - Emphasize the need to answer questions.
  - Repeat questions.
  - Ask about chronology and causality.
  - Conduct a long interview.
  - Ask "Why" questions.

9. Children Do Not Like "Why" Questions

"Why" questions imply that children need to tap into their analytical skills and come up with a logical answer. These questions force young children to make an effort to explain the reason for answers that they give to the interviewer's questions. Children feel put on the spot and from a child's perspective this is like being tested. Young children, therefore, do not like these questions. Interviewers working with young children might be familiar with answers, such as "Because," "I don't know," or a shoulder shrug to "Why" questions.

When faced with these responses, interviewers should not repeat "Why" questions as they might lead to children asking, "How many more questions?" or "When are we done?" The need for the intellectual effort involved in responding to recurrent "Why" questions can make young children uncomfortable and resistant to subsequent questions. In fact, similar to "When" and "How often" questions, these responses to "Why" questions herald the beginning of the end of the interview.

Yet, interviewers often need to ask children (rather than their parents) what might account for their symptoms, particularly those related to emotions and behavior and in situations where emotional factors and/or stressors might exacerbate physical symptoms. Rather than posing "Why" questions, interviewers can obtain information on causality by asking young children "What" questions. For example, instead of asking, "Why are you sad?" to which most children shrug their shoulders, one can ask, "What things make you sad?" Since all children have something that makes them sad, they answer this question. And the answer provides the interviewer with a reason the child feels sad.

Sometimes, however, it might be difficult for a child to talk about the things that make the child sad and the child avoids or resists answering a "What" question. The interviewer can then offer the child several choices, "Do the things that make you sad have anything to do with your family, school, or your friends?" It is important that the interviewer carefully choose these options without putting words into the child's mouth. When offering choices, the interviewer should pause for an answer after each choice.

Thus, "What" questions yield similar information to "Why" questions and require less intellectual effort from the child as they tap the child's memory not reasoning. For example, rather thank asking a child "Why are you scared to go to the doctor?" one can ask the child, "What does your doctor do that is scary?" or "What is scary about your doctor?" Similarly, the question, "Why are you crying?" can be replaced by, "What things make you cry?"

"How" questions can be useful as long as they do not require the child's reasoning. By diversifying the format of the questions, the interview sounds less repetitive and boring for the child. For example, in lieu of the question, "Why do you hit your sister?" the interviewer could ask, "How does your sister bug you and make you want to hit her?" The answer to this question is similar to "What does your sister do that bugs you?" However, asking a child who refuses to go to school, "How does being at school bother you?" taps into reasoning and is similar to the question, "Why are you bothered by going to school?" In contrast, the question "What don't you like at school?" asks the child for facts and, therefore, does not appear to require the child's reasoning.

The interviewer should also use "What" and "How" questions to help the child elaborate on a topic. For example, if a child answers, "Work," to the question, "What don't you like about school?" the interviewer can find out more about the topic by asking, "What work at school do you hate?" In response to the question, "What makes you angry?" a child responds "My brother." The question, "How does he bug you?" assists the child in providing information on triggers for the child's anger.

It is almost second nature for interviewers trained in taking histories and making differential diagnoses to ask "When" and "Why" questions. Interviewers of young children need to consciously avoid "Why" questions and identify causality through use of "What" questions and where appropriate "How" questions. The examples presented in the different chapters of the book demonstrate how to apply this guideline and use "What" and "How" questions to inquire about causality and help children provide more information on specific topics.

Summary
- Children are reluctant to answer "Why" questions.
- "What" and, where appropriate, "How" questions can provide interviewers of young children with information about the conditions and causes that are related to their symptoms.
- They also help children elaborate on the topic of conversation.

10. "Yes/No" Questions Yield Minimal Information

When adults are presented with a "Yes/No" question during an interview, they usually elaborate on their answer. For example, an adult might reply to an orthopedic doctor's "Yes/No" question, "Are you feeling better?" with the answer, "Yes. My back doesn't hurt anymore. I completed a 12-week physical therapy course and now get in and out of my car and bed, and I also move around quite freely without pain." However, consistent with their immature communication skills, young children do not engage in spontaneous speech with adult strangers, such as professionals who work with children. They also do not spontaneously elaborate on their "Yes" or "No" answers.

Given the constraints on the length of an interview with a young child, interviewers should minimize use of "Yes/No" questions because they necessitate subsequent questions to validate if the child is experiencing the symptom or not. Additional questions are also needed to obtain information on symptom severity and conditions under which the symptom occurs. Since we are used to asking "Yes/No" questions to get information, interviewers need to make a concerted effort to avoid asking these questions.

Stella is a 10-year-old girl whose mother thinks she has migraines that run in the family. Stella first started having headaches three months before visiting her nurse practitioner, Ms. Holmes. She came home in the middle of the school day after spending most of the morning in the school nurse's office because of a bad headache. In the following example, Ms. Holmes asks Stella twenty questions: 10 (underlined) "Yes/No" questions, 9 (in bold) "What," "How," "Which," and "Where" questions, and one question that presents multiple "Yes/No" options (question 16).

"Yes/No" vs. "What" Questions

MS. HOLMES: **What's been bothering you?** *(1)*

STELLA: *My head.*

MS. HOLMES: <u>Does it hurt?</u> *(2)*

STELLA: *Yes.*

MS. HOLMES: <u>Do you have a headache now?</u> *(3)*

STELLA: *No.*

MS. HOLMES: **Where does it usually hurt?** *(4)*

STELLA POINTS TO HER FOREHEAD.

MS. HOLMES: <u>Do you have a lot of pain?</u> *(5)*

STELLA: *Yes.*

MS. HOLMES: **How bad does it get?** *(6)*

STELLA: *It hurts.*

MS. HOLMES: *If 0 is no headache and 10 is very bad pain,* **what number would you give your headaches?** *(7)*

STELLA: *8.*

MS. HOLMES: <u>Does it hurt for a long time when it starts?</u> *(8)*

STELLA: *Yes.*

MS. HOLMES: **What is a long time?** *(9)*

STELLA: *The whole day.*

MS. HOLMES: <u>Do you take any medicine for it?</u> *(10)*

STELLA: *Yes.*

MS. HOLMES: **What do you take?** *(11)*

STELLA: *My mom knows the name.*

MS. HOLMES: <u>Does it help?</u> *(12)*

STELLA: *No.*

MS. HOLMES: <u>Do you know when you head is going to start hurting?</u> *(13)*

STELLA: *Yes.*

MS. HOLMES: **How do you know?** *(14)*

STELLA: *I see lights.*

I MS. HOLMES: <u>Do you mean flashes?</u> *(15)*

STELLA: *Yes.*

MS. HOLMES: <u>Do you have nausea, vomiting, or both?</u> *(16)*

STELLA: *Yes.*
MS. HOLMES: **Which one?** *(17)*
STELLA: *Vomiting.*
MS. HOLMES: <u>Do you know what makes your headache better?</u> *(18)*
STELLA: *No.*
MS. HOLMES: *When you have a headache,* <u>does anything make it better?</u> *(19)*
STELLA: *No.*
MS. HOLMES: **What do you usually do to make it better?** *(20)*
STELLA: *I lie down and make my room dark.*

In the interview below, Ms. Holmes obtained the same information from Stella with fewer questions (11 vs. 20) by avoiding "Yes/No" questions, and by asking "What" and "How" questions and two questions with choices (3 and 5).

Avoiding "Yes/No" Questions

MS. HOLMES: **What's been bothering you?** *(1)*
STELLA: *My head.*
MS. HOLMES: **What's not feeling good in your head?** *(2)*
STELLA: *It hurts.*
MS. HOLMES: *Is it hurting now or when you were at home? (3)*
STELLA: *Not now.*
MS. HOLMES: *Show me where does it usually hurt?*
Stella points to her forehead.
MS. HOLMES: *If 0 is no headache and 10 is very bad pain,* **what number would you give your headaches?** *(4)*
STELLA: *8.*
MS. HOLMES: *Does it hurt for the whole day or just for part of the day? (5)*
STELLA: *The whole day.*
MS. HOLMES: **What medicine makes it feel better?** *(6)*
STELLA: *My medicine doesn't help.*
MS. HOLMES: **What do you take?** *(7)*
STELLA: *My mom knows the name.*
MS. HOLMES: **How do you know when you head is going to start hurting?** *(8)*
STELLA: *I see lights.*
I MS. HOLMES: **What do they look like?** *(9)*
STELLA: *Flashes.*
MS. HOLMES: **What else doesn't feel good when you head hurts?** *(10)*
STELLA: *Vomiting.*
MS. HOLMES: *When you have a headache,* **what makes it better?** *(11)*
STELLA: *I lie down and make my room dark.*

SUMMARY

- "Yes/No" questions are often unnecessary when interviewing young children because of the need to validate their symptoms through "What" and, where indicated, "How" questions.
- Given the limited time a young child will tolerate questions by an interviewer, it is best to use "Yes/No" questions only when this is the most effective method to obtain the required information.

11. Use Simple Sentences to Ask Short, Focused Questions

Most adults are unaware that they use complex sentences that include more than one question when talking to children, as in the following example: "Do you have a headache, mainly in your forehead and at night, and does it hurt when you play soccer or other sports?" This question included five separate questions: (1) Does the child have a headache? (2) Does it occur mainly in the forehead? (3) Is the headache at night? (4) Does it occur when playing soccer? and (5) Does the child also have a headache during other sports?

In contrast to a young child, an older child might elaborate on the topic and answer, "Yes," and indicate that her head hurts mainly in the evening. Alternatively, if the question was too long and complicated, the older child might ask the speaker to remind her of all of the options presented. Due to their relatively short attention span, children in the 5–10 year old age range might only focus on the fourth question in their "Yes" or "No" answer. Without further clarification, the interviewer might conclude that the answer addresses all four options presented. Ideally, the interviewer should ask five separate questions. Alternatively, the interviewer should clarify which option the child addressed in her "Yes" or "No" answer.

Examples throughout the book demonstrate the use of questions that contain short, focused single-clause sentences. Interviewers need to be mindful of their use of complex sentences and learn how to simplify their questions.

SUMMARY
- Young children respond well to questions made of short simple sentences.
- When an interviewer uses complex sentences to ask a question, a child's response might address only part of the question.
- When complex sentences are used, follow-up validation questions are necessary to:
  - Determine to which part of the question the child responded.
  - Prevent the interviewer from reaching erroneous conclusions.

12. Work on Understanding

Since most interviewers have not been trained in developmental linguistics or psychology, they need to work to understand what children are saying to them during an interview. To do this, an interviewer should, first and foremost, listen and pay attention to every word the child says during the interview. This enables the interviewer to get a sense of a child's developmental level. If the interviewer has some difficulty comprehending what the child is saying, the interviewer should explain to the child that understanding everything the child says is important for the interviewer to help the child. The interviewer should also ask if the child is willing to help with this. Children are happy to help adults as they usually are in the reverse role, and they need adults to help them. Appointing the child as the interviewer's "helper" strengthens the rapport between the child and the interviewer and emphasizes the interviewer's motivation to help the child.

Furthermore, in trying to comprehend what the child is actually communicating, the interviewer should have no preconception of what the child should be saying in answer to a question. This is particularly relevant when the child's communication appears off topic. For example, in response to the question, "What do you like to eat?" most children will respond with one word or a longer list of foods they like. However, a child who has lost a lot of weight might answer, "I don't like to eat when other people are watching." The interviewer should not repeat the question or indicate that the child is off topic by saying, "I asked you, what do you like to eat." Rather, the interviewer should recognize the message that the child is trying to convey by responding, "Oh, so does that mean that when someone watches you eat, you don't like to eat at all, even your favorite foods?" Thus, when faced with what appears to be derailment to an unrelated topic of conversation, the interviewer should always determine whether:

a. The child is trying to provide the interviewer with information that the child deems important.
b. The child is avoiding the topic of conversation because it is emotionally loaded.
c. The child's pragmatic linguistic difficulties underlie the unpredicted digression to an unrelated topic.

If a child's answer to a question is far from clear, the interviewer should not conclude that this means that the child is unfocused or not listening to the question. The interviewer should ascertain if the child's unclear communication reflects difficulty understanding how the interviewer phrased the question, the child's language or cognitive difficulties, or both.

Children in this age range usually do not volunteer, "I don't understand what you are saying or asking me." The interviewer should ask the child if it was difficult to understand what was just asked. Alternatively, for those children who are embarrassed to acknowledge any difficulties, the interviewer might add, "I think I wasn't saying that very well. Let me try and do a better job." Most children will nod their head in agreement or say, "Okay." This response demonstrates to the child that the interviewer is really motivated and interested in what the child is saying. By stating that she might not have done well, the interviewer has also normalized difficulty and modeled for the child that even adults might not do everything correctly. This is particularly relevant for children with language or cognitive problems who try to hide and cover up their deficits.

Interviewers frequently ask how they can identify children's linguistic or cognitive difficulties without objective standardized testing. Listening to every word the child says and how the child responds to the interviewer's questions can help identify these deficits. An interviewer should consider that a child might be experiencing linguistic or cognitive problems—or both—if the child appears to struggle to understand questions (evident by repeated "Yes," "No," or "I don't know" answers), even when the interviewer speaks in short and simple sentences devoid of abstraction. In addition, grammatical errors, incorrect word choice, and/or unclear reference might imply that the child has expressive difficulties, while the speech of children with cognitive difficulties might appear immature and without the linguistic errors found in the speech of children with impaired language (Table 1–4).

Although these "soft" signs of problems with language and cognition need confirmation through standardized testing, their presence should guide the interviewer

Table 1–4. EXAMPLES DURING AN INTERVIEW OF POSSIBLE LANGUAGE PROBLEMS

Interviewer Questions	Child Response (*italics indicate language errors*)
Is it easy or difficult for you to sleep at night?	Difficult
So when you get into bed, it is hard to fall asleep?	No
What do you do when you get into bed at night?	Sleep
Sounds like you are a good sleeper	Yes
And then do you sleep until the morning?	*Morning is get up and night is sleep*
Oh, I get it. You sleep at night and wake up in the morning.	Nods
Who lives with you in your house?	Andrew, Mathew, Sarah
Are these your brothers and sister?	*He's 13 now*
Who is 13?	Andrew
Are Andrew and Mathew your brothers?	*He's really strong*
Do you mean Andrew?	I already *said it*
Thanks, now I get it. How do you get along with Andrew, Mathew, and Sarah?	We *go the long way*
To where do you go the long way?	School
Are Andrew, Mathew, and Sarah nice to you?	*No nice for me*, only bad, bad, bad

on the need to speak at a level commensurate with the child's apparent linguistic or mental age. Early identification of these difficulties will help the interviewer rephrase rather than repeat unanswered questions using concrete and literal language in short and focused sentences. This will prevent the child from becoming tense because of a sense that he/she is not pleasing the interviewer by not answering the questions. It will also ensure that the child does not say "How many more questions?" or "When are we going to be done?"

SUMMARY
- The interviewer should act as the young child's communication assistant.
- As such, the interviewer needs to work to understand what the child is communicating. This involves:
  - Listening to every word the child says.
  - Using a developmental approach to interpret a child's concrete communication.
  - Making an effort to clarify what the child is saying.
  - Recruiting the child's help when the child does not appear to be answering a question.
  - Consolidating the rapport between the interviewer and the child by thanking the child for this help.
- If the child, rather than the interviewer, is the source of the communication breakdown, the interviewer should determine if the child has difficulties with language, cognition, or both.

Table 1-5. DEVELOPMENTAL GUIDELINES: BRIEF HOW TO DO IT LIST

Guidelines	How to Do It
CHILDREN	INTERVIEWER SHOULD
Are not little adults	Use a developmental approach
Have little spontaneous speech	Help the child communicate
Use nondiscursive speech	Use validation questions
Have poor perception of chronology	Avoid asking "When?" "How long?" and "How often?"
Are concrete thinkers	Use concrete action-based language Understand ideas behind children's concrete language
Like to please adults	Formulate questions that help young children provide the needed information Provide positive feedback
Figure out what interviewer wants to hear	Ask balanced questions not leading questions that emphasize pathology and put words in the child's mouth
Talk if they feel comfortable	Use developmentally appropriate language and questions without repeating questions Introduce sensitive topic(s) late in the interview Allow the child to play/eat Normalize, empathize, and praise the child's efforts to answer questions Avoid emphasizing the need to answer questions and asking chronology and causality questions Limit the length of the interview
INTERVIEWERS SHOULD	
Ask "What" or "How" questions Validate children's answers using "What" and "How" questions	Avoid "Why" questions
Avoid "Yes/No" questions	Reduce inefficient questions that lengthen the interview
Use short, focused sentences	Help the child answer and be motivated to talk
Work on understanding	Be the child's communication assistant

CONCLUSIONS ON DEVELOPMENTAL GUIDELINES

Table 1–5 provides a brief reminder list of how the interviewer should use the developmental guidelines. Armed with these twelve developmental guidelines, interviewers should be mindful that the interview of the young child involves time, patience, and effort. The interviewer needs time to think of how best to formulate questions to obtain valid and reliable information without rushing the child to verbalize and focus on the main complaint or presenting problem. The interview requires patience and considerable effort for both the interviewer and the child.

In the following chapters, the reader will learn how to use these twelve guidelines for the more difficult assessment of emotions, feelings, difficulties, problems, and worries that are often associated with a child's medical illness. Competent evaluation of these abstract (less visible and apparent) topics is necessary for every professional in the transition from novice to expert interviewer of young children.

REFERENCES

Caplan R (1996). Discourse deficits in children with schizophrenia spectrum disorder. In: *Language, Learning, and Behavior Disorders,* JH Beichtman, N Cohen, M Konstantareas, and R Tannock (eds.). Cambridge, UK: Cambridge University Press, 156–177.

Caplan R, Guthrie D, Fish B, Tanguay PE, and David-Lando G (1989). The Kiddie Formal Thought Disorder Rating Scale: Clinical assessment, reliability, and validity. *J Am Acad Child Adolesc Psychiatry* 28: 408–416.

Gogtay N, Giedd J, Lusk L, Hayashi K, Greenstein D, Vaituzis A, Nugent T, 3rd, Herman D, Clasen L, Toga A, Rapoport J, and Thompson P (2004). Dynamic mapping of human cortical development during childhood through early adulthood. *Proc Natl Acad Sci U S A.* 101: 8174–8179.

Hahne A, Eckstein K, and Friederici AD (2004). Brain signatures of syntactic and semantic processes during children's language development. *J Cogn Neurosci* 16: 1302–1318.

Sowell ER, Peterson BS, Thompson PM, Welcome SE, Henkenius AL, and Toga AW (2003). Mapping cortical change across the human life span. *Nat Neurosci* 6: 309–315.

Application of the Developmental Guidelines

Assessment of Emotions and Behaviors in Pediatric Illness

Overview to Part II

In the previous chapter, the reader became familiar with the need for a developmental approach to both speak with and understand young children's communication. The chapter emphasized that young children's language is quantitatively and qualitatively different from that of adult speakers. Speaking to a young child is akin to how one speaks to someone from a different country who has some limited knowledge of the language. Thus, rather than using complex sentences with sophisticated abstract vocabulary, as adults automatically do during conversation, interviewers should carefully plan how they talk with young children using the twelve developmental guidelines.

In chapters 3–9, the reader will learn that communication with young children is further complicated when talking about emotions. This difficulty is developmentally based because emotions are abstract concepts even though they can be accompanied by tangible physiological responses. But the thinking of young children is concrete, not abstract, and the ability to identify and monitor one's emotions matures during late childhood. Thus unlike adolescents and adults, young children usually do not put feelings into words, monitor their emotions, and reflect about the cause or trigger for emotions they experience. In fact, they rarely spontaneously discuss their feelings with anyone. In addition, the external manifestations of emotions and emotional states in children differ from those of adolescents and adults.

The abstract nature of emotions, together with young children's lack of insight into their feelings and their need to talk about them, as well as the communication-related developmental constraints described in the previous chapter, are challenges an interviewer faces when talking to young children about their emotions. The interviewer faces similar obstacles when talking to young children about their behavior. Although behaviors are visible and concrete (crying, hitting), young children do not monitor and think about the causes for their behaviors.

The presence of adversity, such as a medical illness, further increases the interviewer's challenges because young children might not be cognizant of how illness-related adversity affects their emotions and behavior. They also do not spontaneously initiate conversation about their illness. Despite these developmental obstacles, it is important to talk with young, medically ill children to determine if the illness and its treatment negatively impact their functioning.

In fact, a comprehensive examination and diagnosis of a child with a medical illness should include finding out how the illness affects the child and the family. The impact of the child's illness on the child and family has important implications

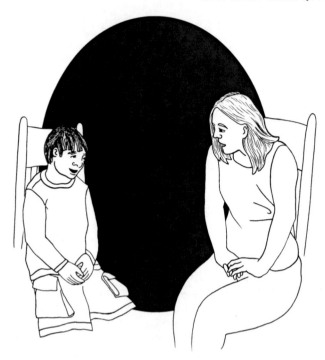

for treatment of the underlying disorder and of associated comorbidities involving mood, irritability, anger, fears, anxiety, attention, aggression, reality testing, judgment, and somatization (experiencing physical symptoms in response to stress).

In contrast to what professionals usually think, the young child is an essential source for information on feelings and behavior. Due to differences in the external presentation of emotions and emotional states between children and adults, parents might be unaware of, not recognize, or misinterpret the emotions their young children experience. Young children might also not share their feelings, particularly those involving negative emotions (sadness, anxiety, anger), with their parents.

Furthermore, children with medical illness often avoid talking with their parents about illness-related negative feelings because they do not want to add to their parent's burden. Some ill children also fear that sharing their negative feelings, such as sadness, anger, and fear, might make their parents angry. While parents are usually good informants about their children's physical symptoms, they might not be a good source of information on their children's emotions (see review in Grills and Ollendick 2002).

To help the interviewer meet the challenges of talking to young, medically ill children about their emotions and behavior, chapters 3–9 present techniques for speaking with children about their feelings and deciding what to talk about. They describe what interviewers should and should not do when asking young children about their illness, mood, anger, irritability, anxiety, fears, aggression/emotional control, attention, reality testing, judgment, and somatization. Through examples, the reader will understand how to make sense of the speech of young children when they talk about their emotions and behavior. In addition, each of these chapters includes a brief review of illnesses commonly associated with these different emotions and behaviors.

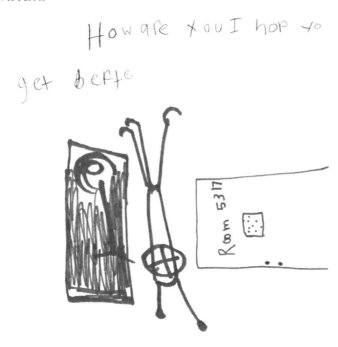

OVERVIEW OF TECHNIQUES

Table 2–1 provides a summary of the "dos and don'ts" during the interview of young children. In terms of the setting, young children should be interviewed separately from their parents in order to obtain valid information on their emotions and behavior. Young children usually agree to do this, but if a child is uncomfortable without his/her parents, the interview should be done with the parents.

The interviewer should explain to the parent that this is the best way to get information needed to help the child. If parents are concerned about this, it is important to clarify these concerns and determine if the parents' fears can be allayed. In most cases, parents are reassured once the interviewer gives them more details about the topics to be addressed with the child. When parents ask if the interviewer will tell them what the child says, the interviewer should let the parents know that she will ask permission from the child to share relevant information with the parent.

The interviewer should let the young, medically ill child know that she would like to understand what it is like for children to have this illness and also talk with the child about how he feels about his school, friends, and family. If the child asks why the parents are not there, she can explain that some children prefer to talk about their illness without their parents. Since young children do not like questions (akin to a testing situation), starting the interview with the statement interviewers typically use, "I am going to ask you questions about … " is counterproductive, as

Table 2–1. INTERVIEW TECHNIQUES: GENERAL SUGGESTIONS

	Actions	
Interview	**Do**	**Do Not**
Setting	Interview the child without parents*	See the child with parents*
Introduction	Tell the child that you want to learn more about the child and his/her illness	Tell the child that you will be asking questions
Activities	Encourage the child to engage in non-distracting activities during the interview	Ask the child to stop activities and focus on the conversation
Hyperactivity	Ignore	Comment on fidgetiness
Encouragement	Provide periodic positive feedback	Say to the child that he/she is not answering what was asked or not talking clearly
Sensitive topics	Only bring up once good rapport is established	Talk about sensitive topics at beginning of the interview Say parent told you about the child's "negative" behaviors
Questions	Provide positive, neutral, and negative options where possible For unanswered questions, check child's understanding, reformulate question, or go on to another question	Do not bias questions towards pathology or ask leading questions Do not repeat questions
Interpretation of answers	Base on information obtained from the child and check with the child to ensure you understand correctly	Do not put words in the child's mouth

* Unless the child cannot separate

it often makes the child quite resistant and leads to the child's inevitable question, "How many more questions?" The interviewer should also avoid introducing each topic or question by saying "I want to ask you … " or "I have another question about.… "

The interviewer should not tell the child that she wants to find out about behaviors the parent described, particularly if they are negative behaviors. Children do not feel good about their negative behaviors. Hearing that the parent is talking about them to others (strangers) is not conducive to making the child feel comfortable or willing to talk.

Reflecting on the developmental guideline, "Children talk if they feel comfortable," the interviewer should prioritize which emotions and behaviors need to be ruled in or out, and determine the order of the questions. In so doing, it is important to leave sensitive topics for later in the interview as time is needed to develop good rapport with the child. For example, if a parent reports that the child has "bad" behavior and has been oppositional, argumentative, angry, or aggressive, the interviewer should not start off by asking questions about these behaviors. Similarly, if the parent describes a child who is unable to separate from the parent or refuses to eat, the interviewer should ask about these difficulties later in the interview.

The interviewer should allow the child to continue to engage in an activity that does not demand the child's full attention as this helps young children get through the interview. Similarly, if the child is fidgety, moving about, and touching objects in the room, the interviewer should not waste time trying to get the child to sit still, as long as the child is talking and responding to the questions.

Bearing in mind the developmental guideline, "Children like to please adults," the interviewer should let the child know that the child is doing a good job or is a good talker periodically during the interview if the child is, in fact, talking. This positive feedback encourages the child to continue to speak. However, negative feedback, even if unintentional, will make the child lose motivation to continue to speak. This can occur if the interviewer tells the child that she cannot understand what the child is saying, that the child is not really answering her question, or that the child's answer appears off topic or makes no sense.

Given the previously mentioned developmental guidelines, "Children like to please adults" and "Children figure out what the interviewer wants to hear," interviewers should be mindful wording the questions they pose to children without biasing the children toward answers that confirm pathology. Two common behaviors by interviewers might inadvertently bias the information obtained from young children. The first is negative or pathological phrasing of questions; the second is misinterpretation of what the child is saying—the tendency to "put words in the child's mouth."

Since interviewers are trained to treat pathology, they gear the questions they ask patients toward identifying abnormalities, often using negative or pathological phrasing. For example a physician might typically ask an adult about headaches or chest pains as part of a general physical history by saying, "Do you have headaches?" or "Do you have chest pains?" Alternatively, to be neutral, a physician could ask, "How does your head usually feel?" or "How do you feel when you walk up a hill?" Similarly when trying to rule out depression or anxiety, a mental health clinician might ask an adult, "Are you sad?" or "Are you anxious?" instead of more neutral questions such as, "Is your mood happy, sad, or in between?" or "Do you takes things as they come or do you worry about them before they happen?" To help readers avoid this tendency, chapters 3–9 provide examples of neutral questions to use when asking young children about their emotions and behavior.

Regarding the tendency to put words in children's mouths, interviewers periodically sum up information they hear from patients while taking a medical history. This ensures that they understand the information they have obtained from the patient. If the interviewer has incorrectly understood what the patient communicated, an adult patient will let the physician know. In contrast, young children are quite timid with adults, particularly with those they do not know well. They also like to please adults and avoid disagreeing with them. As a result, they tend to agree with interviewers' summaries even if they are incorrect. Therefore, an interviewer should always check with the child to make sure that he/she understands what the child is trying to communicate.

Children with language and cognitive difficulties are more prone to do this. Since pediatric professionals have difficulty interviewing these children, they should avoid reaching conclusions that are not based on what the children say or mean to say. This pitfall is also evident when interviewers speak to a young child using language above the child's developmental level. Being cognizant of this tendency, careful monitoring of the language used when speaking to children, and working to understand what children are communicating are strategies that help the interviewer avoid this potential difficulty.

SUMMARY

- Armed with the developmental guidelines and the dos and don'ts for interviews, the reader is now ready to acquire techniques for talking to young children about their emotions and behaviors.
- Knowledge about the impact of medical illness on young children's emotions and behavior and the techniques for talking about this with children is essential for a comprehensive examination.
- Chapters 3–9 provide this information for a wide range of emotions and behaviors.

REFERENCES

Grills A and Ollendick TH (2002). Issues in parent-child agreement: The case of structured diagnostic interviews. *Clin Child Fam Psychol Rev* 5: 57–83.

Mood, Anger, and Irritability

Among the different mood symptoms children experience, depression is prevalent in young children with chronic medical illness (see review in Bursch and Stuber 2004). Early recognition of possible depression is important because of its possible impact on a child's underlying medical illness (Brand et al. 1986; Palermo et al. 2008; Myrvik et al. 2011; Hassan et al. 2006; Wood et al. 2006), as well as on the functioning (Kashikar-Zuck et al. 2001) and quality of life of both the child and the family (Bender et al. 2000; Zeltzer et al. 2009; Baca et al. 2011). However, a diagnosis of major depression is challenging in young children because, unlike adults, young children with depression often do not present with apparent sadness or lack of affect (facial expression of emotions); loss of ability to enjoy things, lack of interest and motivation (anhedonia); or slow and sluggish movements and thinking (Carlson and Kashani 1988).

Although manic mood is rare in young children with medical illness, it can occur as an adverse effect of medications such as steroids. Anger and irritability are often the presenting symptom of a mood disorder in young children, both for depression (Carlson 2000) and mania (Argelinda et al. 2009). Application of the developmental guidelines will help the interviewer identify mood symptoms such as sadness, depression, anger, irritability, as well as other symptoms of mood disorders in young children.

In this chapter, we first present a developmentally based assessment of mood disorder symptoms in young children (see Tables 3–1 and 3–2). We then describes mood disorders associated with medical illness and outline how to differentiate symptoms of a primary medical disorder that might mimic a mood disorder from *de novo* development of a mood disorder.

ASSESSMENT OF MOOD SYMPTOMS IN YOUNG CHILDREN

To detect the presence of a sad mood, the interviewer should word the question without bias (see developmental guideline "Children figure out what the interviewer wants to hear" in chapter 1) by asking, "Do you usually feel happy, sad, or in-between?" or "Are you a happy, sad, or in-between child?" Then, based on the child's answer, the interviewer should validate the mood by asking the child what things make him sad or happy. To rule out possible major depressive disorder (or mania), the interviewer should ascertain if the child also gets sad (or happy) but

Table 3–1. SYMPTOMS OF DEPRESSION AND SCREENING QUESTIONS

Symptoms	Questions
MOOD	
Pervasive mood	Are you happy, sad, or in between?
Sad	What makes you sad (cry)? Are you sad and don't know what makes you sad? Do you cry and don't know what makes you cry?
Irritable	What makes you angry? Are you sometimes angry and don't know at what? Do lots of things bug you?
VEGETATIVE SYMPTOMS	
Sleep onset	Is it easy or difficult to fall asleep (stay asleep)?
Early morning awakening	Do you wake up when it is still dark outside and can't fall asleep again?
Restorative sleep	When you wake up in the morning, do you feel you slept well or not so good?
Appetite/Weight	What do you like/hate to eat? Are your clothes getting small or too big?
Anhedonia	What do you do for fun? Is it still fun now that you have … (current illness)?
Energy/Fatigue	When you want to do fun stuff, do you keep on going or get tired easily?
SUICIDALITY SELF-ESTEEM, AND GUILT	
Thoughts	Do you sometimes think it would be better if you were dead?
Plans	How would you do it?
Acts	Have you ever tried to kill or hurt yourself?
Worthlessness	What do you like/don't like about you? What would you like to change in yourself?
Guilt	How do you feel if you do something wrong? If someone else gets into trouble, how does that make you feel?
ATTENTION	
Concentration	Is it easy or difficult for you to pay attention?

does not know what is making her sad (or happy). Similarly, rather than asking a "Yes/No" question, "Do you cry sometimes?" the interviewer should find out what makes the child cry, and if he sometimes cries but does not know what makes him cry. Even if the child's answer to the initial mood question is "in-between" or "I don't know," the interviewer should proceed to ask all of the above questions.

Rather than sadness, young depressed or manic children often present with irritability and aggressive behavior. Since the word irritable might not be well understood by young children, the interviewer should ask the child what makes him angry, and then ask if he gets angry or grouchy without knowing what is making him mad. If the child says he does not know what makes him angry, the interviewer should clarify if this means that he does not want to talk about it or if he finds it difficult to talk about it.

Table 3–2. Symptoms of Mania and Screening Questions

Symptoms	Questions
Mood Due to poor insight into this condition, obtain parent observations	You told me your mood is happy. Is it sometimes so happy that you don't know what is making you happy?
Elevated, expansive Due to poor insight into this condition, obtain parent observations	When that happens, are you so happy that other people say "What's making you *so* happy?"
Irritable Due to poor insight into this condition, obtain parent observations	How about getting angry? What makes you angry? What bugs you? Are these big things like getting punished or little things like your brother's/sister's voice?
Grandiosity	Some kids have special powers. What special powers do you have? What can you do with them? What can you do that other kids can't? Are you better or smarter than other kids or just like them? How do you know that you have special powers (are better, smarter than other kids, etc.)?
Decreased need for sleep Best determined by parent report in children with mania	Is it easy or hard for you to go to sleep at night? Is that because you don't get tired … are too hyper … just want to play … ?
Pressure to talk Best determined by observation	Do people say you talk too little or too much?
Flight of ideas Best determined by observation	Do you sometimes feel that you have so many thoughts in your head you don't know which one to think about?
Distractibility Best determined by observation	Is it easy or hard for you to pay attention? When you are busy doing something, if you hear noise or other kids talking, can you still pay attention?
Psychomotor agitation Best determined by observation	It looks like you are having a hard time staying still. Is it easy or hard for you to sit without moving?

Some children are embarrassed to talk about what they do when angry. If the interviewer provides examples of what children do when angry—shout, hit, cry, go to their room, sulk, pound on something—this helps to normalize anger, and young children are more willing to describe how they express their own anger.

To assess irritability, the interviewer should clarify whether the child feels that a lot of things "bug" him and make him angry, even little things that might not be important. She should ask the child for examples of what makes him angry to determine if this is, in fact, irritability. Even if the child denies irritability, the

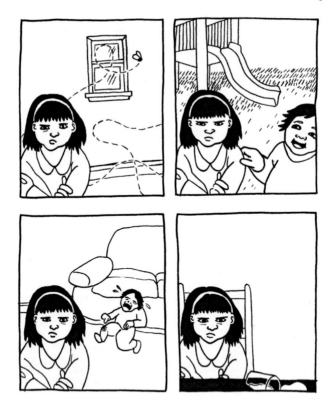

interviewer should provide examples of little things that irritate children to ensure that the child understands what the interviewer means by irritability (annoyance at how people talk to him, what they say, noise they make or laughing, and the like).

The child's answers to the "What" questions on mood help validate if he is, in fact, experiencing being sad, happy, angry, or irritable, and whether these emotions reflect environmental or internal causes. Learning about the circumstances in which the child experiences these feelings also provides the interviewer with important information on the child's psychosocial environment and its relationship with his symptoms.

The two dialogues below highlight how exploring the circumstances that trigger the child's mood symptoms gives the interviewer relevant diagnostic information. They demonstrate that obtaining this diagnostic information is contingent on use of the developmental guidelines. In contrast to the second dialogue, the first dialogue yielded little information from the child because the interviewer did not apply the developmental guidelines.

An 8-year-old girl, Malu, treated for repeated episodes of pain associated with sickle cell anemia, is watching television from her hospital bed when Dr. Harris comes in for morning rounds.

Technically Flawed Dialogue
DR. HARRIS: *Good morning, Malu. Why do you look so sad?* [Why question]
MALU (looking down at the floor): *Because.*
DR. HARRIS: *Do you still have pain?* [Yes/No question]

MALU: *No.*

DR. HARRIS: *So that means you are feeling better?* [Puts words in child's mouth]

MALU (looking down): *I don't know.*

Despite its brevity, this dialogue between Dr. Harris and Malu had several technical problems. First, Dr. Harris asked Malu a "Why" and a "Yes/No" question, and both questions yielded minimal information. Second, she did not use validation questions to clarify what Malu meant by saying "Because." Third, she tried to put words in Malu's mouth by telling her that she is feeling better. Fourth, Dr. Harris did not clarify what Malu's "I don't know" really meant. Alternatively, the interview might have proceeded as follows:

Developmentally Based Dialogue

DR. HARRIS: *Good morning, Malu. What is making you look so sad?*

MALU (looking down): *I don't know.*

DR. HARRIS: *Yesterday the pain was bothering you; is it still hurting?*

MALU: *No.*

DR. HARRIS: *So does that mean that the pain is not making you sad, but something else is?*

MALU (looking down): *Maybe.*

DR. HARRIS: *I am going to try guess what it is so we can figure this out. I don't see your mother. She usually is here early in the morning.*

MALU (looking at Dr. Harris, with anger in her voice): *She's at my brother's school.*

DR. HARRIS: *And how does that make you feel?*

MALU: *Really mad, she should be here with me at the hospital.*

In the second dialogue, Dr. Harris's "What" rather than "Why" question leads to an "I don't know" answer from the child. She clearly expresses empathy for Malu by indicating that she remembers her pain from before and then asking if she still has pain. Rather than putting words in Malu's mouth, she uses Malu's answer that she has no pain to look for additional clues as to why Malu might be looking sad. In this way, Dr. Harris lets Malu know that she is working on trying to understand her. Young children clearly appreciate it when they feel the physician is actively trying to figure out how to help them. By telling Malu that she will try to guess, Dr. Harris also indicates to her that she realizes from her, "I don't know" response that Malu does not want to talk about what is making her sad.

Essentially this approach strengthens rapport with the child and increases Malu's trust in Dr. Harris. Malu's subsequent eye contact with Dr. Harris and full sentence answer confirm that Dr. Harris guessed correctly. As a result, when Dr. Harris asks her how her mother's absence makes her feel (not a "Yes/No" question such as, "Does that make you angry?" to which children might say "No" due to embarrassment), Malu clearly verbalizes her anger. Through this process, Dr. Harris understands that Malu's sadness and anger have something to do with how the mother allocates her time between Malu and her brother. This topic clearly needs to be further clarified separately with both Malu and her mother.

In addition to questions on mood, the interviewer should inquire about anhedonia, even though it is rare phenomenon in young children. To do this, the interviewer should ask what the child likes to do for fun and then find out if the child always and/or currently enjoys these things. It is important to make sure that the child's lack of joy or interest in activities is not due to physical constraints associated with medical illness or external causes. For example, a child with acute exacerbation of rheumatoid arthritis might say she no longer enjoys running. A child who loves watching television might say that now she does not enjoy watching her favorite show. However, further questioning reveals that this is because there is one television in the house and her older sister wants to look at another show that airs at the same time. Similarly, if a child reports she no longer enjoys school, this might reflect increasingly difficult course work within the context of an underlying learning disorder rather than anhedonia.

Questions about having fun can also be good when beginning to talk to young children with a medical illness about their mood, as the illness might limit activities the child enjoys. Most people do not talk with young, medically ill children about feelings associated with illness-related restrictions. In addition to developing or strengthening rapport with the child, these questions help identify possible sources of sadness, anger, or irritability.

Young children with depression might also have thoughts about death, dying, and suicide. It is particularly important to talk with young children about their concerns that they might die due to their illness, because usually no one discusses this topic with them. In addition, helping the child talk about concerns and thoughts about possible death can alleviate this emotional burden and address misconceptions the child might have about his illness and death. Young children do not typically initiate a direct conversation because they might be scared that if they say thoughts out loud, they might die (magical thinking). Although young children do not want to make their parents more worried by sharing these thoughts with them, they might bring up the topic in an indirect manner.

To initiate conversation about fears of death, the interviewer might mention that children often tell her that they worry that they might die. She should then ask the child if he has had similar thoughts. While asking these questions, the interviewer should carefully monitor the child's nonverbal expressions, as children who are scared to talk about these thoughts might respond through gestures, such as a nod of the head or a shift in eye contact. Using a "What" question, the interviewer should find out what thoughts the child has had, if he has shared them with anyone, and what fears he might have if he does talk about these thoughts.

To learn about suicidal behavior, the circumstances that trigger this behavior, and whether the child is in imminent danger of hurting himself, the interviewer should ask the child "Have you felt that it would be better to be dead?" "What made you feel like that?" "When that happened, did you think about doing something to make yourself die?" "What did you think about doing?" "Did you do that?" "How did you feel afterwards?" "If you die, how would that help?" "Do you still feel you want to die?" "Who did you tell about these feelings?" "What did they do?" Similar questions can be asked about self-injurious behavior. Of note, the initial suicidal question is a "Yes/No" question rather than a "What" question, which could suggest suicidal behavior to a child.

Disturbances of appetite, weight, energy level, and sleep (known as vegetative signs) can also accompany depression or mania. Decreased appetite, weight loss, and low energy level due to a medical illness or its treatment need to be differentiated from the vegetative signs found in depression and schizophrenia. If, however, a child's medical illness is inactive or well controlled, development of these symptoms emphasizes the need to rule out depression. Children with mania may have a high energy level associated with poor appetite and weight loss due to over-activity and lack of time to eat. They may also have difficulty falling asleep at night and be awake until very late.

The parents' report on the chronology of the development of vegetative symptoms is essential to determine if these symptoms reflect the underlying medical illness, depression, or both. Similarly, parents are the best informants for confirming the decreased need for food in a manic child and its association with the child's over-activity and "lack of time to eat."

When presenting the child with questions about appetite or weight, the interviewer should ensure that the child understands abstract words, such as appetite and weight, and should formulate questions that include both the normal and abnormal options. Examples of appetite questions include: "Are you the type of kid who likes to eat?" "What is your favorite food?" "Do you always like eating … [favorite food]?" These questions can also shed light on anhedonia if, unrelated to a medical illness or its treatment, a child says he has a favorite food that he no longer wants to eat. For weight questions, the interviewer should inquire if the child's clothes fit him or if they have become too small or too big. If, unrelated to a primary medical illness or medication side effect, the child says he is too fat or getting too fat, has no appetite or too much of an appetite, or has experienced recent weight loss, the interviewer also needs to rule out an eating disorder.

Regarding energy levels (an abstract concept), interviewers should obtain this information from the parents, as young children do not monitor their energy level very well. However, they are good reporters on their sleep. In fact, parents might not be aware of the number of times a child wakes up in the night, nor of the child's perception of whether his sleep is restorative or not (as in depression).

When asking a young child about sleep difficulties, the interviewer should remember to avoid putting words into the child's mouth. Rather than asking the child a leading "Yes/No" question, such as, "Is it difficult for you to sleep at night?" or "Do you have problems sleeping at night?" she should try using some of the following questions: "Is it easy or difficult to fall asleep?" "Are you a good sleeper or not a very good sleeper?" "Do you stay asleep the whole night or do you wake up in the night?"

The interviewer should also remember that young children do not estimate time and duration of time well, so it is best to avoid "When" and "How long" questions such as, "When do you fall asleep at night?" or "How long does it take you to fall asleep?" In fact, a young child might state that it takes a while to fall asleep, but validation questions on what makes it difficult to fall asleep might reveal that he falls asleep shortly after getting into bed. If the child reports difficulty falling asleep, this could be due to conditions listed in Box 3–1.

Use of "What" questions will help the interviewer rule out these diagnostic possibilities. Alternatively, one can present the child with different options of "What makes it difficult for children to sleep" and have the child decide if any of the options apply to him. For example, some children can't sleep when they keep on remembering scary things that happened to them when they were in the hospital; get scared in the dark and cannot sleep; think they might have bad dreams; feel something bad might happen to them or to their parents if they are not together

---

Box 3–1.

CONDITIONS ASSOCIATED WITH INSOMNIA IN YOUNG CHILDREN

- Depression
- Mania
- Excessive environmental stimulation
- Fear of being alone at night because of separation anxiety
- Worries related to a general anxiety disorder
- Trauma (see chapter 4)
- Activation at night of psychotic phenomena, such as hallucinations or delusions (see chapter 7)
- Adverse effects of medications
  - Steroids
  - Vasopressors
  - Antihistamines
  - Decongestants
  - Stimulants

---

in the night; think about what they will be doing the next day; feel hyper; think about everything that happened during the day; cannot stop thinking; or feel their imagination plays tricks on them.

If the child picks one of these options, the interviewer should then use "What" questions for further validation and/or empathize with the child to help him talk more about the topic, as in the following example of a 7-year-old child with asthma since age 3:

Insomnia

INTERVIEWER: *Joe, is it easy or difficult for you to fall asleep at night?*
JOE: *Hard.*
INTERVIEWER: *What happens when you get into bed and try to fall asleep?*
JOE: *The doctors and nurses push me down and yell, "Don't move."*
INTERVIEWER: *They did that?*
JOE: *They also stuck me with needles.*
INTERVIEWER: *How scary for you.*
JOE: *And they put a tube up my nose and I couldn't even breathe.*
INTERVIEWER: *Oh, wow. Was that at the hospital or at home?*
JOE: *At home.*
INTERVIEWER: *Do they come to your house and do that?*
JOE: *At the hospital they did all of that.*
INTERVIEWER: *And when you are at home now and try fall asleep …?*
JOE: *I told you. They push me and yell.*
INTERVIEWER: *Oh, I get it now. You remember all that when you try to go to sleep?*
JOE: *They also made my mother leave.*
INTERVIEWER: *That must have been very scary for you.*
JOE: *I never want to go back to the hospital.*

This dialogue illustrates how the interviewer worked out what the child was communicating through use of empathy, restating what the child said to help the child continue the conversation, careful interpretation of the child's concrete thinking, concrete action-based language, and a "What" question. The interviewer's empathic response focused on how the child felt and encouraged him to talk about his traumatic experiences in the hospital.

By responding that the medical staff forced the mother out of the room, the child acknowledges that he was scared. His concrete action-based statement that they made his mother leave suggests that his fear was made even worse by the separation from his mother. The interviewer's empathic responses, "They did that?" "How scary!" "Oh, wow!" and "That must have been very scary for you" verbalize the child's feelings, and further encourage him to talk about his traumatic experience. When the interviewer makes this last statement, the child responds that he will never go back to the hospital. The content of the conversation and the child's last concrete statement suggests that Joe is experiencing on-going trauma symptoms subsequent to his hospitalization. (See chapter 15 for a detailed discussion of trauma symptoms induced by medical procedures.)

From the diagnostic perspective, children with depression who have difficulty falling asleep might have negative thoughts with self-deprecatory or angry content, or they might only describe not being able to fall asleep. Children with hyperactivity or mania acknowledge difficulty settling down and feeling too hyper to fall asleep.

Answers to questions about poor self-esteem are sometimes a first clue about a child's mood and can be phrased as follows: "What do you like about yourself?" "What do you not like about yourself?" "What things about you would you like to change?" Finding out what other children (friends) like about the child or like to do with him also taps into the child's self-esteem. It is important to corroborate the child's answers regarding friends with information from the parent to determine if feelings of not being liked by peers are objective or distorted (as found in depression). An exaggerated self-esteem is found in children with mania who also feel there is nothing they cannot do and that they are good at everything.

Questions on feelings of helplessness and hopelessness are important given the relationship between these negative feelings and the course of pediatric medical illnesses (Lernmark et al. 1999). A child's answers to these questions also inform the interviewer about the severity of the child's mood (depression or mania) and the risk of suicidal behavior. The interviewer should ask if the child feels that the problems he has shared thus far will get better, stay the same, or get worse. Based on the child's answer, the interviewer should then ascertain why the child feels like this by asking, "What will make things get better [get worse, stay the same]?" The child's answers to these questions will validate whether he feels optimistic (or hopeless) and also indicate if the child feels some control over events in his life (internal locus of control) or powerless (external locus of control) and helpless, as often found in children with a medical illness (Brand et al. 1986) and in depressed children with epilepsy (Dunn and Austin 1999). In contrast, manic children are over-optimistic about their situation, even in the face of a medical illness.

Assessment of feelings of guilt is important as it might be an overlooked symptom in young children with depression. Children with a chronic illness may feel guilty because of the burden their parents and family endure due to their illness.

Table 3–3. EXAMPLES OF QUESTIONS ABOUT FEELINGS OF GUILT

Interviewer's Questions	Child's Response	Validation Questions	Child's Response
Are you the type of kid that feels okay or not so good after doing something that you think is bad?	Not good	What makes you feel like that?	When I shout at my mom
When you shout at your mom, do you feel bad a lot or a little?	A lot	Do you keep on feeling like that or quickly forget about it?	Sometimes I forget about it
What helps you forget?	I go and play	And then you don't think about it again?	Not any more
What other things do you do that you think are bad?	I don't let my sister play with my friends	And then you feel you did something wrong?	Well, she tells my parents
If something bad happens to someone else, do you feel that you made it happen?	Yes	What happened?	My sister has no friends
Who do you blame for all the problems you have told me about?	Me	How are you to blame?	I need to be better
Kids like you with [NAME OF ILLNESS] feel they make problems for their parents. How about you?	They fight about my medicine	What about the medicine makes them fight?	My mom says it makes me more sick and my dad says no
Who do you tell about feeling you did something wrong?	No one	How about your parents?	They will be mad at me

Yet, children with depression or chronic medical illness, or both, often do not talk about their guilt feelings to their parents. Table 3–3 presents questions that can help interviewers ask young children about feelings of guilt.

Finally, poor attention, aggression, and psychotic symptoms, such as hallucinations, delusions, and disorganized thinking (formal thought disorder), could be signs of depression, mania, or bipolar disorder in children. Details on how to apply the developmental guidelines to interview young children about these symptoms are presented in chapter 7.

SUMMARY
- Young children with depressed or manic mood typically do not present with symptoms similar to those of depressed or manic adolescents or adults.
- Due to the internalizing nature of depression and sadness, the young child (rather than the parents) is often the best source of this information.

- Parents are usually the best informants of vegetative signs and manic behavior in young children.
- Review Tables 3–1 and 3–2 for main mood symptom screening questions.

DEPRESSION IN YOUNG CHILDREN WITH MEDICAL ILLNESS

Pediatric illnesses associated with depression include type 1 diabetes mellitus (Wodrich et al. 2011), asthma (Goodwin et al. 2005; Blackman and Gurka 2007), cystic fibrosis (Cruz et al. 2009), sickle cell anemia (Jerrell et al. 2010), epilepsy (Caplan et al. 2005), and multiple sclerosis (Weisbrot et al. 2010). Studies of depression in pediatric disorders, such as type 1 diabetes (Garrison et al. 2005), asthma (Blackman et al. 2007), and inflammatory bowel disease (Greenley et al. 2011), have been conducted mainly on adolescents. Epidemiological studies in the general child population also indicate that depression is more prevalent in adolescence (Kessler et al. 2001).

The lack of depression studies in young children with medical illness probably represents the age-related increase in the prevalence of the disorder (Costello et al. 2002), as well as the previously described problems diagnosing depression in young children (Carlson et al. 1988). More specifically, since young children with depression might present with anger and irritability rather than with sad affect, as typically found in adolescents and adults, children in this age group are more likely to be labeled "bad," poorly behaved, or oppositional by their parents and medical personnel. Additionally, young children are more vulnerable to medically induced trauma symptoms (Rennick et al. 2002) and may deny symptoms of depression due to traumatic avoidance (Erickson and Steiner 2000).

Of note, unless children with medical illness demonstrate marked anger and irritability, their parents usually talk to health professionals about the medical symptoms rather than about their children's behavior (Briggs-Gowan et al. 2000). Furthermore, children with illnesses other than those already described might also become depressed. Clinicians should, therefore, ask parents of young children with any chronic illness about anger and irritability symptoms. They should also include depression in the differential diagnosis of young children whose parents report anger and irritability. A developmentally sensitive interview of the child will help determine if the child's anger and irritability are associated with a diagnosis of depression.

In contrast to under-diagnosis of depression in young children with medical illness, children who are listless and have no energy or motivation for daily activities as part of their primary disorder might be incorrectly diagnosed with depression. A large number of commonly used medications can induce mood symptoms, particularly anger and irritability, in young children. These include hormones (steroids, estrogen, progesterone); barbiturates; new generation antiepileptic drugs (topiramate, levetiracetam, zonisamide); tacrolimus; interferon; and baclofen.

Young children are less able to monitor mood or behavior changes after taking a new medication or following an increase in the dose of their medication than are older individuals. Interviewers should consider side effects if parents describe the onset of mood symptoms shortly after the child begins to take a drug or after a dose increase. The following example demonstrates how a sensitive developmentally based interview of a young child helps determine if the child's symptoms represent depression, the child's medical illness, adverse medication effects, or a combination of these factors.

The father of Naomi, a 9-year-old girl with epilepsy, reports to Dr. Tran that he thinks Naomi might be depressed because she keeps to herself; she is not interested in doing the usual things she enjoys, including school; she sleeps a lot; does not eat her favorite foods; and she cries quite easily. Dr. Tran asks the father when this began and whether it was related to any medication changes or an increase in Naomi's seizures. The father says that he cannot remember when this began and that his wife, Naomi's stepmother, knows about the medication but was unavailable today. He adds that he thinks Naomi is having fewer seizures, but he is not sure about that. He gives Dr. Tran a note from his wife with his daughter's current daily medications: valproic acid 1500 mg (53mg/kg), levetiracetam 1500 mg (53mg/kg), and primidone 300 mg.

Depression or Adverse Medication Effects

DR. TRAN: *Hi, Naomi. I understand that you haven't been feeling too good.*

NAOMI (very slowly, without eye contact): *I'm okay.*

DR. TRAN: *Does okay mean you are not having any seizures?*

NAOMI (after a pause, slowly): *I think I had one yesterday.*

DR. TRAN: *And before that?*

NAOMI (very slowly): *I don't remember.*

DR. TRAN: *When you have a seizure, do you sleep afterwards?*

NAOMI: *A lot.*

DR. TRAN: *And is it difficult for you to remember things?*

NAOMI: *Sometimes*

DR. TRAN: *Besides your seizures, how are you feeling?*

NAOMI: *Tired.*

DR. TRAN: *Are you tired right now?*

NAOMI: *Yes.*

DR. TRAN: *I can see you look tired. And you are sleeping a lot.*

NAOMI: *Yes.*

DR. TRAN: *Even in the day?*

NAOMI: *Yes.*

DR. TRAN: *How about at school?*

NAOMI: *I miss the bus, because I wake up too late in the morning.*

DR. TRAN: *So are you not going to school?*

NAOMI: *I missed a lot of days.*

DR. TRAN: *How does that make you feel?*

NAOMI: *My teacher is mad at me.*

DR. TRAN: *How about fun things? What are you doing for fun?*

NAOMI: *Nothing.*

DR. TRAN: *Is that because you don't want to do anything fun?*

NAOMI: *I just want to sleep.*

DR. TRAN: *How about your appetite?*

NAOMI: *My dad makes me eat.*

DR. TRAN: *So it sounds like you don't feel like eating?*

Naomi nods yes.

DR. TRAN: *Would you say you are happy, sad, or in-between right now?*

NAOMI (with tears in her eyes): *Tired.*

DR. TRAN: *What things make you cry?*

NAOMI: *When they don't let me sleep.*

DR. TRAN: *Who isn't letting you sleep?*

NAOMI: *My mom and dad say I sleep too much.*

DR. TRAN: *Do you think things will get better or stay the same for you?*

NAOMI: *I don't know.*

DR. TRAN: *What would you like to get better?*

NAOMI: *Not being so tired.*

DR. TRAN: *Naomi, you have done a great job explaining to me the problem. I will see what I can do to make sure you won't be so tired. Okay?*

NAOMI (smiling): *Okay.*

Dr. Tran used empathy and balanced (not biased) "What" and "How" questions. She worked on understanding Naomi's difficulties and checked with her to make sure that this is what the child was communicating and feeling. Dr. Tran needed to determine if the child's seizures, depression, medication, or a combination of these factors accounted for her apathy. She was unable to determine the chronology of symptom evolution because the father did not have the necessary information. The father also had minimal knowledge about the child's seizures, so he could not help Dr. Tran ascertain if the child's tiredness was due to an increase in Naomi's seizure frequency, fatigue following seizures, medication changes, or a combination of these factors.

Nevertheless, through her developmentally sensitive interview with the child, Dr. Tran could infer that Naomi did not meet criteria for depression because Naomi confirmed tiredness but not sadness, anhedonia, and hopelessness. She also found out that Naomi's tiredness was continuous rather than occurring mainly after seizures. Naomi's poor memory regarding how many seizures she had was age appropriate; in an older child, not knowing when she had her last seizure could be due to memory difficulties associated with poorly controlled ongoing seizures.

Two of Naomi's medications, levetiracetam (Delanty et al. 2012) and primidone (Lopez-Gomez et al. 2005), can cause depression in children with epilepsy. Rather than depression, the relatively high doses of the three antiepileptic drugs most probably contributed to the child's main complaint, tiredness. The child's first smile when she heard Dr. Tran say that she would find a way to decrease her tiredness confirmed Dr. Tran's diagnostic conclusion and ruled out depression.

Finally, noncompliance with medical recommendations and poor medication adherence might be due to the severity of depression in pediatric disorders such as diabetes (Garrison et al. 2005) and cystic fibrosis (Cruz et al. 2009). Since noncompliance could represent a child's difficulty coping with illness and related depression, clinicians should rule out the possibility of depression in these children.

SUMMARY

- Interviewers should include depression in the differential diagnosis of young children with medical illness, particularly if the parents report anger and irritability, as well as poor adherence to treatment.

- A developmentally sensitive interview of the child is essential to determine the definitive diagnosis.
- Interviewers should always also ask parents about these symptoms and determine if they reflect depression, symptoms of the underlying illness, adverse medication effects, or family factors.

REFERENCES

Argelinda B, Jessica RL, David AL, Kenneth ET, and Ellen L (2009). Practitioner review: The assessment of bipolar disorder in children and adolescents. *J Child Psychol Psychiatry* 50: 203–215.

Baca C, Vickrey BG, Caplan R, Vassar D, and Berg AT (2011). Psychiatric and medical comorbidity and quality of life outcomes in childhood-onset epilepsy. *Pediatrics* 128: 1532–1543.

Bender BG, Annett RD, Ikle D, DuHamel TR, Rand C, and Strunk RC (2000). Relationship between disease and psychological adaptation in children in the childhood asthma management program and their families. Camp Research Group. *Arch Pediatr Adolesc Med* 154: 706–713.

Blackman JA and Gurka MJ (2007). Developmental and behavioral comorbidities of asthma in children. *J Dev Behav Pediatr* 28: 92–99

Brand A, Johnson JH, and Johnson SB (1986). Life stress and diabetic control in children and adolescents with insulin-dependent diabetes. *J Pediatr Psychol* 1: 481–495.

Briggs-Gowan M, Horwitz SM, Schwab-Stone ME, Leventhal JM, Leaf PJ (2000). Mental health in pediatric settings: distribution of disorders and factors related to service use. *J Am Acad Child Adolesc Psychiatry* 39: 841–849.

Bursch B and Stuber M (2004). Pediatrics. In: *Textbook of Psychosomatic Medicine*, JL Levenson (ed.). Arlington, VA: American Psychiatric Publishing, Inc.

Caplan R, Siddarth P, Gurbani S, Hanson R, Sankar R, and Shields WD (2005). Depression and anxiety disorders in pediatric epilepsy. *Epilepsia* 46: 720–730.

Carlson G (2000). The challenge of diagnosing depression in childhood and adolescence. *J Affect Disord* 61, Supplement 1: S3–S8.

Carlson GA and Kashani JH (1988). Phenomenology of major depression from childhood through adulthood: Analysis of three studies. *Am J Psychiatry* 145: 1222–1225.

Costello E, Pine DS, Hammen C, March JS, Plotsky PM, Weissman MM, Biederman J, Goldsmith HH, Kaufman J, Lewinsohn PM, Hellander M, Hoagwood K, Koretz DS, Nelson CA, and Leckman JF (2002). Development and natural history of mood disorders. *Biol Psychiatry* 52: 529–542.

Cruz I, Marciel KK, Quittner AL, and Schechter MS (2009). Anxiety and depression in cystic fibrosis. *Semin Respir Crit Care Med* 30: 569–578.

Delanty N, Jones J, Tonner F (2012). Adjunctive levetiracetam in children, adolescents, and adults with primary generalized seizures: Open-label, noncomparative, multicenter, long-term follow-up study. *Epilepsia* 53: 111–119

Dunn D and Austin J (1999). Behaviour issues in pediatric epilepsy. *Neurology* 53: S96–S100.

Erickson SJ and Steiner H (2000). Trauma spectrum adaptation: Somatic symptoms in long-term pediatric cancer survivors. *Psychosomatics* 41: 339–346.

Garrison MM, Katon WJ, and Richardson LP (2005). The impact of psychiatric comorbidities on readmissions for diabetes in youth. *Diabetes Care* 28: 2150–2154.

Goodwin RD, Messineo K, Bregante A, Hoven CW, and Kairam R (2005). Prevalence of probable mental disorders among pediatric asthma patients in an inner-city clinic. *J Asthma* 42: 643–647.

Greenley RN, Hommel KA, Nebel J, Raboin T, Li S-H, Simpson P, and Mackner L (2011). A meta-analytic review of the psychosocial adjustment of youth with inflammatory bowel disease. *J Pediatr Psychol* 35: 857–869.

Hassan K, Loar R, Anderson BJ, and Heptulla RA (2006). The role of socioeconomic status, depression, quality of life, and glycemic control in type 1 diabetes mellitus. *J Pediatr* 149: 526–531.

Jerrell J, Tripathi A, and McIntyre RS (2010). Prevalence and treatment of depression in children and adolescents with sickle cell disease: a retrospective cohort study. *Prim Care Companion CNS Disord* 13.

Kashikar-Zuck S, Goldschneider KR, Powers SW, Vaught MH, and Hershey AD (2001). Depression and functional disability in chronic pediatric pain *Clin J Pain* 17: 341–349.

Kessler RC, Avenevoli S, and Ries Merikangas K (2001). Mood disorders in children and adolescents: An epidemiologic perspective. *Biol Psychiatry* 49: 1002–1014.

Lernmark B, Persson B, Fisher L, and Rydelius PA (1999). Symptoms of depression are important to psychological adaptation and metabolic control in children with diabetes mellitus. *Diabet Med* 16: 14–22.

Lopez-Gomez M, Ramirez-Bermudez J, Campillo C, Sosa AL, Espinola M, and Ruiz I (2005). Primidone is associated with interictal depression in patients with epilepsy. *Epilepsy Behav* 6: 413–416.

Myrvik MP, Campbell AD, Davis MM, and Butcher JL (2011). Impact of psychiatric diagnoses on hospital length of stay in children with sickle cell anemia. *Pediatr Blood Cancer* 58: 239–243.

Palermo TM, Riley CA, and Mitchell BA (2008). Daily functioning and quality of life in children with sickle cell disease pain: Relationship with family and neighborhood socioeconomic distress. *J Pain* 9: 833–840.

Rennick J, Johnston CC, Dougherty G, Platt R, and Ritchie JA (2002). Children's psychological responses after critical illness and exposure to invasive technology. *J Dev Behav Pediatr* 23: 133–144.

Weisbrot DM, Ettinger AB, Gadow KD, Belman AL, MacAllister WS, Milazzo M, Reed ML, Serrano D, and Krupp LB (2010). Psychiatric comorbidity in pediatric patients with demyelinating disorders. *J Child Neurol* 25: 192–202.

Wodrich DL, Hasan K, Parent KB (2011). Type 1 diabetes mellitus and school: A review. *Pediatr Diabetes* 12: 63–70.

Wood BL, Miller BD, Lim J, Lillis K, Ballow M, Stern T, and Simmens S (2006). Family relational factors in pediatric depression and asthma: Pathways of effect. *J AmerAcad Child Adolesc Psychiatry* 45: 1494–1502.

Zeltzer LK, Recklitis C, Buchbinder D, Zebrack B, Casillas J, Tsao JCI, Lu Q, and Krull K (2009). Psychological status in childhood cancer survivors: A report from the childhood cancer survivor study. *J Clin Oncol* 27: 2396–2404.

Fears and Anxiety

FEARS

Fear is a normal developmental phenomenon that does not denote psychopathology in young children. Despite prevalent fears in 49% of children aged 8–13 years, only 22.8% of the children in a community survey had an anxiety disorder (Muris et al. 2000). However, in addition to different anxiety disorders, children's fears can be associated with medical illness as well as other forms of emotional difficulties and conditions, such as psychosis and delirium (see chapter 7).

To help the reader both understand how to talk with young children and make sense of what they mean when they talk to adults about fear, this section first describes "normal" fears found in young children. In the subsequent section, the reader will learn how to ask children questions about anxiety and, in doing so, determine when fears are associated with an anxiety disorder. Techniques for talking with young, medically ill children about fears and associated anxiety disorders related to their illness are briefly presented here and in more detail in chapters 11–12 (on epilepsy) and chapters 14–16 (on pain, iatrogenic trauma symptoms, and terminal illness). Chapter 7 (on insight, judgment, and reality testing) describes how to determine when fears are signs of psychosis and delirium.

Type of Fears

The fears of young children reflect their developmental stage, understanding of the world around them, ability to differentiate reality from fantasy, and sense of control of the source of fear (Jones and Jones 1928; Bauer 1976; Ollendick and Horsch 2007). Fears commonly found in children include spiders, burglars breaking in, accidents, death, bombs, darkness, being kidnapped or home alone, getting lost, snakes, difficulty breathing, thunderstorms, frightening movies, becoming seriously ill, falling from a high place, and fires (Muris et al. 2000).

The type of fear changes with age. Younger children typically harbor fears about imaginary sources of danger: monsters and ghosts, scary dreams, animals, or being abandoned (Bauer 1976). These fears occur when darkness obscures visual perception at bedtime (Bauer 1976). Older children, however, have realistic fears about bodily injury and physical danger (Bauer 1976). As described by Bauer (1976), young children with fears equate physical characteristics, such as "His face looks

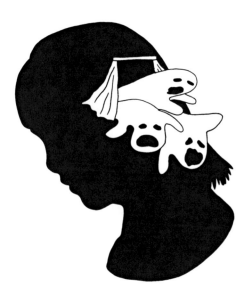

ugly" and "He has big ears" with potential threatening actions. With older children, actions are the source of their fears, as in fear "that he would kill me" or "I guess he would have choked me or something."

Whereas age is related to the types of fears found in children, gender is associated with the expression of these fears. Girls are more likely than boys to report or confirm fears, which is related in part to the social stereotype that boys are not afraid (Ollendick et al. 2007). Fears in both young girls and boys might only be activated when they are separated from their parents, as when they go to bed at night, go to school, are left alone at the hospital, or left at home with a babysitter. Parents might, therefore, not be aware of their children's fears, particularly if they are boys. Recent evidence suggests that parents are aware of physical complaints rather than fears in their children (Kushnir and Sadeh 2010). This finding is relevant for the assessment of young, medically ill children, because an increase in physical complaints might suggest that a child is experiencing fears.

Medical Fears

Children with and without an illness have medical fears (Ollendick 1983) such as fears of injections, needles, and medical procedures (see review in Forsner et al. 2009). It is common for these fears to go unaddressed, because the medical team focuses on children's medical symptoms and might have difficulty understanding and managing children's fears and their related fearful behavior.

From their analysis of the narratives of children 7–11 years old with identified medical fears, Forsner and colleagues (2009) note that children in contact with medical care feel as if they are "being threatened by a monster," are aware of danger, fear being hurt, feel unsafe due to the unknown, and fear doctors and nurses. They also feel unfairly treated, disregarded, violated, forced, and overpowered by the adults (medical staff and parents who do not listen to the child or empathize with the child's feelings). Children are also overwhelmed by feelings, fearing they might get out of control, feeling trapped in despair, and wishing for rescue and protection from medical situations.

Due to the possible impact of fear on the course and treatment of an illness, as well as on the child's emotional well being, it is important for interviewers to help young children talk about fears related to their illness and treatment, even if they are covert rather than apparent (Gupta et al. 2001). A child's opposition to required medical examinations, procedures, or treatment negatively affects the treatment of the illness. The subsequent negative response (anger, disappointment, criticism) of the medical team and/or the parents toward the child intensifies the child's distress. This distress, in turn, triggers a vicious cycle of increasing fears and fantasies about the dangers of the procedures, treatment, and medical team, and escalates to avoidant behavior and feelings of despair (Forsner et al. 2009). Of note, medications such as benzodiazepines (Graae et al. 1994), sometimes given to relax young children before a medical procedure, can disinhibit some young children and make them feel more out of control and unable to use cognitive coping strategies.

Summary
- Evaluation of fears is relevant in young children with a medical illness due to:
  - The possible impact of fear on the treatment and course of the illness.
  - The possibility that the parents might be unaware of the child's fears.

How to Talk with Children about Their Fears

A similar approach to the one taken when talking with young children about fears of death and fears that might present when trying to fall asleep (see chapter 3) can be used to begin the conversation about fears in general and about specific medical fears.

While being aware of possible cultural restrictions to speaking about fears, particularly in boys, the interviewer should let the child know, "Everyone, children and adults, are scared of different things. What things scare you?" To determine if the fear the child describes impacts functioning and coping, the interviewer should follow up the child's answer with "What do you do when ... (e.g., you think there might be a burglar in the backyard)?" followed by, "And how does that help?" The interviewer should then find out, "What other things make you scared?" and continue with the same follow-up questions. If, as often happens, the young child denies having fears, the interviewer should tell the child about fears that other children of a similar age and cultural background have, and ask if the child has any of these fears. Once the child confirms a fear, the interviewer should follow up with the previously described validation questions.

Sometimes the child does not mention any medical fears or fears related to a specific illness, because it is difficult for young children to verbalize what they think might happen to them as a result of their illness. When this occurs, the interviewer should tell the child that children with the same illness say they are scared of different things that might happen to them because of their illness. In describing fears that children with the same illness experience, the interviewer should wait for the child's response and clarify the child's concerns about specific fears before describing additional fears.

In the conversation below, Dr. Gomez demonstrates how to query Preston, a 6-year-old boy with a moderately malignant brain tumor and seizures, about illness-related fears.

Illness Related Fears

DR. GOMEZ: *When I speak to other children with the same problem you have in your brain, they tell me they are scared about different things that might happen to them because of this problem.*

PRESTON: *What things?*

DR. GOMEZ: *Some say they think they might become stupid.*

PRESTON: *Not me. Well … sometimes I am kind of stupid.*

DR. GOMEZ: *That's not a good feeling.*

PRESTON: *Yes, my dad says they talk to me and I don't answer.*

DR. GOMEZ: *Did your dad tell you this or you remember that this happened?*

PRESTON: *He told my mom.*

DR. GOMEZ: *And how did that make you feel?*

PRESTON: *Stupid.*

DR. GOMEZ: *Not a good feeling. What did you tell your mom and dad?*

PRESTON: *Nothing.*

DR. GOMEZ: *And how does that help?*

PRESTON: *They won't be mad that I heard them speaking.*

DR. GOMEZ: *What other things don't you like about having this brain tumor and seizures?*

PRESTON: *I don't know.*

DR. GOMEZ: *How about I tell you what other kids with a brain tumor and seizures have told me they are scared of?*

PRESTON: *Okay.*

DR. GOMEZ: *Some say they are scared of what the doctors want to do to their brain.*

PRESTON: *You mean cut off all their hair?*

DR. GOMEZ: *Yes. What don't you like about that?*

PRESTON: *I will be ugly (pointing to an area above his left ear).*

DR. GOMEZ: *That's not a lot of fun at all.*

PRESTON: *No one will play with me.*

DR. GOMEZ: *Wow, it sounds like this tumor and the seizures are really not making you feel very good about yourself. What else are this tumor and the seizures doing to you?*

PRESTON: *I want to throw up this disgusting medicine. Tomorrow they are going to stick me right here. See all the black marks. Every day shots, shots, shots.*

DR. GOMEZ: *This illness is causing a lot of trouble for you. What would you say is the very worst part of it all?*

PRESTON: *The shots and the medicine.*

DR. GOMEZ: *Preston, let's see if I understood everything you said because I want to figure out how to help you with all of this. If something I say is not exactly right, then please tell me, okay?*

Preston nods yes.

DR. GOMEZ: *The brain tumor is making you scared about quite a few things, like acting stupid, having some of your hair shaved off, getting shots, and throwing up your medicine.*

PRESTON: *Wrong for taking the medicine.*

DR. GOMEZ: *Oh, but I thought you throw up from the medicine.*

PRESTON: *No, I might.*

DR. GOMEZ: *Now I get it, you are scared you might throw up.*

Preston nods yes.

DR. GOMEZ: *Wow, Preston, you have done an amazing job explaining all that to me. Would it be okay if I speak with your mom and dad about the things you told me about?*

PRESTON: *Why?*

DR. GOMEZ: *I think they need to understand how bad the tumor and seizures are making you feel.*

PRESTON: *But they will be mad at me.*

DR. GOMEZ: *About what?*

PRESTON: *Because I don't take my medicine and don't want any more shots.*

DR. GOMEZ: *What if I also tell them that lots of kids feel this way? That might help them not be mad.*

PRESTON: *Okay.*

As described above, the combination of short, concrete "What" questions, validation of the child's answers through "What" questions, the interviewer's empathy for what the child is experiencing, and only one "Yes/No" question at the end of the conversation encourage the child to speak. Preston's answers inform Dr. Gomez about illness-related fears and the parents' negative response to what they interpret as Preston's "bad" or uncooperative behavior. It is important to find out with whom the child shares his fears and how this person responds. These questions will inform the interviewer as to whether the parents (or someone else) are helping the child deal with these problems.

Armed with this information and the child's permission to share it with the parents, Dr. Gomez can help the parents understand that, like themselves, the child also has fears related to his illness. His fears, however, are commensurate with the developmental stage when children are primarily scared about the external aspects of disease (looking stupid and ugly, shots, and vomiting). Dr. Gomez can then guide the parents on how to help the child cope with his fears.

Sometimes, despite prompts to talk about fears, a child does not mention any illness-related fears. When this occurs, the interviewer can use alternative strategies as in the example below of David, an 8-year-old boy with asthma who made no eye contact with Dr. Williams during the interview.

Denial of Fears

DR. WILLIAMS: *David, what is the worst thing about having asthma?*

DAVID: *I don't know.*

DR. WILLIAMS: *Sometimes when kids say, "I don't know," they mean they don't want to talk about something. Does your "I don't know" mean that you don't want to talk about this or that you really don't know.*

DAVID: *I don't know.*

DR. WILLIAMS: *Some kids think doctors shouldn't ask silly questions and that they should know all of this if they are good doctors.*

David smiles and looks at Dr. Williams.

DR. WILLIAMS: *So I am one of the silly ones, right?*

David smiles and nods again.

DR. WILLIAMS: *Ok, so can I tell you what I would be afraid of if I had asthma.*

DAVID NODS YES.

DR. WILLIAMS: *The scariest thing for me would be that I can't catch my breath and might die.*

DAVID (making eye contact again with Dr. Williams): *What else?*

DR. WILLIAMS: *Well, I would really be scared that the doctors and nurses make my mom wait outside.*

DAVID: *Last time I was in the ER, they did that.*

DR. WILLIAMS: *Those doctors really didn't understand how scared you were.*

DAVID: *I told you they are stupid.*

DR. WILLIAMS: *What did you tell your mom?*

DAVID: *Nothing.*

DR. WILLIAMS: *So she didn't know that you were scared you might die and wanted her near to you.*

DAVID: *She should have known that herself.*

DR. WILLIAMS: *And how did you feel because she didn't know that?*

DAVID: *I don't know.*

DR. WILLIAMS: *Does that mean you don't want to talk about this?*

DAVID: *Yes.*

DR. WILLIAMS: *It could help her understand if you tell her.*

DAVID: *No, she'll start crying.*

DR. WILLIAMS: *Should we do it together?*

DAVID: *You tell her and also those stupid doctors and nurses.*

This example demonstrates the need to recognize that comments such as "I don't know" or "I don't care" might mean, "Help me figure out a way how to talk about this." If the interviewer acts as the child's communication assistant, the interviewer will usually figure out a way to get the child to speak about even highly emotional fears. Giving the child examples of fears the interviewer would have in a situation similar to that of the child is another helpful strategy for children who appear unable to talk about their fears. This strategy normalizes fears and helps children express their scary thoughts and feelings.

SUMMARY

- Although fears are a normal component of child development, interviewers should assess fears and their impact on young children's functioning.
- Embarrassment about having fears and/or magical thinking might make children unwilling to talk about their fears.
- Techniques for helping children talk about their fears include:
  - Using short concrete "What" and "How" questions.
  - Validating the child's answers.
  - Normalizing fears through examples of what other children experience.
  - Expressing empathy for the child's fears.
  - Acting as the child's communication assistant and working on understanding.
- Table 4–1 provides a checklist of what to assess and how to speak to young ill children about their fears.

Table 4–1. FEAR CHECKLIST FOR YOUNG CHILDREN WITH MEDICAL ILLNESS

Interviewer Should Assess	Technique
Child's age-related fears	Use concrete action based "What" questions
Medical fears	Explain that kids who are sick get scared of different things
Illness effects	Find out what about child's illness is scary
Death, disfigurement, disability	Describe fears of other children with same illness, and ask child what fears he/she has
Procedures	Ask child about the different tests he/she needs. Determine which tests are scary and what is the worst part about these tests
Medicine	Find out what is the worst thing about having to take the medicine(s)
Medical personnel	Inquire if the people treating the child are nice (not so nice), and what nice (not nice) things they do
Parents' responses to child's behavior	Ask what the parents do when child has to have tests, take medicine, etc.
With whom child shares fears and their response	If no one, find out what could happen if the parents know about the child's fears What do your mom and dad do when you are scared to … ? How does that make you feel? Encourage child and/or get child's permission to tell parents about child's fears

ANXIETY

Using Barlow's concepts, Craske and colleagues (2009) describe anxiety as a "possible mood state associated with preparation for upcoming negative events" and fear as "an alarm response to present or imminent danger." Thus, young fearful children feel an imminent danger and need to escape the source of danger or be with someone who can protect them. Anxious children, however, are in a state of mind that they try to avoid because the mood state in itself is unpleasant or the upcoming event is negative. This state of mind might be associated with physical symptoms of autonomic arousal (pounding heart, sweating, or shortness of breath).

Despite prevalent fears in 49% of children aged 8–13 years in the study described earlier, only 22.8% of those with fears met diagnostic criteria for an anxiety disorder (Muris et al. 2000). Regarding the type of anxiety disorder, 4.5%–7.9% had specific phobias, 5.5% had generalized anxiety disorder, 4.8% had separation anxiety disorder, and 7.2% had more than one anxiety disorder (Muris et al. 2000). Since this study did not include questions on posttraumatic stress disorder in children, the association of fears with anxiety disorder diagnoses might be higher.

In terms of the assessment of anxiety symptoms, anxious adolescents and adults are usually aware of their worries, speak about them, and express their need to get rid of their worries, as well as the associated negative emotions and physical symptoms. In contrast, young children are unable to identify and verbalize the negative feelings experienced in this state and typically act them out. In addition, some cultures discourage verbal expression of emotions, particularly negative emotions and children might be embarrassed to talk about anxiety symptoms.

Therefore, anxious children might present as overactive or agitated, whiny, demanding, irritable, oppositional, and aggressive. They might easily cry, lose their temper, or shout. At the doctor's office, they might resist being examined, touch every object in the room, and run in and out of the room while the parent provides the history. In the hospital, they might start crying when an interviewer enters the room.

Similar to parents' mislabeling of the mood state of depressed children, parents might perceive the behavior of anxious children as "bad," "spoiled," "demanding" or "hyperactive," rather than anxious. In addition, interviewers who are unfamiliar with the developmental presentation of anxiety disorders in young children might misdiagnose these children based on the parents' report as having attention deficit/hyperactivity disorder (ADHD), oppositional defiant disorder, or bipolar disorder. When highly anxious children's behavior becomes quite regressive and/or disorganized, they might be labeled psychotic. Thus, anxiety in young children can present as a broad range of behavioral and emotional symptoms.

In addition to misinterpretation of behaviors that reflect anxiety in young children, parents are often unaware of their children's anxiety-related internalizing symptoms, as described previously for depression and fears. In fact, 236 children, aged 8–13 years, who completed a self-report anxiety symptom instrument, the Screen for Child Anxiety Related Emotional Disorders (SCARED), while waiting for their primary care visit had significantly higher scores than their parents' SCARED ratings (Wren et al. 2004). This excess, accounted for by somatic/panic and separation anxiety items, was found mainly in the younger subjects and in girls.

It is essential, therefore, for the interviewer to be mindful that young children have limited insight about their emotions and limited ability for verbal formulation and expression of abstract concepts such as anxiety symptoms. Interviewers should also be aware of the variety of abnormal behaviors representing anxiety symptoms in young children and that parents might misinterpret their children's anxiety symptoms. These limitations emphasize that interviewers must apply the developmental guidelines to obtain reliable and valid information from young children on anxiety symptoms. The next section presents the reader with techniques to meet the challenges of this task.

How To Identify Anxiety Disorder Symptoms in Interviews of Young Children

GENERALIZED ANXIETY DISORDER
Children with generalized anxiety disorder have excessive anxiety and worry (apprehensive expectation) about a number of events or activities (school performance, friends) and difficulty controlling their worry. In addition, they have problems concentrating or their mind goes blank. They can be irritable, sleep poorly, become easily fatigued, and feel restless, keyed up or on edge. The anxiety, worry,

or associated symptoms cause clinically significant distress and impairment in important areas of the child's functioning.

Young children might not understand the words "worry" and "anxiety." Therefore, the interviewer should explain that worry means that one thinks a lot about things or events before or after they happen. And then the interviewer should give the child examples, such as thinking a lot about a test before or after it takes place, or about homework or a difficult school project.

The interviewer should wait for the child's response after each example and follow up with "What" questions to determine if, in fact, the child is worrying and cannot control his thoughts. If the child participates in extracurricular activities that might also be competitive, such as sports, dancing, music, or acting, the interviewer can use these as examples of possible sources of worry. In addition, the interviewer should determine if the child repeatedly thinks about what friends, peers, siblings, teachers, coaches, or parents say or think about the child. The interviewer should also ask if the child repeatedly questions if what he/she has said or done is okay, and if the child needs approval from others (teacher, parents) and to be told that he/she is doing a good job.

If the child confirms worry about any of these topics, the interviewer should determine what additional things or events concern the child. To obtain a sense of the distress the child experiences from these different worries, the interviewer should ask if the child likes or is bothered by these thoughts, what he does to make the thoughts stop, and how this helps.

If the interview includes questions about mood (see chapter 3), the interviewer might have already asked the child questions about irritability, concentration, and sleep. As described under the developmental guideline, "children talk if they feel comfortable" (see chapter 1), the interviewer should not repeat these questions. Repetition of questions make the child angry and resentful because it lengthens the interview, and the child feels that the interviewer has not paid attention to his answers.

But the interviewer might need to ascertain if the child is irritable, distracted, and sleepless due to excessive worries. The interviewer should tell the child that, although they spoke about getting angry easily, the interviewer wants to check if the "worrying" thoughts also bug the child. Similarly, the interviewer should inquire if the concentration difficulties the child mentioned happen when these "worry" thoughts keep on coming into his head. This same approach should be used if the child previously mentioned difficulties falling asleep or staying asleep during the night.

Inquiring if these thoughts come into his head when he should be paying attention at school or while doing homework also yields information on how well the child can or cannot control his worries. The interviewer should avoid using the term "mind going blank" as it is an abstract concept. Similarly, most young children are not aware of feeling keyed up, muscle tension, or fatigue.

Finally, the interviewer should assess the child's perception of the severity of the problem by asking the child if he thinks a lot or a little about the worries he mentioned to the interviewer. To validate the child's answer (whether a lot or a little), the interviewer should inquire if that means the child thinks about it when he eats breakfast, when he is at school, when he comes home in the afternoon, when he plays with his friends, or when he goes to sleep. Again, as previously recommended, the interviewer should wait for an answer after each one of these options.

Summary

- Anxiety, worrying, difficulty controlling thoughts, and the mind going blank are abstract concepts.
- Young children usually do not have the insight to perceive and verbalize feelings associated with muscular or nervous tension, and fatigue.
- Use of short "What" and "How" questions, concrete language, and examples of what make other children worry help the interviewer determine if the child has generalized anxiety disorder and its severity.
- The checklist in Table 4–2 presents the two main questions on generalized anxiety disorder symptoms.

Table 4–2. SCREENING QUESTIONS FOR ANXIETY DISORDER SYMPTOMS

Disorder/Symptoms	Questions
Generalized Anxiety Disorder	Do you think a lot or a little about:
Worry/Apprehension	things that are going to happen, like tests, homework, or school projects? what friends think about you? what you said to other people (friends, teacher, parents)?
Uncontrolled	What do you do to make the thoughts stop? How does that help?
Separation Anxiety Disorder	Is it easy or difficult for you not to be with your parents?
Worry	What can happen? Are you scared something bad might happen to them or to you?
Distress	Do you think about that a little or a lot? How does it make you feel when you can't be with your parents? What do you do?
Refusal	Are you scared to go to school because something bad might happen to you or to your parents?
Nightmares	Do you have bad dreams about not being with your parents?
Panic	
Fear of an unknown source	Do you ever get a feeling of being very scared but don't know what you are scared of?
Physical symptoms	Does your body sometimes feel not good and you suddenly feel: Your heart beating? It is hard to breathe? You sweat a lot? You get very cold or very hot? Dizzy? Any other bad feeling?

Table 4–2. (CONTINUED)

Disorder/Symptoms	Questions
Phobias	Fear + avoidance
Specific	What things are you scared of? What do you do when … ?
Agoraphobia	Is it easy or difficult for you to go to places with lots of people? Do you feel okay or scared? Do you go to or stay away from places with lots of people?
Social	Is it easy or difficult for you to be with kids you do not know or just know a little?
Obsessive Compulsive Disorder	
Obsessions: thoughts, images, impulses	Do thoughts (pictures, strong feelings to do something dangerous) come into your head again and again even if you do not want to think about them? Does that make you feel good or not so good? How do you stop the thoughts?
Compulsions: behaviors, mental acts	Do you feel you have to do things again and again that you cannot stop like, for example, washing your hands, jumping over cracks, counting things, checking food for germs? Does that make you feel good or not so good?
Posttraumatic Stress Disorder	
Traumatic event	Did something scary happen to you or did you see that happen to someone else?
Recurrent recollections	Do you think about that again and again?
Recurrent nightmares	Do you have dreams about that?
Physiological reactivity	Do you scare easily when there is a loud noise or someone comes up behind you?

SEPARATION ANXIETY DISORDER

Children with this disorder have developmentally inappropriate or excessive anxiety concerning separation from the individual to whom the child is attached (parent, caretaker) evidenced by the symptoms presented in Table 4–3.

In contrast to the abstract nature of generalized anxiety disorder symptoms—anxiety and worry—the interviewer's task is easier when assessing young children for separation anxiety disorder, because the questions are easily formulated in concrete action-based language. The interviewer should first tell the child that children often get scared if they are not with their parents and ask if that also happens to the child. Irrespective of the answer, the interviewer could then say, "When you are not with your parents, what do you get scared of?" followed by "What" questions to determine if the child is scared something might happen to the parents and/or to the child. The interviewer should also determine if the child's separation fears and

Table 4–3. SYMPTOMS OF SEPARATION ANXIETY DISORDER

Distress When Separation Is Anticipated
When separated, worries about losing or possible harm befalling • a major attachment figure or • the child
Anticipation of an event that will lead to separation, such as: • getting lost • kidnapped
Because of fear of separation, persistent reluctance or refusal to: • go to school (or elsewhere) • be alone or without major attachment figure at home • go to sleep without being near a major attachment figure
Nightmares involving themes of separation from attachment figure
Repeated complaints of physical symptoms when anticipating separation, including: • headaches • stomachaches • nausea • vomiting
Symptoms can cause significant impairment in functioning as in: • school attendance • play dates • sleep over

worries occur at night or during the day by asking the child, "If you cannot be with your parents, is it worse more difficult during the day, the night, or both?"

To determine if the child worries about separation, and the extent of his worry, the interviewer should clarify, "Do you sometimes think that something bad might happen to your parents or to you even when you are together with them?" followed by "And then do you think about it in the morning before school [WAIT FOR ANSWER], at school [WAIT FOR ANSWER], when you come home [WAIT FOR ANSWER], or at night [WAIT FOR ANSWER]?" A question on what makes these thoughts go away provides the interviewer both with a sense of the severity of the child's separation worries and what helps the child cope with them.

Regarding refusal behaviors because of fear of separation, the interviewer should ask, "What do you like to do without your parents?" If the child provides no examples of what he does without his parents, the interviewer should then ask, "Do you sometimes not want to go to school because you think something bad might happen to your mom and dad or to you?" and "How about when you have play dates at other kids houses?" The interviewer should also establish if the child is able to be alone in a room at home by asking, "In which rooms of the house do you feel okay to be by yourself?" and "In which rooms do you not feel okay by yourself?" The interviewer should then clarify how this varies in the day and in the evening, "When is it okay for you to be in a room by yourself in the daytime or at night?"

If the interviewer obtained information on separation fears at bedtime when inquiring about mood (see chapter 3) or about fears, the interviewer should not repeat questions on this topic. But if not, the interviewer should find out, "What is scary for you about going to sleep by yourself without mom and dad?" If the child says, "I don't know," the interviewer should ask if the child is concerned that something bad happening to the parents or to him, and follow up by asking, "What can happen?" Even if the child endorses no fears, the interviewer should inquire where the child sleeps at night, who else sleeps in the same room, and if the child is able to sleep alone in the room.

The interviewer might have obtained information on nightmares when previously asking the child about bedtime fears or insomnia in the depression section of the interview (see chapter 3). If so, the interviewer should differentiate them from nightmares associated with separation anxiety disorder that specifically involve separation themes. To do this, the interviewer should say, "I know you told me before that you have (don't have) bad dreams about ..., but I was wondering if you also have bad dreams about not being with your mom and dad?" If the child says, "Yes," the interviewer should find out the content of the nightmares to make sure that they, in fact, involve separation fears.

Regarding physical symptoms, anxious children might be quite suggestible. Cognizant that children like to please the interviewer and tell the interviewer what he/she wants to hear, the interviewer should avoid biasing the child toward answers that confirm pathology. This is important in ill children whose symptoms involve headaches, stomachaches, nausea, and vomiting. The interviewer should find out about physical symptoms specifically associated with separation anxiety by asking, "When you are scared or think that your parents might leave you or that you have to leave them, does any part of your body not feel good?"

The information the interviewer obtained previously on school refusal and participation in play dates without parents help evaluate the impact of separation fears on the child's functioning. Use of "What" questions that inquire into what the child likes and does not like about sleeping over at other children's houses, sleepaway camp, or extracurricular activities involving separation from parents will shed light on the extent of dysfunction associated with the child's separation fears.

Summary
- The most challenging aspect of separation questions is to avoid "Yes/No" questions, because children who are embarrassed by their separation fears might simply say "No" to all these questions.
- The following techniques help the interviewer obtain valid information on separation anxiety symptoms:
  - Normalization of separation fears by indicating that other children have similar experiences
  - Use of "What" and "How" questions even if the child does not confirm separation fears
- See screening questions for separation anxiety disorder in Table 4–2.

Phobias

Phobias are fears that are associated with significant impairment in the child's functioning or with marked distress about having the fear. Specific phobias involve animals or insects, the natural environment (storms, heights, tornados, water), blood-injection-injury-medical procedures (discussed above under fears), and being in situations, such as on elevators, airplanes, public transportation, tunnels and bridges, or in enclosed places. The essential feature of social phobia, also called social anxiety disorder, is marked and persistent fear, as well as avoidance of social or performance situations. Agoraphobia involves fear about being in places or situations from which escape might be difficult or embarrassing.

SPECIFIC PHOBIAS

A child with a specific phobia has a marked and persistent fear that is excessive or unreasonable and cued by the presence or anticipation of a specific object or situation. Exposure to the phobic stimulus provokes an immediate anxiety response that can be expressed by crying, tantrums, freezing, or clinging. The child avoids the phobic situation or else endures it with intense anxiety or distress. The avoidance, anxious anticipation, or distress caused by the feared situation interferes significantly with the child's normal routine, school, or social activities.

To assess the presence and severity of specific phobias, the interviewer should present the child with a list of different things children fear. After each item on the list (insects, dogs, other animals, heights, riding in elevators, blood, and the like), the interviewer should pause and wait for the child's answer. If the child confirms a fear, the interviewer needs to use concrete action-based questions to determine if the child avoids the phobic stimulus, responds with anxiety and agitation when exposed to the stimulus, and repeatedly thinks about the stimulus with apprehension, as presented in the example below.

Phobia

INTERVIEWER: *So now I am going to tell you about things children are scared of, and you tell me if you are also scared of any of these things.*
VICTOR: *OK, but I'm not scared of anything.*
INTERVIEWER: *Well, how about insects?*
VICTOR: *No, I just kill them.*
INTERVIEWER: *What about animals?*
VICTOR: *No, but I don't want a tiger or lion for a pet.*
INTERVIEWER: *Are you scared of them?*
VICTOR: *Of course, everyone is.*
INTERVIEWER: *What about elevators?*
VICTOR: *I'm not scared; I never go on one.*
INTERVIEWER: *Did you ever try go in one?*
VICTOR: *Only once.*
INTERVIEWER: *What happened when you went in that elevator?*
VICTOR: *When the door started to close, I started to scream, "Get me out of here."*
INTERVIEWER: *And then what happened?*
VICTOR: *My dad put his hand in the door and it opened.*
INTERVIEWER: *And how did you feel when you got out of the elevator?*
VICTOR: *I never ever want to go back in one.*
INTERVIEWER: *Sounds like that was scary for you.*
VICTOR: *I guess so.*
INTERVIEWER: *So when you have to go a building with an elevator what happens?*

VICTOR: *I tell my mom that I am not going on the elevator.*
INTERVIEWER: *And what does she say?*
VICTOR: *But we have to go the doctor's office on the 6th floor.*
INTERVIEWER: *And how does that make you feel?*
VICTOR: *I tell her she can't make me go in the elevator. When I start to cry, she says, "Okay we will go up the stairs."*

In this example, the interviewer used action-based and concrete "What" and "How" questions, and continued to ask Victor about fears even though he denied having fears. The interviewer communicated to the child that his action-based statement, "I never want to go back in one," meant that he is scared. The interviewer's reflection, "Sounds like that was a scary thing for you," helped the child acknowledge his fear. However, if the interviewer had responded, "So you *are* scared of elevators," he would have put words in the child's mouth and challenged Victor's prior statement that he is fearless. Since young children talk if they feel comfortable (see this developmental guideline in chapter 1), this response by the interviewer would not have encouraged the child to talk.

SOCIAL PHOBIA

A child with social phobia has a marked and persistent fear of one or more social or performance situations, including being exposed to unfamiliar people or to possible scrutiny by others. Exposure to the feared situation provokes anxiety that may take the form of crying, tantrums, freezing, or shrinking from the social situation or unfamiliar people. The child avoids the social or performance situation or endures it with intense anxiety. The avoidance, anxious anticipation, or distress in the feared situation interferes significantly with the child's normal routine, school, or social activities.

However, fear or avoidance of social engagements due to a medical condition, such as disfigurement from chemotherapy, surgery, burns, or injury, is not considered to be a social phobia. Other conditions that need to be included in the differential diagnosis of social phobia include social skill deficits and social withdrawal in young children with depression, psychosis, and autism spectrum disorders (see chapters 3, 7, and 9).

The interviewer should also inquire about agoraphobia by asking if the child is able to be in a place with a lot of people, such as a mall or movie house, or on public transportation. If not, the interviewer should clarify if the child actively avoids these situations, what the child experiences when in a crowded place, as well as what the child fears might happen in these situations. The interviewer should be aware that children with separation anxiety disorder might confirm fear of being in a mall. However, their answers to validation questions indicate that the fear is one of getting lost rather than fear of crowds.

To interview a child about possible social phobia, the interviewer should ask the child if it is easy or difficult for him to talk or play with children that he does not know from before. The interviewer should also ask similar questions about doing things in public places, such as going to a public bathroom, eating in a restaurant, answering a teacher's question in front of the whole class, or going on stage. As for specific phobias, the interviewer should clarify if the child actively avoids these situations, worries about them before they happen, and feels distressed if in this situation.

In addition to working on formulation of the questions and validation of the child's answers, making a concerted effort to understand what the child says is essential to help the interviewer distinguish between social phobia and shyness. In contrast to the child with social phobia, a shy child does not demonstrate the avoidance, anxious anticipation, or distress in the feared situation, as in the example that follows of social phobia.

Risha is a 5-year-old girl seen by Dr. Weinberg because of stomachaches that occur every morning. Dr. Weinberg found no abnormalities on Risha's physical exam and began to talk with her about school and her social life.

Social Phobia vs. Shyness

DR. WEINBERG: *So your stomach hurts you real bad every morning. On which days of the week is it the worst?*

RISHA: *I don't know.*

DR. WEINBERG: *What happens on Saturday mornings?*

RISHA: *I watch my favorite show on TV.*

DR. WEINBERG: *And when you wake up on Sunday mornings?*

RISHA: *I have another favorite on TV.*

DR. WEINBERG: *After you watch TV, what do you usually do?*

RISHA: *Eat breakfast.*

DR. WEINBERG: *What about Monday morning?*

RISHA: *I have to go to school.*

DR. WEINBERG: *Oh, so then you don't get to watch TV?*

RISHA NODS YES.

DR. WEINBERG: *What do you like about school?*

RISHA: *Going home.*

DR. WEINBERG: *What don't you like about school?*

RISHA: *Recess.*

DR. WEINBERG: *What is bad about recess?*

RISHA: *No one plays with me.*

DR. WEINBERG: *That's not nice of them.*

RISHA: *In my old school, the kids were my friends.*

DR. WEINBERG: *Oh, you changed schools.*

RISHA: *Yes.*

DR. WEINBERG: *How do the new kids know you want to play with them?*

RISHA: *I stand and watch them.*

DR. WEINBERG: *What do they say when you tell them you want to play?*

RISHA: *I don't tell them.*

DR. WEINBERG: *So how do they know you want to play?*

Risha shrugs her shoulders.

DR. WEINBERG: *What would happen if you say, "Can I play?"*

RISHA (shaking her head from side to side): *I don't know.*

DR. WEINBERG: *It sounds like it is difficult for you to make friends with kids you don't know.*

RISHA (nodding with a shy smile): *But not if they want to play with me.*

DR. WEINBERG: *Oh, so if they say, "Come play," you feel okay even if you don't know them from before.*

RISHA: *Yes.*

DR. WEINBERG: *So are you shy to start talking to them?*
RISHA: *Yes.*
DR. WEINBERG: *Do you think about this during class before recess?*
RISHA: *Only when I stand next to the kids and before school.*
DR. WEINBERG: *And then is there any part of your body that doesn't feel good?*
RISHA: *My tummy hurts.*
DR. WEINBERG: *So your tummy hurts when you are thinking about being shy?*
RISHA: *Yes.*
DR. WEINBERG: *I understand. How about speaking in class? Is it easy or difficult for you to speak up when the teacher asks you a question in front of all the kids?*
RISHA: *If I know the answer, easy.*
DR. WEINBERG: *How about using the restroom at school? Is that easy or difficult?*
RISHA: *Easy.*
DR. WEINBERG: *What about eating in a restaurant?*
RISHA: *I love Mexican food.*
DR. WEINBERG: *You are so helpful and such a good talker. Now I think I understand what we need to do to help your tummy aches.*

In this dialogue, Dr. Weinberg applied the developmental guideline of speaking to Risha about the identified problem (stomachache) only after establishing good rapport with the child. Dr. Weinberg obtained the information needed to understand the difficulties Risha experienced at school by asking concrete "What" questions. Dr. Weinberg expressed empathy for the child's difficulties and checked with the child to make sure he correctly understood what Risha was communicating. These interview techniques helped Dr. Weinberg determine that Risha is shy and does not have social phobia.

SUMMARY

- Asking young children about specific phobias is less challenging than symptoms of anxiety disorders because of the concrete nature of these symptoms.
- Posing questions on social phobia, however, is more difficult because of the need to differentiate social phobia from:
  - Shyness
  - Social withdrawal associated with:
    - Depression
    - Psychosis
    - Autism spectrum disorder
    - Disfigurement due to medical illness or its treatment
- See screening questions for phobias in Table 4–2.

Panic Disorder

A panic attack is a discrete period in which there is an abrupt onset of intense apprehension; fear of an unknown source; terror with a sense of impending doom; or sudden onset of physical symptoms, including palpitations, sweating, trembling, the sensation of shortness of breath, chest pain, dizziness, nausea, chills or hot flushes, and numbness or tingling.

Most young children are not able to verbalize the associated fear of a lack of escape or possible panic attack. The interviewer should ask if the child sometimes feels very scared but does not know what is making him scared. If the child confirms this feeling, the interviewer should inquire if, when the child has this feeling, parts of his body also do not feel good without suggesting which parts. The interviewer should then find out which physical symptoms the child experiences. Since children with the physical symptoms of a panic attack typically present in medical settings, it is important to differentiate their symptoms from those of children with an underlying medical illness or a conversion disorder (see chapter 8). This is particularly difficult because these children might not acknowledge anxious thoughts in addition to their physical symptoms.

Summary
- Panic attacks are rare in young children.
- Nevertheless, they should be included the differential diagnosis of children who present with physical symptoms to medical settings.
- See screening questions for panic disorder symptoms in Table 4–2.

Obsessive Compulsive Disorder

Obsessions involve recurrent and persistent thoughts, impulses, or images that are experienced as intrusive and inappropriate and that cause marked anxiety or distress, but are not worries about real life problems. The individual attempts to ignore, suppress, or neutralize (through another thought or action) these recurrent and persistent thoughts, impulses, or images.

Compulsions are repetitive behaviors or mental acts that an individual feels driven to perform in response to an obsession or according to rigidly applied rules. These behaviors or actions prevent or reduce distress, or prevent a dreaded event or situation. Both obsessions and compulsions cause marked distress, are time consuming, and significantly interfere with a child's functioning.

To identify obsessions, the interviewer should tell the child that some children complain about thoughts that come into their head again and again even if they do not want to think about them. The interviewer should then ask the child, "How about you?" Although young children sometimes say this happens to them, validation questions, such as "What are these thoughts about?" reveal that they are talking about an anticipated enjoyable event, such as an upcoming birthday party. In other cases, the answers to validation questions indicate that the children are actually talking about the worries of generalized anxiety disorder or delusions of psychosis (see chapter 7).

Young children might be embarrassed to talk about their obsessions. As the child's communication assistant, the interviewer should describe commonly found obsessions that bother some children and ask if any of these bother the child. These include thoughts about hands being dirty, germs in food and other objects, a need for symmetry or to check that a back pack has everything in it or is closed, collecting things, and hearing recurring tunes, phrases, and words. However, frequent hand washing and awareness of germs in food and on objects would not be considered obsessions in hospitalized children or in children whose immune system is compromised. The interviewer should also be aware that a germ "obsession" in young children might actually be a delusion (see chapter 7). Likewise, hoarding or repeated thoughts about specific topics, such as trains, planes, numbers, bus schedules and the like, might reflect the circumscribed preoccupations of young children with autism spectrum disorders (see chapter 9).

The interview should also determine if the child experiences recurrent pictures or impulses. A child who confirms seeing repeated images that do not go away may actually be experiencing visual hallucinations (see chapter 7) or posttraumatic disorder symptoms (described in the next section). Obsessions in the form of repeated impulses often involve dangerous actions, such as stabbing someone with a sharp knife or jumping out of a tall building. Young children do not understand what impulses mean. Therefore, the interviewer can ask the child if thoughts come into his head again and again that he has to do something that is wrong or dangerous, like hurting someone or jumping out of a window in a tall building. If a young child acknowledges experiencing repeated impulses, the interviewer should rule out the possibility of command auditory hallucinations, such as a voice that tells the child to stab someone with a knife or jump out of a building (see chapter 7).

Rather than asking if the child can control these thoughts (pictures, impulses), an abstract concept, the interviewer should use concrete action-based language and find out, "So do the thoughts (pictures, strong feelings to do something you can't stop) come back again and again and bug you?" followed by "What do you do to make the thoughts go away?" and "How does that help?" The interviewer should also ascertain if the child experiences distress associated with the repeated thoughts and images by asking, "Do you like having these thoughts (pictures, strong feelings) come in your head again and again or not like it?" Unlike obsessions, circumscribed preoccupations of children with autism spectrum disorder do not distress the child. To evaluate the extent of impairment associated with obsessions, the interviewer should ask if these thoughts bother the child when the child is in class, watching TV, going to sleep, or playing with friends.

After evaluating the presence of obsessions, the interviewer can use similarly phrased questions to determine if the child is experiencing compulsions. Examples include hand-washing, counting, touching with both hands (for symmetry), carrying out bedtime rituals, jumping over cracks on the sidewalk, checking, erasing, and the like. While parents might be unaware of their child's obsessions, they may be a better source of information on compulsions than the young child who might be too embarrassed to talk about these behaviors.

Summary

- Since children might be embarrassed to talk about their obsessions and compulsions, the interviewer needs to use the developmental guidelines to help the child talk about these symptoms.
- Parents are usually a more reliable source of information on compulsions and the associated functional disturbances than their children.
- The interviewer should differentiate obsessions and compulsions from symptoms such as:
  - Circumscribed preoccupations in autism spectrum disorder
  - Repeated worries in generalized anxiety disorder
  - Delusions and hallucinations
- See screening questions for obsessions and compulsions in Table 4–2.

Posttraumatic Stress Disorder (PTSD)

The symptoms of PTSD occur when children experience or witness an event that involves fear, helplessness, or horror, and they reexperience the event in a recurrent manner (Table 4–4). To find out if a child has had any of these symptoms, the interviewer can start off by asking if the child was ever in or saw an accident, fire, storm, earthquake, tornado, or any other traumatic event, or if the child saw or heard the noise of a fight in which people or family members were hurt. The interviewer should ask if anyone has hurt the child in any part of his body by hitting, beating, whipping, or touching him in private parts. If the child says, "Yes," to any of these questions, the interviewer should find out what the child experienced, how that made the child feel, who caused the trauma, who the child told about the event(s), and that person's response. If further prompting is needed, the interviewer should inquire what is the worst thing that ever happened to the child.

Since young children might avoid all thoughts about the trauma and not speak about it, assessment of most of the PTSD symptoms is sometimes best made based on the parent report unless the parent(s) are the perpetrators. However, the child, not the parent, might be aware of an exaggerated startle response. To ask a young child about this symptom, the interviewer should find out if it is easy or difficult to scare the child

Table 4–4. FEATURES OF POSTTRAUMATIC DISORDER

A traumatic event is reexperienced as recurrent or intrusive distressing recollections or play of the event through: <ul><li>images</li><li>thoughts</li><li>perceptions</li><li>dreams of the event or nightmares without recognizable content</li><li>reenactment of the event</li></ul>
Intense psychological distress or physiological reactivity at exposure to internal or external cues that symbolize or represent the event
Persistent avoidance of stimuli associated with the trauma and numbing of general responsiveness as evident by the following: <ul><li>avoidance of thoughts</li><li>feelings, conversations</li><li>activities, places, or people associated with the trauma</li><li>markedly diminished interest or participation in significant activities</li><li>detachment or estrangement from others</li><li>restricted range of affect</li><li>sense of foreshortened future</li></ul>
Persistent de novo onset of symptoms of arousal including: <ul><li>insomnia</li><li>irritability or anger outbursts</li><li>difficulty concentrating</li><li>hypervigilance</li><li>exaggerated startle response</li></ul>
Significant impairment of functioning

by things such as loud noises, screaming, sirens, and someone unexpectedly walking into the room or coming up behind the child. Chapter 15 provides the reader with a detailed description of pediatric iatrogenic (medically induced) trauma symptoms and clinical examples that demonstrate how best to help children talk about the traumatic event(s) and associated behavioral and emotional symptoms. It is also important to note that inattention, hyperactivity, and impulsivity are found in children who were sexually abused and have PTSD (Weinstein et al. 2000).

SUMMARY
- Young children might experience or witness a broad range of traumas.
- Unless parents are perpetrators or protect the perpetrator, they are usually the best informants as young children avoid thinking and talking about the trauma.
- See screening questions for PTSD in Table 4–2.

How to Identify Symptoms of Anxiety Disorders: Main Points to Remember
- Young children do not understand the word "anxiety," an abstract word. They are more likely to understand what scares them.
- Young children are not aware of their feelings in the same way as adults.
- Interviewers can best access information on anxiety disorder symptoms in young children through:
  - Concrete action based "What" and "How" questions.
  - Understanding the emotions represented by children's action-based concrete language.
  - Expressing empathy for children's experiences and feelings that represent anxiety.

Anxiety Disorders in Young Children with Medical Illness

Whereas the rate of anxiety disorders in the general population of children is about 9%, it is about 20% in children with chronic illness based on studies of diabetes mellitus (Davies et al. 2003), chronic urticaria (Hergüner et al. 2011), asthma (Ortega et al. 2002), cystic fibrosis (Cruz et al. 2009), hyperandrogenism (Mueller et al. 2010), and sickle cell anemia (Myrvik et al. 2011). The association of anxiety disorder with the number and length of hospitalizations in children with asthma (Ortega et al. 2002) and in those with sickle cell anemia (Myrvik et al. 2011), together with the high rate of chronic medical illness in children with anxiety disorders (Chavira et al. 2010) implies a two-way relationship between having these illnesses and anxiety disorder. This is especially apparent in the high rates of comorbid anxiety in pediatric pain disorders (Campo et al. 2004).

A two-way relationship between medical illness and anxiety disorders underscores the importance of careful assessment of anxiety disorder symptoms in children with chronic illness for several reasons. First, exacerbation of the child's underlying illness can trigger anxiety symptoms. Second, a longer time in the hospital because of multiple admissions or long hospitalizations increases the likelihood of hospital-related trauma. Third, the behavioral and cognitive adverse effects of medications, such as corticosteroids, can trigger symptoms of anxiety disorders.

Fourth, children with anxiety disorders have somatic complaints that might mimic the symptoms of their underlying medical disorder. Fifth, the presence of anxiety disorder symptoms could have a negative impact on treatment adherence. Sixth, the quality of life of children with medical illness is adversely impacted by anxiety.

When the interviewer assesses anxiety symptoms in young children, the interviewer should differentiate symptoms of the child's illness and its treatment from anxiety disorder symptoms. This section of the chapter describes techniques that help the interviewer meet this challenging task.

Type of Anxiety Symptoms

Although young children with anxiety disorders can present with a wide range of somatic (physical) symptoms, they most commonly report abdominal pain (Campo et al. 2004) and headache (Greholt et al. 2003). Therefore, anxiety disorders should always by part of the differential diagnosis of young children presenting with these types of pain. The three examples that follow demonstrate how to talk to young children with these symptoms and how to differentiate "functional" somatic symptoms from those of a medical illness. In the first case, the child's abdominal pain and apparent separation anxiety disorder are exacerbated by the child's fear of dying from his neurological illness. In the second case, what appears to be exacerbation of a child's liver disorder is, in fact, undiagnosed obsessive-compulsive disorder. The third case demonstrates how symptoms of generalized anxiety disorder caused by an adverse effect of prednisone are mislabeled as "bad behavior."

Harry, aged 5, has Panayiotopoulos syndrome (Koutroumanidis 2002), a benign form of childhood epilepsy, with early onset of benign seizures, that manifests mainly with autonomic seizures such as nausea, vomiting, retching, pallor, cyanosis (turning blue), dilation or narrowing of pupils, increased heart rate, and incontinence of urine (see Table 10–1 in chapter 10). These seizures occur in the day or night. Children with this disorder have occipital or extra occipital spikes on an electroencephalogram (EEG). During the day Harry suddenly pales, says, "I want to throw up," and vomits. When he has a seizure at night, he either wakes up with similar complaints or is found vomiting. He also experiences intense recurrent abdominal pains before going to sleep and wakes up in the night with these pains. Harry's babysitter sometimes calls Harry's mother to come home from work because of these pains, and on occasion Harry has had to leave school. The interviewer, Dr. Dal Santo, does not think Harry's "attacks" of stomachache represent seizures, and found no abnormalities during his physical exam.

Stomach Pains vs. Anxiety

DR. DAL SANTO: *So help me try figure out how to help you with these bad tummy aches. When your tummy hurts at night, what makes it better?*

HARRY: *My mom or my dad.*

DR. DAL SANTO: *How about during the day, what makes it better?*

HARRY: *My mom.*

DR. DAL SANTO: *And when you are at school?*

HARRY: *I go home.*

DR. DAL SANTO: *How do your mom and dad make it better?*

HARRY: *They read me a story.*

DR. DAL SANTO: *And when the story is done?*

HARRY: *They say its time to go to sleep.*

DR. DAL SANTO: *Is that easy or difficult for you?*

HARRY: *Easy in their bed*

DR. DAL SANTO: *So where is it difficult?*

HARRY: *In my bed.*

DR. DAL SANTO: *Some kids who don't sleep in their bed tell me that they are scared at night. What are you scared of?*

HARRY: *Throw up.*

DR. DAL SANTO: *So let me understand, is the throwing up scary or can something bad happen if you throw up?*

HARRY: *Something bad.*

DR. DAL SANTO: *Something bad, like what?*

HARRY: *I don't know. Where's my mom?*

DR. DAL SANTO: *Is talking about this also kind of scary?*

HARRY (putting both his hands on his stomach, and bending forward): *Where's my mom?*

DR. DAL SANTO: *Let's call your mom from the waiting room so she can help us figure out the bad thing that can happen from throwing up.*

Harry and mother return and Harry sits on her lap.

DR. DAL SANTO: *Thank you for joining us. Harry told me that throwing up makes him scared that something bad will happen. But Harry seemed to get scared talking about this, and wanted you to be with him. Has he ever told you that he is scared to throw up?*

MS. GOLDEN: *No, I thought he was dealing very well with the seizures. He never talks about them. Actually, after he says, "I want to be sick" just before his seizure, he usually blanks out. So I thought he wasn't aware of throwing up.*

HARRY: *You said my bed was full of throw up, yuck.*

MS. GOLDEN: *Yes Harry, but then we clean it up and change the sheets,*

DR. DAL SANTO: *So Harry you feel your bed is yucky?*

HARRY: *It also smells.*

MS. GOLDEN: *We always open the windows to air out the room and if it's cold we just spray some deodorizer.*

HARRY: *My room smells.*

DR. DAL SANTO: *So is the smell the bad thing that can happen from the throw up or something else?*

HARRY: *I don't know*

DR. DAL SANTO: *Well, I know that kids who have seizures are scared that something really bad can happen to them when they have a seizure.*

HARRY: *What are they scared of?*

DR. DAL SANTO: *The scariest thing for most kids is that they think a seizure might make them die.*

Harry looks at Dr. Dal Santo and then hugs his mother.

DR. DAL SANTO: *Is that the bad thing that can happen from throwing up?*

HARRY NODS.

DR. DAL SANTO: *Do you think about this all the time or only when you are not with your mom and dad?*

HARRY: *Not with mom and dad.*

DR. DAL SANTO: *Harry, you have really helped us figure out a lot of stuff, but I want to make sure I understand.*

HARRY NODS.

DR. DAL SANTO: *You really don't like throwing up, and the worst is that your bed gets yucky and there is a bad smell. That doesn't make you scared but you feel it is yuck, right?*

HARRY NODS.

DR. DAL SANTO: *But you are afraid that if you throw up, you might die, right?*

HARRY NODS.

DR. DAL SANTO: *What other bad things can happen from the seizures or the throw up?*

HARRY: *Nothing.*

DR. DAL SANTO: *You have been so helpful and I think we can make this all better. Let me talk with your mom now and explain to her how we are going to do that while you play in the waiting room.*

By asking "What" and "How" questions and normalizing fears in children with seizures, Dr. Dal Santo finds out that the child's abdominal pain is associated with separation anxiety triggered by Harry's fear of death due to his seizures. In addition, physical aspects of throwing up repelled him and made him apprehensive of falling asleep in his bed. The mother is quite unaware of the child's fears and thought that his not talking about seizures meant he is coping well with the illness (a common clinical finding among parents of children with epilepsy). To tease out possible triggers of the child's abdominal pain, Dr. Dal Santo asks simple concrete "What" questions to clarify the conditions under which his stomachaches occur. Dr. Dal Santo understands that the child is communicating how difficult it is for him to talk about the "bad" thing throwing up can cause by saying, "I don't know" and asking where his mother was. Dr. Dal Santo helps the child by verbalizing and normalizing Harry's fear of death. Dr. Dal Santo also understands that by hugging his mother, Harry confirms this fear.

Furthermore, Dr. Dal Santo asks Harry if the summary of their conversation is correct to avoid putting words in the child's mouth. Dr. Dal Santo's empathic approach and efforts to make sense of what the child is saying help the child trust Dr. Dal Santo and encourages him to speak. Dr. Dal Santo achieves this by giving Harry positive feedback during and at the end of the conversation, as well as by providing him with hope that his problem can be solved.

Sarah is a 10-year-old girl who has Wilson disease in which there is progressive copper accumulation in the liver, central nervous system, cornea, kidney, bones, and joints because of a mutation in a gene that encodes a copper-transporting enzyme, ATPase. Sarah was diagnosed with Wilson disease when increased liver transaminase was found by chance in a blood test done because of diarrhea, vomiting, and dehydration. The diagnosis was confirmed by low plasma ceruloplasmin levels (<20 mg/dL) but increased levels of basal urinary copper (>100 μg/24 hours), her urinary copper level after a penicillamine challenge test (PCT; >1575 μg/24 hours), and her liver copper (>250 μg/g of dry weight), as well as a positive family history, the presence of Kayser-Fleischer (KF) rings, and Coombs' negative hemolytic anemia (Nicastro et al. 2011).

There is no evidence of involvement of organs other than the liver in Sarah's Wilson disease. Her parents reported to Dr. Hyman that Sarah has not been doing well in school recently and that her teacher complained that she was daydreaming and not paying attention. Sarah stopped eating meat and poultry and has lost about 5 pounds over the past few months. About a month ago, she began to use only paper straws to drink, and she carefully unwraps a new straw and places it in a glass or cup every time she drinks something. Her parents were concerned that her inattentiveness at school, lack of appetite, and weight loss might reflect increased liver damage from her Wilson disease.

Wilson Disease vs. Obsessive Compulsive Disorder

DR. HYMAN: *Hi, Sarah. Since I last saw you, what got better?*

SARAH: *I don't get blood tests all the time.*

DR. HYMAN: *That's good. What else got better?*

SARAH: *Nothing.*

DR. HYMAN: *What didn't get better?*

SARAH: *Nothing.*

DR. HYMAN: *What got worse?*

SARAH: *School.*

DR. HYMAN: *What is not going well at school?*

SARAH: *My teacher gets angry with me.*

DR. HYMAN: *That probably doesn't make you feel too good.*

SARAH: *She says I am not paying attention.*

DR. HYMAN: *What do you think about that?*

SARAH: *I try.*

DR. HYMAN: *So when you try to pay attention to what the teacher is saying, do you start thinking about different things?*

SARAH: *No.*

DR. HYMAN: *Do kids around you talk and you try and listen to what they are saying?*

SARAH: *No.*

DR. HYMAN: *Is it difficult to understand what the teacher is talking about?*

SARAH: *No.*

DR. HYMAN: *So let me see if I got it right. You can hear the teacher talking, but you are not listening to her or not thinking about anything.*

SARAH: *Yes.*

DR. HYMAN: *And it's not the kids being noisy or the work being too hard?*

SARAH NODS YES.

DR. HYMAN: *Huh, so I wonder what you are doing during that time?*

SARAH: *Oh, just counting.*

DR. HYMAN: *Counting what?*

SARAH: *Different things.*

DR. HYMAN: *Like what?*

SARAH: *Windows, bricks, pictures, desks, posters, almost anything in the classroom.*

DR. HYMAN: *Where else do you count things?*

SARAH: *Everywhere.*

DR. HYMAN: *So do you have to count to a certain number or a certain number of times?*

SARAH: *If I have to stop before 3 or 5, I start again.*

DR. HYMAN: *Do you enjoy counting or does it bother you?*

SARAH: *When I can't do it, it bothers me.*

DR. HYMAN: *What happens then?*

SARAH: *I think about it, and that bothers me.*

DR. HYMAN: *How's your appetite?*

SARAH: *Fine, but I don't like to meat or chicken.*

DR. HYMAN: *What's not good about meat or chicken?*

SARAH: *Germs.*

DR. HYMAN: *What germs?*

SARAH: *I saw on TV how the chicken and cows all live close together and it's so dirty, yuck!*

DR. HYMAN: *But the meat and chicken are cooked?*

SARAH: *I don't want to get sick from disgusting germs.*

DR. HYMAN: *Do your parents know how you feel about this?*

SARAH: *They said I am being stupid so I don't tell them.*

DR. HYMAN: *How did you feel when they said that?*

SARAH: *I shouldn't have told them.*

DR. HYMAN: *What do they say about the counting?*

SARAH: *They don't know.*

DR. HYMAN: *Is it because of the same reason you don't talk to them about the germs?*
Sarah nods yes.

DR. HYMAN: *So it looks like you got thinner? Did you want that to happen?*

SARAH: *No.*

DR. HYMAN: *Well, what do you like to drink?*

SARAH: *Milk, juices, soda.*

DR. HYMAN: *Are those okay?*

SARAH: *As long as I drink them from a straw.*

DR. HYMAN: *What's good about drinking from a straw?*

SARAH: *No one used it before so there are no germs.*

DR. HYMAN: *Oh, so now I get it you really are quite worried about germs. This might sound like a stupid question but what are you scared germs might do to you?*

SARAH (looking at Dr. Hyman): *You're a doctor, you should know.*

DR. HYMAN: *You know, kids who worry about germs tell me different things. And I would like to understand what you think germs might do to you.*

SARAH: *They can make me sick.*

DR. HYMAN: *That is a scary thought. Do you mean get a new sickness or make the one you have worse?*

SARAH: *Make the one I have worse.*

DR. HYMAN: *Sarah you are a really good talker, thank you very much. I now understand what things are bothering you. Do you want to not have to count, drink from a straw, and not eat meat and chicken?*

SARAH: *Well if my teacher would stop yelling at me and my Wilson's go away, that would be good.*

DR. HYMAN: *Can I talk with your parents about the counting and germs and explain to them that you are not being stupid?*

SARAH: *If it will help. They're mad at me and want me to eat meat and chicken and stop wasting straws.*

DR. HYMAN: *I think they should also know that you are scared that germs will make the Wilson worse.*

SARAH: *Won't it?*

DR. HYMAN: *No, germs have nothing to do with Wilson's disease.*

SARAH: *Okay, but germs are disgusting and I don't want any.*

DR. HYMAN: *If the counting is making it difficult for you to pay attention in class, shouldn't we figure out how to help you count less?*

SARAH: *Then maybe my teacher will not yell so much at me.*

DR. HYMAN: *Good idea. Thanks Sarah for all your help and let's talk with your parents.*

In this conversation Dr. Hyman applies the developmental guidelines using simple "What" questions to determine if the child's "attention" problems are because of distractibility, difficulty with the schoolwork, or a change in state of consciousness as found in a seizure. Although Sarah clearly was not forthcoming about her counting, Dr. Hyman proceeds slowly in clarifying the nature of Sarah's "daydreaming." Dr. Hyman is sensitive to the cues the child gives that suggest she does not want to talk about this topic, such as her "Nothing," and other one-word answers. Furthermore, Dr. Hyman does not repeat questions when the child indicates she is unwilling to talk about the topic. Dr. Hyman uses the same approach to understand Sarah's reluctance to eat meat and chicken, as well as her fear of germs.

It is also important to note that Dr. Hyman enlists Sarah's help and consent for information that Dr. Hyman can share with Sarah's parents. Dr. Hyman also ascertains if Sarah is motivated to be treated for her counting behavior. By making it clear to Sarah that Dr. Hyman is working with her rather than only with Sarah's parents, Dr. Hyman establishes the girl's trust.

Based on this interview, Sarah meets criteria for obsessive-compulsive disorder. In the absence of evidence for central nervous system involvement by her Wilson disease, Sarah's obsessive-compulsive disorder appears to be a separate disorder. Although Sarah's obsession with germs was related to her parents' fear of possible worsening of her Wilson's disease, the conversation clearly demonstrates that she has obsessions (germs) and compulsions (drinking from straws, abstaining from meat and poultry) unrelated to her fear of making her illness worse.

Cody is a 7-year-old boy with nephrotic syndrome (Eddy and Symons 2003) with marked reduction of his edema, hyperlipidemia counting, and proteinuria, as well as improved kidney functions on a treatment regimen of 60 mg/day of prednisone for 8 weeks and 40 mg/day for 4 weeks. Dr. Salas is seeing him for follow-up and he has one week left of treatment with 40 mg/day of prednisone. The parents report that he seems to be much better, he is less puffy, and he has more energy. Dr. Salas asks why Cody's hand is bandaged and the parents answer that he physically attacked his twin brother claiming that his brother was distracting him from doing his homework. The parents add that Cody's behavior has been difficult to manage. He has been angry, argumentative, and oppositional, particularly about going to sleep at night. He has also been spending a lot of time doing his homework, and Cody is angry with his teacher for giving so much work. He complains that everyone in the family makes too much noise when he needs to do homework. The parents felt that all their efforts to placate him have failed.

Steroid-Induced Anxiety

DR. SALAS: *Cody, you are looking much better than when I saw you last. How are you feeling?*

CODY: *Fine.*

DR. SALAS: *What happened to your hand?*

CODY: *Nothing.*

DR. SALAS: *Looks like you don't want to talk about it.*

CODY: *Yeah.*

DR. SALAS: *How is school going for you?*

CODY: *Too much work.*

DR. SALAS: *Has it been too much the whole year or only now?*

CODY: *My teacher gave me lots of work sheets.*

DR. SALAS: *Is that since you were in the hospital?*

CODY: *She said I have to catch up.*

DR. SALAS: *Oh that's not easy. Does that mean you have to do everything the others did while you were in the hospital and all the new work as well?*

CODY: *Everything*

DR. SALAS: *Did you tell anyone that you feel this is too much for you?*

CODY: *My parents.*

DR. SALAS: *What did they say?*

CODY: *My brother can help me. But he just plays video games and his music.*

DR. SALAS: *What do your parents say about that?*

CODY: *I didn't tell them because then my brother will get real mad at me.*

DR. SALAS: *Sounds like you feel no one can help you now.*

CODY: *He doesn't have to play his music so loud.*

DR. SALAS: *So he gets to have all the fun while you were sick, in the hospital, on medicine, and now you also have all this work to do.*

CODY: *It's just not fair.*

DR. SALAS: *Also sounds like your brother makes you angry.*

CODY: *I got punished, but I'm glad I punched him in the nose.*

DR. SALAS: *Oh, so that's why you have a bandage. Did you hurt yourself real bad?*

CODY: *Yes, he ducked and I hit the closet.*

DR. SALAS: *Ouch, that must have really hurt and made you even more angry with him.*

Cody looks at Dr. Salas.

DR. SALAS: *And it also seems that your schoolwork is very important to you.*

CODY: *It's too much work.*

DR. SALAS: *Maybe your parents should explain to your teacher that you worry a lot about the catch-up work?*

CODY: *Then she won't like me.*

DR. SALAS: *I am hearing that you think a lot about people not liking you and being mad at you. Did I understand that correctly?*

CODY: *Yes.*

DR. SALAS: *Is this a new thing for you to feel like this?*

CODY: *A little.*

DR. SALAS: *So before you went to hospital were you also thinking that people don't like you or will be mad at you?*

CODY: *No.*

DR. SALAS: *How about getting angry at things like loud music?*

CODY: *No.*

DR. SALAS: *Some kids tell me that when they think a lot about their schoolwork and get angry easily with people it bothers them. How about you?*

CODY: *I guess so.*

DR. SALAS: *For you, which are worse, thinking about how much work you have to do or getting angry?*

CODY: *Thinking.*

DR. SALAS: *Ok, thank you very much for explaining that to me and I will see how we can help you feel better. Will it be ok if I tell your parents what you told me?*

CODY: *Yes. But I don't want to miss any more school.*

DR. SALAS: *Oh, so you mean that you also had to miss school today to come see me?*

CODY: *Yes, and now I will have more catch up work.*

DR. SALAS: *I really appreciate you coming to see me today. I think it was important because you helped me understand what is bothering you. Now I can also explain that to your parents and we can figure out how to help you.*

CODY: *I don't want them to be mad at me.*

In this conversation, Dr. Salas uses several strategies to talk with Cody about a topic he was not interested in talking about, his bandaged hand. Dr. Salas does not repeat questions when the child was unwilling to talk about something. Although the child appears to provide indirect answers to the questions, Dr. Salas works on understanding the feelings the child is expressing (anger toward brother, worry about not being able to catch up with his work, feeling that people will be angry at him and that no one can help him) in his short action-based sentences. Cody's marked change in behavior appears to reflect an increase in worrying about his schoolwork which exacerbated his poor regulation of emotions (temper outbursts and aggressive behavior). His "bad" behavior includes symptoms of an iatrogenic generalized anxiety disorder induced by the prednisone. If Dr. Salas had based the assessment on the parents' report, without the child's interview, Dr. Salas would not have reached this diagnosis.

SUMMARY

- Children with medical illness can present with anxiety symptoms that are:
  - Similar to those of their primary disorder
  - Secondary to an anxiety disorder
  - Adverse effects of the treatment of their underlying disorder
  - All of the above
- Careful interviewing of the child using the developmental guidelines will help the interviewer reach a definitive diagnosis.

REFERENCES

Bauer DH (1976). An exploratory study of developmental changes in children's fears. J *Child Psychol Psychiatry* 17: 69–74.

Campo JV, Bridge J, Ehmann M, Altman S, Lucas A, Birmaher B, Lorenzo CD, Iyengar S, and Brent DA (2004). Recurrent abdominal pain, anxiety, and depression in primary care. *Pediatrics* 113: 817–824.

Chavira D, Accurso EC, Garland AF, and Hough R (2010). Suicidal behaviour among youth in five public sectors of Care. *Child Adolesc Ment Health* 15: 44–51.

Craske MG, Rauch SL, Ursano R, Prenoveau J, Pine DS, and Zinbarg RE (2009). What is an anxiety disorder? *Depress Anxiety* 26: 1066–1085.

Cruz I, Marciel KK, Quittner AL, and Schechter MS (2009). Anxiety and depression in cystic fibrosis. *Semin Respir Crit Care Med* 30: 569–578.

Davies S, Heyman I, and Goodman R (2003). A population survey of mental health problems in children with epilepsy. *Dev Med Child Neurol* 45: 292–295.

Eddy AA and Symons JM (2003). Nephrotic syndrome in childhood. *Lancet* 362: 629–639.

Forsner M, Jansson L, and Soderberg A (2009). Afraid of medical care: School-aged children's narratives about medical fear. *J Pediatr Nurs* 24: 519–528.

Graae F, Milner J, Rizzotto L, and Klein RG (1994). Clonazepam in childhood anxiety disorders. *J Amer Acad Child Adolesc Psychiatry* 33: 372–376.

Greholt E-K, Stigum H, Nordhagen R, and Kohler L (2003). Recurrent pain in children, socioeconomic factors and accumulation in families. *Eur J Epidemiol* 18: 965–975.

Gupta S, Mitchell I, Giuffre RM, and Crawford S (2001). Covert fears and anxiety in asthma and congenital heart disease. *Child Care Health Dev* 27: 335–348.

Hergüner S, Kılıç G, Karakoç S, Tamay Z, Tüzün Ü, and Güler N (2011). Levels of depression, anxiety and behavioural problems and frequency of psychiatric disorders in children with chronic idiopathic urticaria. *Br J Dermatol* 164: 1342–1347.

Jones H and Jones MC (1928). A study of fear. *Childhood Education* 5: 136–143.

Koutroumanidis M (2002). Panayiotopoulos syndrome. *BMJ* 324: 1228–1229.

Kushnir J and Sadeh A (2010). Childhood fears: Neurobehavioral functioning and behavior problems in school-age children. Child Psychiatry Hum Dev 41: 88–97.

Mueller SC, Ng P, Sinaii N, Leschek EW, Green-Golan L, VanRyzin C, Ernst M, and Merke DP (2010). Psychiatric characterization of children with genetic causes of hyperandrogenism. *Eur J Endocrinol* 163: 801–810.

Muris P, Merckelbach H, Mayer B, and Prins E (2000). How serious are common childhood fears? *Behav Research Ther* 38: 217–228.

Myrvik MP, Campbell AD, Davis MM, and Butcher JL (2011). Impact of psychiatric diagnoses on hospital length of stay in children with sickle cell anemia. *Pediatr Blood Cancer* 58: 239–243.

Nicastro E, Ranucci G, Vajro P, Vegnente A, and Iorio R (2011). Re-evaluation of the diagnostic criteria for Wilson disease in children with mild liver disease. *Hepatology* 52: 1948–1956.

Ollendick TH (1983). Reliability and validity of the revised fear survey schedule for children (FSSC-R). *Behav Res Ther* 21: 685–692.

Ollendick TH and Horsch LM (2007). Fears in clinic-referred children: Relations with child anxiety sensitivity, maternal overcontrol, and maternal phobic anxiety. *Behav Ther* 38: 402–411.

Ortega A, Huertas SE, Canino G, Ramirez R, and Rubio-Stipec M (2002). Childhood asthma, chronic illness, and psychiatric disorders. *J Nerv Ment Dis* 190: 275–281.

Weinstein D, Staffelbach D, and Biaggio M (2000). Attention-deficit hyperactivity disorder and posttraumatic stress disorder: Differential diagnosis in childhood sexual abuse. *Clin Psychol Rev* 20: 359–378.

Wren FJ, Bridge JA, Birmaher B (2004). Screening for childhood anxiety symptoms in primary care: Integrating child and parent reports. *J Am Acad Child Adolesc Psychiatry* 43;1364-1371.

Attention

Attention involves the ability to focus selectively on a selected stimulus, sustain that focus, and shift it at will. Differential impairment of these components in different childhood disorders reflects the localization and extent of brain regions affected by the underlying illness. Attention deficit/hyperactivity disorder (ADHD) involves all three components and both the anterior and posterior attention systems in the brain, including fronto-striatal, fronto-parieto-temporal, fronto-cerebellar and fronto-limbic regions and networks (Bush 2011; Cubillo et al. 2012).

Treatment of pediatric cancer, namely intrathecal chemotherapy for acute lymphoblastic leukemia and cranial radiation for brain tumors (particularly medullolastoma) (Maddrey et al. 2005; Peterson et al. 2008; Kahalley et al. 2011), primarily impacts sustained attention (Butler et al. 2008). Impairment in both the shift and focus of attention are related to the severity of traumatic brain injury (Park et al. 2009) and to thinning of the posterior brain attention system in children with shunted hydrocephalus (Brewer et al. 2001). Although children with epilepsy (see review in Caplan 2010), multiple sclerosis (Portaccio et al. 2010), and neurofibromatosis (Hyman et al. 2006) have attentional impairment, studies to date have not examined the specific components involved (focus on stimulus, sustained attention, and shift of focus) and their associated brain regions and networks.

Teachers and parents are good informants about problems with attention in young children, particularly when they are associated with observable behaviors, such as distractibility, in which the child's attention is drawn from the task at hand to irrelevant stimuli. But, children with disorders involving internalizing symptoms, such as depression, anxiety disorders, or psychosis, might also appear to be distracted. In addition, children with language difficulties or with other learning difficulties might not pay attention (give up concentrating) due to these learning problems. From the teacher's perspective, however, children with impaired attention associated with depression, anxiety disorders, psychosis, language disorders, and learning disorders might all appear to be distracted.

This is particularly important because the problem of mislabeling or misinterpretation of young children's behavior is further complicated by the popular misconception that young children are not reliable informants about their thoughts and feelings (see review in Grills and Ollendick 2002). For young children to be reliable informants, they need the interviewer's help. To address this popular misconception, this chapter informs the reader how to find out from young children if

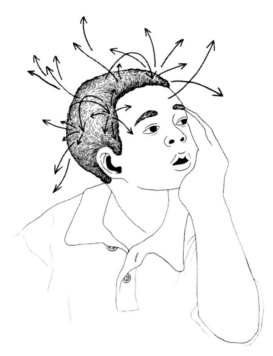

they have problems with attention. We then describe how to use this knowledge to determine if difficulties with attention are associated with a diagnosis of ADHD or another psychiatric disorder, a medical illness, adverse effects of medication(s), or a combination of these factors in young children.

SUMMARY
- Attention involves selectively focusing on a stimulus, sustaining the attention, and volitional shifting of the focus to another stimulus.
- Attention is impaired in medical, neurological, and psychiatric disorders.
- Parents and teachers are good informants on inattention and distractibility in young children.
- Other problem behaviors and emotions might be mislabeled as impaired attention.

TALKING TO CHILDREN ABOUT ATTENTION

When talking to children about attention, the first task at hand is to ensure that the child understands what the interviewer means by the word "attention." As early as preschool, children repeatedly hear teachers or parents use the word attention when they say, "I need you all to pay attention," "You are not paying attention," or "All look at me and pay attention to what I am saying." From the young child's perspective, paying attention means listening to what a teacher or parent is saying. For some young children, however, this could mean "being good" or "doing what the teacher says."

To inquire about the child's ability to focus selectively on a selected stimulus, the interviewer should first find out if the child finds it easy or difficult to listen when the teacher is talking. If the child says that it is easy, the interviewer should validate this by clarifying if, when the teacher speaks, the child finds himself thinking about what the teacher says or about other things. The interviewer should also inquire if the teacher often tells the child to pay attention or says that the child is not listening.

If the child says it is difficult to listen to the teacher or that the teacher frequently tells the child to pay attention, the interviewer should ask the child what makes it difficult to pay attention. The child's response to this question might be concrete, such as "The way she talks," "She talks funny," "She talks too softly," or it might be vague, as in, "I don't know." A follow-up question to any one of these responses can help the interviewer clarify the child's difficulty. For example, in response to the child stating "It's just how she (the teacher) talks," the interviewer can ask, "So is it her voice or what she talks about that makes it difficult?" The child might reply, "Her voice bugs me," or "It's what she says." The interviewer can then determine, "Is it difficult to understand what she is talking about?" If the child says, "Yes," or repeats his prior answer, "I told you it's what she says," the interviewer should clarify if this difficulty occurs across the board or for specific subjects by asking, "So does she talk funny all the time or only in reading [WAIT FOR RESPONSE], math [WAIT FOR RESPONSE], social studies [WAIT FOR RESPONSE], or science [WAIT FOR RESPONSE]."

Invoking humor strengthens the rapport with the child and encourages him to talk. The interviewer might consider responding to the child's claim that the teacher talks funny by jokingly asking the child, "Does that mean funny silly or funny weird?" Based on the child's response, the interviewer could inquire, "So is it silly (weird) because it is hard to understand what she is talking about?" and then proceed as above to clarify if the child has difficulty attending to the lessons for a specific subject or for all subjects.

Whether the child confirmed a problem with attention or not, the interviewer should also determine if the child is distractible or has a problem sustaining the focus of his attention. This is best done by use of concrete, action-based questions, such as "When kids around you in class are talking, do you stop listening to the teacher and listen to what they say?" or "If different kids are making a noise in the class, do you listen to them or to the teacher?" It is important to note that most young children are distracted if their friends are the ones chatting or if there are disruptive children in the class. If the child confirms distractibility, the interviewer should clarify if the child experiences this difficulty in all or specific subjects.

Another way to probe for distractibility includes asking, "When you play, do you play with one toy or game until you are done [WAIT FOR ANSWER], go from one toy to another [WAIT FOR ANSWER], or play lots of things at one time?" The interviewer should validate the child's answer by requesting examples of what occurs to make sure the child understood the concept of going from one toy or game to another or playing with several toys or games at the same time.

A child's difficulty in shifting his attention at will to a new focus is sometimes misinterpreted by teachers and parents as distractibility. It can be a handicap in a classroom setting when the teacher wants to go on to the next topic. One can rule in or out problems with disengagement by asking the child, "Let's say the teacher teaches math and then says put away your math sheets and open up your reading book. Do you still think about the math or are you ready to go on to the reading?" Alternatively, the interviewer can ask, "Does you teacher have to then tell you to pay attention?" or "Does she say, I told you we are now reading?"

Table 5–1 presents additional features of poor attention and symptoms found in children with ADHD (see reviews in Pliszka 2000; Reiff and Stein 2001; Cunningham and Jensen 2011). These include frequent careless mistakes; avoidance, dislike, or reluctance to engage in tasks that require sustained mental effort; lack of follow-through on instructions and failure to finish homework, chores, or duties; difficulty organizing tasks or activities; losing things necessary for tasks and activities; and forgetfulness in daily activities. The interviewer should assess carelessness with the following question, "Does your teacher sometimes say that you are not checking your work [WAIT FOR ANSWER] or that you make careless mistakes?" To determine if the child avoids doing homework, the interviewer might say, "So are you the type of kid who likes or hates doing homework?" If the child confirms that he hates homework, the interviewer should ascertain whether the child feels this way for all subjects or only for certain subjects. Regarding chores and following instructions, the interviewer should ask, "What chores do you do at home?" [WAIT FOR

Table 5–1. SYMPTOMS OF ADHD

ATTENTION

Attention
• Lack of focus
• Distractibility
• Difficulty shifting attention
• Carelessness
• Avoidance of sustained mental effort
• Lack of follow-through for:
  ▪ instructions
  ▪ homework
  ▪ chores
  ▪ duties

FORGETFULNESS
DISORGANIZATION
IMPULSIVITY
• Blurts out answers • Has difficulty waiting a turn • Interrupts • Intrudes
HYPERACTIVITY
• Fidgets • Squirms • Goes from one object, activity, or game to another • Leaves seat in class • Talks too much

ANSWER] "Do you always do them or sometimes try not to do them?" "How about at school?" "Do you do exactly what the teacher asks or does the teacher say that you are not following instructions?"

For disorganization, the interviewer should find out "What's your room like at home? Do you keep your stuff neat and tidy or all over the place?" and "How about your desk (locker) at school or your backpack—are they neat or a mess?" The interviewer should also ask the child if it is easy or difficult to remember to take things from home that he needs for school or to take work from school that he needs for homework. In addition, the interviewer should find out if the parents often say he loses things.

For children who acknowledge difficulties focusing, sustaining attention, doing homework and chores, following instructions, and being organized, the interviewer should ascertain the severity by asking the child if the teacher or parents remind him about these things a lot or a little. To clarify how much these acknowledged difficulties disturb him, the interviewer could ask, "Would you like to get help so it will be easier for you to pay attention [WAIT FOR ANSWER], and to listen to what the teacher is saying even when other kids are chatting or making a noise [WAIT FOR ANSWER], and to do you homework and chores [WAIT FOR ANSWER], and to do what the teacher tells you [WAIT FOR ANSWER], so you don't lose things [WAIT FOR ANSWER], and so you remember to take home your work and bring it to school in the morning?"

"Yes" answers to these questions confirm that the child is having problems with attention. If the child answers, "No," even though he previously acknowledged these difficulties, it is possible that the child might not have understood all the questions on attention. The interviewer should then clarify what the child might not have understood. For example, she could state, "Help me out. I am a little confused and maybe I messed up. Tell me if what I am saying is right or wrong. Before you said … " The interviewer should slowly repeat each of the above signs of impaired attention and wait to hear if she understood correctly or incorrectly.

The attentional difficulties of children with ADHD are associated with impulsivity and hyperactivity. An impulsive child blurts out answers before the teacher (or others) finishes asking the questions, has difficulty waiting for a turn, interrupts and/or intrudes on others. Since young children might not understand the abstract term, impulsivity, the interviewer should use concrete language when inquiring about this behavior. It is helpful to ask a young child, "Are you the type of kid who thinks about things before you do them, like looking left and right before crossing the street [WAIT FOR ANSWER], or do you start crossing and then look to see if a car is coming?" If the child says that he looks before crossing, the interviewer should validate this by asking, "How about with other things? Do you think first and then do them or first do them and then think that you shouldn't have done that?" If the child responds that he does not think before he does things, the interviewer should validate his answer by requesting examples.

Inquiring whether the child waits until called on or talks out of turn in class, blurts out an answer without raising his hand, and has difficulty waiting in line will provide information on impulsivity. Aware that "children figure out what the interviewer wants to hear" (see developmental guidelines in chapter 1), the interviewer should present the child first with the "normal" behavior, and then the problem behavior, when asking these questions.

The interviewer should also determine if the child is hyperactive, an additional sign of the combined type of ADHD. A hyperactive child fidgets with his hands and feet or squirms in his seat; he often leaves his seat in classroom or in other situations in which remaining seated is expected; he runs or climbs excessively in situations in which it is inappropriate; he is "on the go" or acts as if "driven by a motor," and he talks excessively.

In severe cases of hyperactivity, the interviewer can readily observe that the child is fidgety, squirming, or distracted by different objects in the room. However, in milder cases this might not be apparent, particularly if the child is not faced with the scholastic demands of the classroom. In such cases, the interviewer should ask the child "Is it easy or difficult for you to sit still in class?" If the child says it is difficult, the interviewer should find out if this is the case throughout the school day or only for specific subjects. If the child answers that he fidgets only in specific subjects, the interviewer should find out the difficulties the child encounters with that subject using "What" questions. Young children might answer that their difficulty is "The work!" In these cases, the interviewer should clarify if the child is having difficulty with the reading, writing, or the listening (attention) part of the work.

The interviewer should also ask the child "Do your teachers or parents often say you are talking too much or just sometimes?" If the child says the parents say he talks too much, the interviewer should clarify under what circumstances this occurs. If this occurs when the child and siblings are all trying to talk to their parents at the same time, this would not qualify as talking excessively. Finally, the interviewer should assess the severity of hyperactivity and if it has a negative impact on the child's life by asking if the teacher or parents often tell him to stay seated or stop moving and whether the child wants help with these behaviors.

As noted in previous chapters, the interviewer should also ascertain if the child's fidgetiness and/or excessive talking are signs of anxiety disorders, including post-traumatic stress disorder (see chapter 4), or mania (see chapter 3) rather than ADHD, using the guidelines provided in those chapters. In addition, the interviewer needs to consider movement disorders, such as Tourette's syndrome, chorea and others; medication induced hyperactivity; neurological and metabolic disorders, as well as psychosocial factors in the differential diagnosis of ADHD-like symptoms (see review in Cunningham and Jensen 2011).

SUMMARY

- Inattentiveness is a feature of ADHD and presents with or without hyperactivity and impulsivity.
- Children with a learning and/or language disorder might be inattentive due to comorbid ADHD, or because of an attention problem secondary to their underlying learning difficulties.
- Children with mood (depression, mania, bipolar disorder), anxiety, and psychotic disorders might also be inattentive.
- Parents, teachers, and children are essential informants on attention.
- Interviewers' concrete, action-based questions on attention should address:
  - Primary inattentiveness
  - Inattention secondary to a language or learning disorder
  - Distractibility

- Carelessness
- Forgetfulness
- Disorganization
- Lack of carry-through
- Avoidance of tasks involving mental effort
- Parents and teachers are also reliable informants on hyperactivity and impulsivity found in ADHD.

IMPAIRED ATTENTION AND MEDICAL ILLNESS

ADHD can occur in children with medical disorders, such as cystic fibrosis (Georgiopoulos and Hua 2011), hyperandrogenism (Mueller et al. 2010), asthma (Blackman and Gurka 2007), type 1 diabetes mellitus (Gelfand et al. 2004; Wodrich et al. 2011), celiac disease (Zelnik et al. 2004), and sickle cell disease (Hijmans et al. 2009), as well as in disorders of the central nervous system, including epilepsy (Dunn et al. 2003; Hesdorffer et al. 2004; Sherman et al. 2007), traumatic brain injury (Levin et al. 2007), multiple sclerosis (Banwell and Anderson 2005), neurofibromatosis (Hyman et al. 2006), pediatric cancer (Butler and Copeland 2002), and delirium/encephalopathy (see review in Bursch and Stuber 2004). In ADHD associated with a primary medical illness involving the central nervous system, such as epilepsy, the attentional rather than the hyperactivity and impulsivity components (Dunn et al. 2003), as well as slowed reaction time, are consistent findings (Dunn et al. 2010; Berg et al. 2011). Therefore, when interviewing the young, medically ill child with a central nervous system disorder, interviewers should focus on the previously described questions on attention.

As mentioned in chapter 4, anxiety disorders might also occur in asthma (Ortega et al. 2004), epilepsy (Caplan et al. 2005; Jones et al. 2007), traumatic brain injury (Luis and Mittenberg 2004), and celiac disease (Cruz et al. 2009), among other disorders. In addition, anxious or scared children might appear both inattentive and hyperactive. Similarly, children with depression might appear inattentive, and several of the disorders mentioned above are also associated with depression, namely diabetes (Wodrich et al. 2011) asthma (Ortega et al. 2004), cystic fibrosis (Cruz et al. 2009), multiple sclerosis (Weisbrot et al. 2010), and epilepsy (Caplan et al. 2005; Jones et al. 2007).

Therefore, it is essential to determine if inattention in young children with these illnesses reflects ADHD, an anxiety disorder, illness-related fears, or depression. This can be done by asking sensitive developmentally-based questions as described in chapters 3–4 on depression, fear, and anxiety disorders, as well as those described earlier in this chapter on attention.

Furthermore, children with acute or chronic illnesses that have not been well studied might also develop behavioral and emotional responses to these disorders that appear to be inattention, hyperactivity, or impulsivity. In fact, recent evidence demonstrates significantly higher rates of medical illness in children with psychiatric disorders, such as anxiety disorders (Chavira et al. 2008), than in the general population. Children with unexplained chronic pain also have higher rates of undiagnosed affective, anxiety, and disruptive disorders (ADHD) (Knook et al. 2011). The presence of these comorbidites is related to increased severity of the medical illness and caregiver strain (Chavira et al. 2008).

These findings emphasize the importance of early evaluation, diagnosis, and treatment of comorbidities in medically ill children. As evident from the clinical example that follows, these findings also underscore the need for interviewers to collect information on attention from parents and teachers and to carefully interview young children with medical and neurological illness about attention and its association with symptoms of disorders such as ADHD, mood disorders, anxiety disorders, and psychosis.

Darla is a 10-year-old girl with type 1 diabetes with onset at age 4 years. Her parents requested that her nurse practitioner, Ms. Davis, evaluate her because of frequent temper tantrums and aggression toward her younger sister, as well as recent arguments with her friends at school.

Type 1 Diabetes and Aggression

MS. DAVIS: *Hi, Darla. You have grown so much taller since your last visit. Are you one of the tallest kids in your class?*

DARLA: *Yes, but some are taller than me.*

MS. DAVIS: *How are things at school?*

DARLA: *Not good.*

MS. DAVIS: *What's not good?*

DARLA: *Kids say I'm weird.*

MS. DAVIS: *That must make you feel bad.*

DARLA: *They call me druggie and junky because I prick my finger to check my sugar before the insulin.*

MS. DAVIS: *You are doing a good job taking care of your diabetes at school and they call you that? Which kids are doing this?*

DARLA: *Different ones.*

MS. DAVIS: *Your friends or other kids?*

DARLA: *Other kids, but some friends when they get mad at me.*

MS. DAVIS: *What do you do when they tease you like this?*

DARLA: *Nothing.*

MS. DAVIS: *Nothing?*

DARLA: *I told the teacher. She said I am old enough to fight my own battles.*

MS. DAVIS: *What do your mom and dad say?*

DARLA: *They spoke to the teacher. She said I bug the kids.*

MS. DAVIS: *How?*

DARLA: *I tell on them when they talk during class and I can't concentrate.*

MS. DAVIS: *Is it difficult for you to concentrate only when they are chatting or also when it is quiet?*

DARLA: *It's hard, but when they talk I can't do any work.*

MS. DAVIS: *Is it hard to concentrate in all the subjects?*

DARLA: *Only for math.*

MS. DAVIS: *So what do you do?*

DARLA: *My sister is really good at math.*

MS. DAVIS: *How does that help you?*

DARLA: *I ask her to help with my math homework, but she's a show-off.*

MS. DAVIS: *What does she say?*

DARLA: *Sugar brains can't do math.*

MS. DAVIS: *How does that make you feel?*

DARLA: *Mad.*

MS. DAVIS: *So what do you do?*

DARLA: *Hit her.*

MS. DAVIS: *Does that help?*

DARLA: *She makes me so mad. She has all the fun, friends, eats what she wants, no shots.*

MS. DAVIS: *Do your parents know how angry she makes you?*

DARLA: *They just listen to her. She's a big crybaby and a liar, too.*

MS. DAVIS: *Do mom and dad know that it is difficult for you to concentrate on math?*

DARLA: *I told them. They say I need to try harder because I am smart.*

MS. DAVIS: *How does that make you feel?*

DARLA: *Mad.*

MS. DAVIS: *Hmm, sounds like things are really tough for you at school and at home, with school work, your friends, the teacher, and your family.*

Darla starts to cry.

MS. DAVIS: *How about we talk with your parents about all these problems?*

DARLA: *They won't understand.*

MS. DAVIS: *Well, sometimes parents are so worried about the diabetes that they don't think about these problems you have told me about. Can I explain all this to them first and then you will join us and tell them how you feel?*

DARLA: *If you think it will help.*

MS. DAVIS: *Before I talk with them, I want to understand better what is not going well between you and the friends that tease you.*

DARLA: *I told the teacher on two of them because they talk all the time in class, and in math they don't let me concentrate.*

MS. DAVIS: *Oh, so they teased you because you told the teacher on them.*

DARLA (with tears in her eyes): *Yes.*

Sensitive to the fact that Darla is having problems in the home environment (as per the parents' report), Ms. Davis began the conversation about school. She conducted a developmentally sensitive interview with action-based and concrete "What" and "How" questions, empathy for the child, and making sure Darla agreed with what Ms. Davis understood from Darla's responses to the interview questions. It became clear that children at school are teasing Darla about her diabetes. In addition, she has problems with concentration and some learning difficulties, as found in children with onset of type 1 diabetes before age 4 (see review in Wysocki et al. 2005). Although Darla mentioned mainly math, she also might have difficulties concentrating in other subjects. This might reflect a primary problem with attention or the subtle learning difficulties and secondary attention problems described in children with early onset diabetes (see review in Wysocki et al. 2005). A detailed interview is needed to determine if Darla has ADHD or symptoms of any of the psychiatric comorbidities in which inattention occurs.

This example demonstrates the importance of obtaining information on attention directly from young children. In this case, the parents were clearly only aware of the child's aggressive behavior. Their lack of awareness that Darla might be inattentive, have learning difficulties, and be experiencing sibling rivalry due to her younger sister's good math skills could have prevented them from understanding the child's increasing anger and frustration.

Finally, Darla's need to do well in math, given her sister's success in this subject, appears to have impaired her social judgment and make her "tell" on her friends who chat during math. The parents' lack of awareness that Darla might be inattentive, have learning difficulties, be experiencing sibling rivalry due to her younger sister's good math skills, and be a target of teasing at school impeded their understanding of the sources of the child's increasing anger and frustration.

SUMMARY

- Inattention with or without hyperactivity and impulsivity is found in a broad range of medical and neurological illnesses.
- These symptoms might reflect the primary illness, its treatment, and/or comorbidities, such as ADHD, mood, anxiety, and psychotic disorders, as well as delirium/encephalopathy.
- Early diagnosis through a developmentally based assessment and treatment are needed to optimize the child's functioning.

ATTENTION IN YOUNG CHILDREN: CONCLUSIONS

Impaired attention is found in young children with disorders that are medical, neurological, and psychiatric. Since young children might be mislabeled as inattentive, direct assessment of the child is essential for accurate diagnosis. Underreporting of problems with attention in children with medical and neurological illnesses underscores the need to ask parents about ADHD symptoms and to conduct individual developmentally based assessments of these children.

REFERENCES

Banwell B and Anderson PE (2005). The cognitive burden of multiple sclerosis in children. *Neurology* 64: 891–894.

Berg AT, Hesdorffer DC, and Zelko FAJ (2011). Special education participation in children with epilepsy: What does it reflect? *Epilepsy Behav* 22: 336–341.

Blackman JA and Gurka MJ (2007). Developmental and behavioral comorbidities of asthma in children. *J Dev Behav Pediatr* 28: 92–99.

Brewer V, Fletcher JM, Hiscock M, and Davidson KC (2001). Attention processes in children with shunted hydrocephalus versus attention deficit-hyperactivity disorder. *Neuropsychology* 15: 185–198.

Bursch B and Stuber M (2004). Pediatrics. In: *Textbook of Psychosomatic Medicine*, JL Levenson (ed.). Arlington, VA: American Psychiatric Publishing, Inc.

Bush G (2011). Cingulate, frontal, and parietal cortical dysfunction in attention-deficit/hyperactivity disorder. *Biol Psychiatry* 69: 1160–1167.

Butler RW and Copeland DR (2002). Attentional processes and their remediation in children treated for cancer: A literature review and the development of a therapeutic approach. *J Int Neuropsychol Soc* 8: 115–124.

Butler RW, Copeland DR, Fairclough DL, Mulhern RK, Katz ER, Kazak AE, Noll RB, Patel SK, and Sahler OJZ (2008). A multicenter, randomized clinical trial of a cognitive remediation program for childhood survivors of a pediatric malignancy. *J Consult Clin Psychol* 76: 367–378.

Caplan R (2010). Pediatric Epilepsy: A Developmental Neuropsychiatric Disorder. In: *Epilepsy: Mechanisms, Models, and Translational Perspectives,* JM Rho, R Sankar, and CE Stafstrom (eds.). Boca Raton, FL: CRC Press—Taylor & Francis Group, 535–549.

Caplan R, Siddarth P, Gurbani S, Hanson R, Sankar R, and Shields WD (2005). Depression and anxiety disorders in pediatric epilepsy. *Epilepsia* 46: 720–730.

Chavira DA, Garland AF, Daley S, and Hough R (2008). The impact of medical comorbidity on mental health and functional health outcomes among children with anxiety disorders. *J Dev Behav Pediatr* 29: 394–402.

Cruz I, Marciel KK, Quittner AL, and Schechter MS (2009). Anxiety and depression in cystic fibrosis. *Semin Respir Crit Care Med* 30: 569–578.

Cubillo A, Halari R, Smith A, Taylor E, and Rubia K (2012). A review of fronto-striatal and fronto-cortical brain abnormalities in children and adults with Attention Deficit Hyperactivity Disorder (ADHD) and new evidence for dysfunction in adults with ADHD during motivation and attention. *Cortex.* 48: 194–215

Cunningham N and Jensen P (2011). Attention deficit hyperactivity disorder. In: *Kliegman: Nelson Textbook of Pediatrics, 19th ed.,* RM Kliegman, BF Stanton, JW St. Geme III, and NF Schor (eds.). St. Louis, MO: W.B. Saunders Company.

Dunn DW, Austin JK, Harezlak J, and Ambrosius WT (2003). ADHD and epilepsy in childhood. *Dev Med Child Neurol* 45: 50–54.

Dunn DW, Johnson CS, Perkins SM, Fastenau PS, Byars AW, deGrauw TJ, and Austin JK (2010). Academic problems in children with seizures: Relationships with neuropsychological functioning and family variables during the 3 years after onset. *Epilepsy Behav* 19: 455–461.

Gelfand K, Geffken G, Lewin A, Heidgerken A, Grove MJ, Malasanos T, and Silverstein J (2004). An initial evaluation of the design of pediatric psychology consultation service with children with diabetes. *J Child Health Care* 8: 113–123.

Georgiopoulos A and Hua LL (2011). The diagnosis and treatment of attention deficit-hyperactivity disorder in children and adolescents with cystic fibrosis: A retrospective study. *Psychosomatics* 52: 160–166.

Grills A and Ollendick TH (2002). Issues in parent-child agreement: The case of structured diagnostic interviews. *Clin Child Fam Psychol Rev* 5: 57–83.

Hesdorffer DC, Ludvigsson P, Olafsson E, Gudmundsson G, Kjartansson O, and Hauser WA (2004). ADHD as a risk factor for incident unprovoked seizures and epilepsy in children. *Arch Gen Psychiatry* 61: 731–736.

Hijmans CT, Grootenhuis MA, Oosterlaan J, Last BF, Heijboer H, Peters M, and Fijnvandraat K (2009). Behavioral and emotional problems in children with sickle cell disease and healthy siblings: Multiple informants, multiple measures. *Pediatr Blood Cancer* 53: 1277–1283.

Hyman S, Arthur E, and North KN (2006). Learning disabilities in children with neurofibromatosis type 1: Subtypes, cognitive profile, and attention-deficit- hyperactivity disorder. *Dev Med Child Neurol* 48: 973–977.

Jones J, Watson R, Sheth R, Caplan R, Koehn M, Seidenberg M, and Hermann B (2007). Psychiatric comorbidity in children with new onset epilepsy. *Dev Med Child Neurol* 49: 493–497.

Kahalley LS, Conklin HM, Tyc VL, Wilson SJ, Hinds PS, Wu S, Xiong X, and Hudson MM (2011). ADHD and secondary ADHD criteria fail to identify many at-risk survivors of pediatric ALL and brain tumor. *Pediatr Blood Cancer* 57: 110–118.

Knook L, Konijnenberg A, van der Hoeven J, Kimpen J, Buitelaar J, van Engeland H, and de Graeff-Meeder E (2011). Psychiatric disorders in children and adolescents presenting with unexplained chronic pain: What is the prevalence and clinical relevancy? *Eur Child Adolesc Psychiatry* 20: 39–48.

Levin H, Hanten G, Max J, Li X, Swank P, Ewing-Cobbs L, Dennis M, Menefee DS, and Schachar R (2007). Symptoms of attention-deficit/hyperactivity disorder following traumatic brain injury in children. *J Dev Behav Pediatr* 28: 108–118.

Luis C and Mittenberg W (2004). Mood and anxiety disorders following pediatric traumatic brain injury: A prospective study. *J Clin Exp Neuropsychol* 24: 270–279.

Maddrey AM, Bergeron JA, Lombardo ER, McDonald NK, Mulne AF, Barenberg PD, and Bowers DC (2005). Neuropsychological performance and quality of life of 10 year survivors of childhood medulloblastoma. *J Neurooncol* 72: 245–253.

Mueller SC, Ng P, Sinaii N, Leschek EW, Green-Golan L, VanRyzin C, Ernst M, and Merke DP (2010). Psychiatric characterization of children with genetic causes of hyperandrogenism. *Eur J Endocrinol* 163: 801–810.

Ortega AN, McQuaid EL, Canino G, Goodwin RD, and Fritz GK (2004). Comorbidity of asthma and anxiety and depression in Puerto Rican children. *Psychosomatics* 45: 93–99.

Park BS, Allen DN, Barney SJ, Ringdahl EN, and Mayfield J (2009). Structure of attention in children with traumatic brain injury. *Appl Neuropsychol* 16: 1–10.

Peterson CC, Johnson CE, Ramirez LY, Huestis S, Pai ALH, Demaree HA, and Drotar D (2008). A meta-analysis of the neuropsychological sequelae of chemotherapy-only treatment for pediatric acute lymphoblastic leukemia. *Pediatr Blood Cancer* 51: 99–104.

Pliszka S (2000). Patterns of psychiatric comorbidity with attention-deficit/hyperactivity disorder. *Child Adolesc Psychiatr Clin N Am* 9: 525–540.

Portaccio E, Goretti B, Zipoli V, Hakiki B, Giannini M, Pastò L, Razzolini L, and Amato M (2010). Cognitive rehabilitation in children and adolescents with multiple sclerosis. *Neurol Sci* 31: 275–278.

Reiff M and Stein MT (2001). Attention-deficit/hyperactivity disorder evaluation and diagnosis: A practical approach in office practice. *Pediatr Clin North Am* 50: 1019–1048.

Sherman E, Slick DJ, Connolly MB, and Eyri KL (2007). ADHD, neurological correlates and health-related quality of life in severe pediatric epilepsy. *Epilepsia* 48: 1083–1091.

Weisbrot DM, Ettinger AB, Gadow KD, Belman AL, MacAllister WS, Milazzo M, Reed ML, Serrano D, and Krupp LB (2010). Psychiatric comorbidity in pediatric patients with demyelinating disorders. *J Child Neurol* 25: 192–202.

Wodrich DL, Hasan K, and Parent KB (2011). Type 1 diabetes mellitus and school: A review. *Pediatr Diabetes* 12: 63–70.

Wysocki T, Buckloh LM, Lochrie AS. and H A (2005). The psychologic context of pediatric diabetes. *Pediatr Clin North Am* 52: 1755–1778.

Zelnik N, Pacht A, Obeid R. and Lerner A (2004). Range of neurologic disorders in patients with celiac disease. *Pediatrics* 113: 1672–1676.

Aggression

Aggression, whether verbal or physical, is a nonspecific symptom that can be associated with a wide range of often interrelated factors, including socioeconomic, family environment, and psychopathology, that are beyond the scope of this book. In this chapter, we will apply the developmental guidelines to the assessment of aggression in young children and provide the interviewer with tools to determine the underlying causes and trigger factors for aggression in young ill children. We then describe aggression in medically ill children and how to determine causes and trigger factors. Identifying trigger factors is essential for determining the appropriate treatment of aggression. Symptomatic or "Band-Aid" treatment of aggression might provide temporary relief, but it does not help the young child and parents deal effectively with the underlying causes and trigger factors.

ASSESSMENT OF AGGRESSION IN YOUNG CHILDREN

Parents are good informants regarding their children's aggression because it is observable and most young children are embarrassed to talk about their aggressive behavior. However, parents might be unaware of the trigger factors for aggression for several reasons. First, parents do not watch their children all the time. Second, young children do not monitor the causes for their feelings. Third, they also often lack the words to express them. Fourth, adults might not understand young children's concrete verbalization of feelings and what made them angry. Fifth, when an angry parent asks a child, "Why did you hit him?" the child might be too scared to tell the parent the reason.

Assessment of the trigger factors of aggression is important. This helps the interviewer identify possible psychosocial causes and, in essence, treatment targets for the child's anger. These triggers might include the child's relationships in the home, at school, or in extracurricular activities. From the diagnostic perspective, understanding the trigger factors also provides the information essential for the interviewer to determine if, despite the maladaptive nature of the aggressive response, the child's anger was "warranted," or if both the child's anger and aggression were excessive.

Identification and psychopharmacological treatment of aggression associated with a psychiatric disorder without assessment of the psychosocial variables that trigger the child's aggression does not address the problem and has at best a

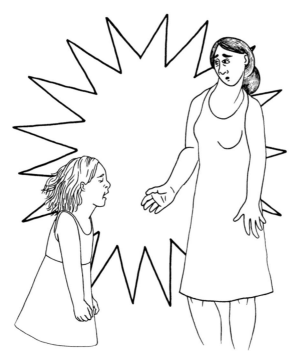

palliative symptomatic effect. Therefore, to help the child deal with causative factors and to prevent recurrent aggression, the interviewer should identify the triggers and determine if the child's aggression is a symptom of a psychiatric disorder.

In terms of diagnosis, aggression is found in children with a wide range of psychiatric disorders. These include externalizing disorders (oppositional defiant disorder, the combined and hyperactive types of attention deficit/hyperactivity disorder [ADHD], and conduct disorder); internalizing disorders (depression, bipolar disorder, anxiety disorders); psychosis; developmental disorders (autism spectrum disorders, developmental language disorder); and intellectual disability. Aggression in children with these disorders can be verbal or physical and directed toward others, property, and/or self.

As for mood, fear, anxiety, and inattention symptoms, young children are usually the best source of information on the trigger factors. However, since children are embarrassed by their aggressive behavior, the interviewer should not start an interview with questions about aggression. (See "Children Talk If They Feel Comfortable" in chapter 1.) Similarly, children do not feel comfortable if the interviewer tells the child that the parent has told him/her about the child's aggressive behavior. This can have a negative impact on the rapport between the interviewer and the child, and make the child even more reluctant to talk about aggressive behavior. To encourage talking about aggressive behavior, it is also important that the interviewer carefully choose words and monitor tone of voice to be nonjudgmental and non-accusatory.

The questions on mood (sad, happy), anger, and irritability described in chapter 3 are good ways to begin an interview and establish rapport with a young child. Through use of "What" questions after statements, such as "Kids tell me different things make them feel sad (angry, mad); what makes you feel like that?" the interviewer normalizes these feelings. As a result, children feel more comfortable talking about them and this helps the interviewer begin to talk about aggression.

Whether the child acknowledges anger and describes its causes or not, the interviewer should ask what the child does when angry. The interviewer should then find out how others react to the child's angry response of verbal or physical aggression and how that makes the child feel. Understanding the context for the anger and aggressive response, the interviewer should echo the child's feelings. This gives the child the message that the interviewer understands and makes the child more willing to talk about other things that induce anger and aggression.

If the child denies getting angry or aggressive, the interviewer should continue saying "When they get angry, some kids shout, use bad language, hit, or bang things; which of those things do you do?" The child might continue to deny aggression. Then the interviewer can ask, "How do your family or friends know you are angry?" If the child then describes what she does when angry, the interviewer should follow up with questions to ascertain the trigger factors for the aggression, the environmental response, and how all this makes the child feel. Whether the child confirms aggression or not, the interviewer should also determine what helps the child stop being angry or aggressive, "So if you are angry or feel like hitting someone, what helps make these feelings go away."

To determine the severity of aggression, the interviewer should ask the child "Do you ever get so angry that you feel you want to hurt someone or even kill them?" The interviewer should then follow up and find out what things occur that make the child feel this way, what the child does when aggressive, what happens afterwards, how that makes the child feel, and the environmental response to the child's aggressive behavior. Finally, it is important to ask if the child wants help with aggression.

The first dialogue below between a new pediatric intern and an aggressive child highlights how *not* to talk to young children about aggression. Dr. Sanders, the pediatric attending, then interviews the child using a developmental approach.

Jacob is a 7-year-old boy seen because of physical aggression toward his siblings and, more recently, verbal aggression toward his parents. The intern obtained a history from the mother who reported that her son has had sudden unpredicted mood changes in which he becomes very angry, curses, and then hits his older and younger siblings. When the parents try to restrain and calm him, he screams and more recently curses. Jacob then goes into his room and slams the door. He later appears to be in a good mood as if nothing ever happened.

Aggression: Technically Flawed Interview

INTERN: *So your mother tells me that you have been aggressive toward your brothers.*

Jacob looks down and does not respond.

INTERN: *Why do you get angry with them?*

Jacob shrugs his shoulders.

INTERN: *Besides hitting them, what else do you do to them?*

JACOB: *Nothing.*

INTERN: *For how long has this been going on?*

JACOB: *I don't know.*
INTERN: *How often do you hit them?*
JACOB: *I don't know.*
INTERN: *How hard do you hit them?*
JACOB: *Not hard.*
INTERN: *When did you first start hitting them?*
JACOB: *I don't know.*
INTERN: *Do you also hit kids at school?*
JACOB: *No.*
INTERN: *So why are you hitting your brothers?*
JACOB: *They hit me.*
INTERN: *If they hit you, why did you come to see Dr. Sanders today?*
JACOB: *My mother brought me.*
INTERN: *Did you ever hit them so hard that they were bleeding or got bruises?*
JACOB: *They did that to me.*
INTERN: *How come?*
JACOB: *They always start with me.*
INTERN: *Is there anything else you want to tell me about your aggressive behavior?*
JACOB: *Are we done?*

The intern told Dr. Sanders that Jacob supplied minimal information and accused his brothers of hitting him. From the outset, the intern made Jacob quite uncomfortable by saying he already knows that Jacob hits his siblings. He further increased the child's resistance as indicated by Jacob's one word or "I don't know" answers with "Why" and "How come" questions. In addition, the intern's approach was judgmental and implied that he believed that Jacob has been hitting his brothers. He also challenged the boy by asking why Dr. Sanders was seeing him and not his brothers.

Aggression: Developmentally Sensitive Interview
DR. SANDERS: *It's been a while since I saw you, Jacob. What grade are you in now?*
JACOB: *Third.*
DR. SANDERS: *Aren't you young for third grade?*
JACOB: *My birthday is in August.*
DR. SANDERS: *That's right, I forgot. How are you liking third grade?*
JACOB: *Good.*
DR. SANDERS: *What do you like best about third grade?*
JACOB: *The work.*
DR. SANDERS: *What don't you like about third grade?*
JACOB: *Nothing.*
DR. SANDERS: *How about home? What's good about home?*
Jacob looks down.
DR. SANDERS: *Sounds like things aren't too good at home.*
Jacob nods yes.
DR. SANDERS: *What's not going well at home?*
JACOB: *Fighting.*
DR. SANDERS: *Who is fighting with whom?*
Jacob shrugs his shoulders.

DR. SANDERS: *Is it your mom with your dad?*

JACOB: *No.*

DR. SANDERS: *Is it your parents with the kids?*

JACOB: *Sometimes.*

DR. SANDERS: *And is it the kids between themselves?*

JACOB: *Sometimes.*

DR. SANDERS: *Sounds like things aren't so good for you with all this fighting.*

Jacob nods yes.

DR. SANDERS: *So which parent is fighting with which kid?*

JACOB: *My mom gets mad because the kids are fighting and then she calls my dad and he gets mad.*

DR. SANDERS: *With both of them mad, you probably don't feel so happy.*

Jacob nods yes.

DR. SANDERS: *So what happens that makes the kids so angry?*

JACOB: *Dan wants to play when my friends come over. When I say "No" he goes to Tom. Tom doesn't want him to bother him when he is doing homework and yells at me. Dan just hangs out with my friends, plays with them. I don't get to do anything with them, and then they have to go home.*

DR. SANDERS: *That's too bad. So what do you do?*

JACOB: *I tell Dan to leave us alone and then he tells my mom. She yells at me in front of my friends and says they can't come over again. Dan laughs when she goes out and I hit him.*

DR. SANDERS: *And then what does he do?*

JACOB: *The crybaby tells my mom and she punishes me.*

DR. SANDERS: *Wow, this all probably makes you feel real bad.*

JACOB: *Now I can't have play dates.*

Dr. Sanders used "What" questions, a nonjudgmental approach, and empathy to get valid information from Jacob about the triggers for his anger and aggressive behavior. In contrast to the mother's report, Jacob's aggression is provoked by his younger brother's intrusive behavior. With this information, Dr. Sanders is in a better position to guide the parents on how to deal with this family problem.

SUMMARY

- To assess aggression in young children, the interviewer should determine:
  - Causes
  - Trigger factors
  - Expression and extent of aggression
- And how:
  - Parents respond to and manage the child's aggression
  - The child feels about being aggressive
- As the child's communication assistant, the interviewer should help young children talk about their aggressive behavior by use of:
  - "What" and "How" questions
  - "Normalizing" anger
  - Examples of how children express aggression
  - A nonjudgmental approach

AGGRESSION IN YOUNG, MEDICALLY ILL CHILDREN

Aggression in a young, medically ill child could reflect difficulty the child has due to the combined effect of the illness, its treatment, and comorbid psychopathology on the functioning and quality of life of the child, the parents, and the family. Among pediatric disorders, children with traumatic brain injury are vulnerable to the development of aggressive behavior post-injury, particularly if they had pre-injury aggression attention problems and anxiety, as well as greater disability after the head trauma (Cole et al. 2008; Dooley et al. 2008). The interviewer should apply the techniques described in the previous section to assess trigger factors for aggression and whether the aggression is related to psychiatric diagnoses found following head trauma (ADHD, posttraumatic stress disorder, and learning disorder) and/or to the impact of illness (neurological, cognitive, and linguistic deficits) on parenting, family functioning, and socioeconomic factors (See example below). The interviewer should also rule out possible iatrogenic effects due to medical procedures and adverse medication effects (posttraumatic stress disorder, delirium, steroid-related aggression, etc.).

This comprehensive approach is applicable to the assessment of aggression in children with any type of chronic illness. In addition, in all cases of aggression in young, medically ill children, the interviewer should also determine how the parents handle the child's anger and aggression for two main reasons. First, parents of young, medically ill children might feel guilty their child is ill or might be concerned that if their child gets angry or is aggressive, this might have a negative or deleterious effect on the child's illness. As a result, parents might refrain from saying, "No," to a child and they might make sure that the child always gets what the child wants. In addition to its negative effect on the non-ill siblings (who do not get what they want), this parental approach does not help the ill child develop and optimize coping skills. The child's outbursts of anger or aggression to get what the child wants, together with the parents' reluctance to set limits, can easily become a vicious cycle and a significant parental challenge.

Second, parents often differ in how they deal with the child's anger and aggression, with one parent being the "disciplinarian" and one the "go-to parent" who always says, "Yes." These different approaches can cause significant marital tension and teach the child to "split" between the parents in order to achieve his or her goals. Overhearing parents argue about their different approaches also increases the child's guilt (and stress) about being sick and the source of arguments between the parents. Therefore, the interviewer should determine if these behavior patterns are evident and explain to parents how such behavior patterns can negatively affect the child, the siblings, and the parental relationships.

Ronny is a 10-year-old boy who is being seen by Dr. Beck because of severe aggression toward his teacher. While crossing the street six months ago, he was hit by a car and sustained a blow out of his left orbit and associated frontal lobe damage. He underwent reconstruction of his orbit and returned to school three months ago. His mother reported increasing frequency of temper tantrums in his special education class in which he has thrown objects and, more recently, hit his teacher. Prior to his accident, he was diagnosed with ADHD and treated with a stimulant.

Aggression and Traumatic Brain Injury
DR. BECK: *Ronny, how are you feeling today?*
RONNY: *Good.*

DR. BECK: *How is school going?*
RONNY: *OK.*
DR. BECK: *Is you teacher nice or not so nice?*
RONNY: *Nice sometimes.*
DR. BECK: *When she's not nice, what does she do?*
RONNY: *She yells.*
DR. BECK: *Whom does she yell at?*
RONNY: *Kids.*
DR. BECK: *What does she yell about?*
RONNY: *To be quiet.*
DR. BECK: *What does she do that makes you angry?*
RONNY: *Nothing.*
DR. BECK: *Does that mean she doesn't make you mad?*
Ronny nods.
DR. BECK: *How about the kids in the class, are they nice or not nice?*
RONNY: *Nice.*
DR. BECK: *So whom does the teacher yell at?*
RONNY: *The kids.*
DR. BECK: *What do they do that makes her angry?*
RONNY: *Make a noise.*
DR. BECK: *Does that bother you?*
RONNY: *No.*
DR. BECK: *I get it so your teacher yells at the kids to be quiet but not at you.*
Ronny nods.
DR. BECK: *Is the work in class easy or difficult?*
RONNY: *Easy.*
DR. BECK: *What work is easy for you?*
RONNY: *All of it.*
DR. BECK: *What is your best subject?*
RONNY: *Recess.*
DR. BECK: *What do you hate to do at school?*
RONNY: *Work.*
DR. BECK: *Is that the reading?*
Ronny nods.
DR. BECK: *How about the writing?*
Ronny nods.
DR. BECK: *And the math?*
Ronny nods.
DR. BECK: *It sounds like it is hard for you in class.*
RONNY: *At home it's good.*
DR. BECK: *Does your teacher know how hard it is for you?*
RONNY: *She yells.*
DR. BECK: *Do mom and dad know how hard it is for you at school?*
Ronny shakes his head.
DR. BECK: *Did you try telling them?*
RONNY: *That she yells.*
DR. BECK: *Oh, so you told them that the teacher yells.*

RONNY: *She did.*
DR. BECK: *You mean the teacher told them?*
RONNY: *I hit her.*
DR. BECK: *She must have made you very angry. What did she do?*
RONNY: *She said I must finish the work.*
DR. BECK: *Was this the hard work?*
RONNY: *Yes.*
DR. BECK: *So it was hard for you to finish it?*
Ronny nods.
DR. BECK: *But the teacher didn't know that and said you must finish.*
RONNY: *Now she won't say that again.*
DR. BECK: *How do you know that?*
RONNY: *I'll hit her.*
DR. BECK: *And if you hit her, what will happen?*
RONNY: *She won't say finish the work.*
DR. BECK: *How did you feel after you hit the teacher?*
RONNY: *Good, now she won't say, "Time to finish the work."*
DR. BECK: *Thanks very much Ronny for explaining all this to me.*
RONNY: *Okay.*
DR. BECK: *Ronny you said that at home it is good. Who makes you feel good at home?*
RONNY: *My mom.*
DR. BECK: *Who bugs you at home?*
RONNY: *No one.*
DR. BECK: *So at home you don't get angry like at school?*
RONNY: *No.*

Despite Dr. Beck's developmentally appropriate approach, Ronny spoke in one-word sentences. The child's constricted laconic speech probably represents the damage sustained to his frontal lobe by the accident and not a resistance to speaking due to a technically flawed interview. In terms of the developmental guidelines, Dr. Beck did not begin the conversation with Ronny by asking questions about aggression. Using indirect questions, Dr. Beck first inquired about possible trigger factors for Ronny's aggression in the classroom including the teacher ("Is your teacher nice?"), the students ("How about the kids?"), and the schoolwork ("What do you hate about school?")

Through these questions, Dr. Beck established that Ronny is having great difficulty with his work and loses his temper when forced to finish his work. The boy's lack of understanding for the implications of his aggression probably also reflects the frontal lobe damage sustained in the accident as children his age have internalized that aggression in general and, in particular to a teacher, is socially unacceptable. Dr. Beck also applied additional developmental guidelines in this interview, including asking unbiased "What" and "How" questions, using concrete action-based language, and giving the child examples from which he could choose to answer the questions.

Interestingly, the mother and Ronny did not report anger or aggression at home. Given Ronny's relatively low frustration level in class, this is surprising. To conduct a comprehensive assessment of the child's aggression and trigger factors, Dr. Beck obtained additional information from the mother on how she, the father, and the siblings cope with changes in Ronny's functioning and behavior since his head injury. She found out that when Ronny first came home from the hospital, he had severe rage attacks when he did not get what he wanted. He would hit family members, break objects, and punch holes in the walls. As a result, no one in the family says, "No," to Ronny, and the mother has stopped working so she can take care of Ronny, as he needs constant supervision.

Although the mother is aware of increasing anger and resentment in her other children toward Ronny, she feels quite helpless to change the situation. The burden of care is entirely on her because Ronny's father has had to take on additional work to cover the salary the mother no longer earns. When he comes home, he is exhausted and has no patience for Ronny or the other children. The mother is concerned that the school will expel Ronny if he has an additional aggressive outburst in the class.

When Dr. Beck told Ronny's mother that Ronny was finding the work at school very hard, the mother was surprised; she thought that Ronny's special education class was addressing his learning difficulties. She also mentioned that the teacher complained that Ronny was not paying attention, and she wondered if he should be on a stimulant to help him with inattentiveness.

This clinical example demonstrates the importance of obtaining information from both the child and the parents to best assess aggression and its trigger factors in young children with an illness. Despite Ronny's cognitive and linguistic handicaps, the interview yielded information about Ronny's cognitive difficulties and lower frustration threshold subsequent to his traumatic brain injury; about what might be the teacher's lack of understanding for the severity of his learning difficulties and his low frustration tolerance due to his head injury; and about the impact of the boy's behavior problems on parenting, on the family budget, and on the siblings.

In the next example, the interviewer Julie, a child life specialist, was asked to help prepare a 7-year-old girl for a bone marrow aspiration. The young girl, Hannah, had no previous medical problems but is now suspected of having leukemia. When a nurse attempted to obtain a blood sample from Hannah, she reacted violently. She screamed, kicked, bit, and hit anyone who came near her. It took 5 residents and nurses to hold her down for the blood draw. Her mother was very distressed by this event and had no idea why her daughter reacted so violently. The following conversation took place the next day.

Trauma
JULIE: *Hi, Hannah. My name is Julie. Want to draw with me?*
HANNAH: *Okay.*
They start drawing.
JULIE: *How are things going in the hospital so far?*
HANNAH: *Bad.*
JULIE: *What bad things happened?*
HANNAH: *Needles.*
JULIE: *Oh yeah. Lots of kids don't like needles. What happened?*

HANNAH: *They held me down.*
JULIE: *That must have been scary for you.*
Hannah nods head yes.
JULIE: *What else happened?*
HANNAH: *I don't remember. They said I kicked someone.*
JULIE: *Sounds like you were mad.*
HANNAH: *Maybe.*
JULIE: *Were you ever scared like that before?*
HANNAH: *Ask my mom.*
JULIE: *Does that mean you don't want to talk about it?*
Hannah nods yes.
JULIE: *That's okay. You did a good job talking with me. Want to play a game?*
Hannah nods yes.

Julies' "How" and "What" questions, concrete language, and offer to draw with Hannah helped the child talk about her difficulties. Julie expressed empathy for the child's traumatic experience in the hospital. Julie was also sensitive to cues Hannah gave that she could not or did not want to answer questions about fear in the past. Hannah provided two helpful pieces of information in this conversation. First, Hannah seemed to think her mother would know when she previously felt very scared, and second, she either did not remember being aggressive or she did not want to talk about it.

When the child life specialist asked Hannah's mother about it, her mother could not think of any prior traumatizing medical events that Hannah had experienced or witnessed. However, when Julie asked the mother about other past traumas, the mother started to cry and described a long history of severe domestic violence witnessed by Hannah. Although Hannah's father had abandoned the family over a year earlier, they had never been evaluated or treated by any mental health professionals for this significant trauma exposure.

It appeared that her past trauma exposure had made Hannah a high risk to be traumatized and respond with aggression during her painful medical experiences as described in more detail in chapter 15 on pediatric iatrogenic trauma. The child life specialist recommended that the oncology team consult with the child psychiatry service to formally evaluate and address Hannah's trauma history.

SUMMARY

- Aggression in young, medically ill children significantly impacts the functioning and the quality of life of the child, the parents, and the siblings.
- Although parents are reliable informants on young children's aggressive behavior, they might be unaware of the trigger factors.
- A developmentally sensitive interview can tease out the role of contributing factors including direct effects of the illness, its treatment and comorbidities, family coping and functioning, as well as socioeconomic factors.
- Early detection of the causes of the aggression and its treatment promote both the child's physical and mental health.

REFERENCES

Cole W, Gerring JP, Gray RM, Vasa RA, Salorio CF, Grados M, Christensen JR, and Slomine BS (2008). Prevalence of aggressive behaviour after severe paediatric traumatic brain injury. *Brain* 22: 932–939.

Dooley JJ, Anderson V, Hemphill SA, and Ohan J (2008). Aggression after paediatric traumatic brain injury: A theoretical approach. *Brain Inj* 22: 836–846.

Insight, Judgment, and Reality Testing

Insight, judgment, and reality testing are three complex cognitive skills that individuals develop with age from middle childhood through adolescence. Insight represents the child's ability to monitor feelings, behavior, and thoughts. Judgment integrates skills involved in making sound, reasoned, and responsible decisions. A child with reality testing differentiates the external from the internal world and the self from the nonself.

Impairment of these skills can produce symptoms such as hallucinations, delusions, and thought disorder that are found in pediatric conditions associated with psychosis. These include psychiatric disorders, such as schizophrenia (Caplan 2011); depression (Ulloa et al. 2000); bipolar disorder (Tillman et al. 2008); dissociative psychosis (Hornstein and Putnam 1992); and substance abuse (Fiorentini et al. 2011); neurological disorders (epilepsy and delirium/encephalopathy) (Caplan et al. 1991; Bursch and Stuber 2004; Caplan et al. 2004); and medical disorders (systemic lupus erythematosus) (Sibbitt et al. 2002). Poor insight, impaired judgment, and *normal* reality testing are evident in children with psychiatric disorders, such as attention deficit/hyperactivity disorder (ADHD), oppositional defiant disorder, conduct disorder, depression, and bipolar disorder, as well as in medically ill children with these comorbidities.

In this chapter, we first describe how to use a developmental approach to assess the triad of poor insight, judgment, and reality testing, and how to determine if young children have hallucinations, delusions, or thought disorder. We will also discuss the need to differentiate these symptoms from what might appear to be symptoms of mood and anxiety disorders in young children. We then identify the challenges of diagnosing psychosis in young children with medical and neurological illnesses. This includes the difficulties involved in identifying symptoms of delirium/encephalopathy.

HOW TO TALK TO YOUNG CHILDREN ABOUT PSYCHOTIC SYMPTOMS

Since psychosis is rare in young children, most interviewers have not seen psychotic children as part of their training or professional experience. Interviewers sometimes use the term psychosis quite loosely to describe children with aggressive,

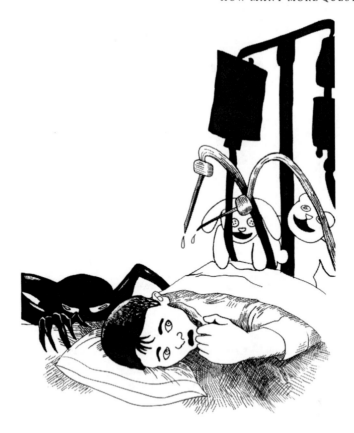

disorganized, and/or regressive behavior, even though children presenting with these behaviors are usually not psychotic. Misdiagnosis of psychosis in young children is of concern given the marked adverse effects, particularly the metabolic syndrome, of treatment with first and second-generation antipsychotic drugs (see review in Correll and Kratochvil 2008).

To identify psychotic symptoms in young children, an interviewer needs to carefully apply the developmental guidelines to help the child talk about symptoms, such as hallucinations and delusions and, most importantly, to understand what the child is communicating. A developmentally based interview also provides the interviewer with speech samples of adequate length to asses thought disorder in young children.

HALLUCINATIONS

A hallucination is the perception of a sensory experience in the absence of an external sensory stimulus. The sensory experience can involve the auditory, visual, tactile (superficial sensation on the skin), olfactory (smell), or gustatory (taste) systems. From age 5 years, most children have reality testing with a good sense of the difference between their internal and external worlds and between self and nonself.

Therefore, they understand that sensory experiences involving these systems are external.

Hallucinations are rare in children under age 7 years (see review in Caplan 2011). Experiencing a hallucination, irrespective of its sensory modality, induces fear for two reasons. First, the child knows this is an abnormal experience. Second, the content of the hallucination is often threatening and scary. Young children will typically share this abnormal experience with their parents because they are afraid, and they seek their parents' comfort and assurance that they are safe.

But parents often respond by telling their children that it is nothing or that this is the child's imagination. This makes children feel that their parents do not believe them or think they are "crazy." As a result, children learn to keep this information to themselves even when hallucinations are recurrent. Young children are also sometimes fearful that if they talk about their hallucinations, the threats or fearful content of the hallucination will become a reality. This fear makes young children reticent to speak to anyone, including their parents and an interviewer, about their hallucinations. Therefore, the interviewer needs to be sensitive and selective in how he or she asks children questions about hallucinations.

In addition, parents might be aware of their children's experiences but attribute fantasies and imaginary friends to normal developmental phenomena and therefore, do not report them to the child's interviewer. Thus, as with mood, fear, and anxiety symptoms, the child, not the parents, are the reliable informants about hallucinations and delusions.

As described under the developmental guidelines (see chapter 1), the interviewer should not begin the interview by asking questions about symptoms that the child may be reticent to talk about, such as hallucinations or delusions. Because children having hallucinations might be perceived as "mad" or "crazy," the interviewer should avoid using words such as "weird," "strange," or "unusual" when posing questions about hallucinations.

For older children aged 9–10 years, the interviewer can first ask a general question, such as "Some kids tell me that their imagination sometimes plays tricks on them; how about you?" Younger children might understand, "Some kids tell me that pretend things are real," rather than the more abstract "imagination plays tricks."

The interviewer should then continue with, "Some kids say they hear sounds or voices that no one else hears; does that happen to you?" Children often say they hear noises in the house at night when they are in bed. To validate if these are hallucinations or not, the interviewer should ask, "When you hear those noises, what do you think they are?" Children typically answer that their parents tell them it is the house settling down, the neighbors, or some external noise, and they appear reassured by this explanation.

Another frequent response is that children think they hear their parents or someone else calling their name, but add that their parents deny it. The interviewer should determine if the child accepts the parents' explanation by asking, "And what do you think when mom and dad say that?" If the child is not reassured by the parents' answers, the interviewer should establish if the child has good reality testing by asking, "What do you think might be making those noises?" or "Who else is calling your name?"

If the child is convinced that the noise is real and appears fearful, the interviewer should empathize, "That sounds scary." The interviewer should then inquire if the child also hears voices that speak to him or about him, threaten him, tell him to do things he thinks are bad, and/or talk to him about others. The interviewer should also ask who the voices belong to, what language they speak in, and what they are saying in order to determine the validity of the child's experience. The interviewer should also find out if the child told his parents or anyone else about his hallucinations and what their response was. If the child did not to tell anyone, the interviewer should ask, "And you didn't tell your parents because … ?" [WAIT FOR RESPONSE].

As previously mentioned, most hallucinations are scary. If the child does not experience distress and makes no effort to stop the hallucinations, this suggests that the child is not really hallucinating. Children with a dissociative disorder who have hallucinations do not appear to have associated subjective distress. Thus for diagnostic purposes, the interviewer should clarify if the child experiences distress while hallucinating and when he recalls the experience, and what he does to try to make the hallucinations go away. To do this, the interviewer can ask, "How does that make you feel when you hear the voices that say you are stupid and dumb?" After hearing how the child feels, the interviewer should ask, "And then what do you do to try make the voices go away?"

To evaluate the child's judgment, the interviewer should ask if the child acts on the basis of hallucination, and what, if anything, he does to avoid carrying out a hallucinatory command, using the following questions: "When the voices tell you to … (beat up your cousins), are you scared that you will do it?" "So what do you do?" "And how does that help?" A child with poor judgment might answer, "No, I'm not scared. I will beat them up and then they will stop talking about me all the time and telling everyone that I'm a retard."

To prevent the child from feeling that the interviewer, like the parents, does not believe him, he should challenge the child's reality testing only after asking all of the above questions. By this time, the child usually feels the interviewer understands his fear about the experience, he is quite relieved to be able to talk with someone about it, and he senses that the interviewer can help rid him of these experiences. Two complimentary approaches help the interviewer assess the child's reality testing. First, the interviewer could ask, "Do your friends also hear these voices talking or does that only happen to you?" Second, the interviewer might ask, "Some kids are not sure when they hear voices if they sound real or not real. How about you?"

To determine the clinical significance of a hallucinatory experience, the assessment of insight, judgment, and reality testing both confirms the experience and provides information on the severity of the symptom. As previously described, when first experiencing hallucinations, children might have partial insight or reality testing, as well as preserved judgment. However, if the child does not think that his hallucination is an abnormal experience (poor insight) or that it is his imagination (impaired reality testing), and if he also says he will act out or be forced to act out a command hallucination (bad judgment), there is a serious safety concern for the child and/or others.

After assessing auditory hallucinations, the interviewer should also find out if the child has visual hallucinations by asking, "Do you sometimes feel that you can see things that other people can't see?" or "Do you sometimes feel that that your eyes are playing tricks on you?" Similarly, to inquire about olfactory, tactile, and gustatory hallucinations, the interviewer should ask, "Do you sometimes smell a bad smell that no one else can smell?" and "Do you ever feel that there is something on your skin or moving on your skin, and when you look there is nothing there?" as well as, "Do you sometimes feel a bad taste in your mouth even when you haven't eaten anything to give you that taste?" The interviewer should then follow up the child's answers to each of these questions separately using questions similar to those used for auditory hallucinations.

Pauline is an 8-year-old girl who had her first seizure at age 8 months. She first developed staring spells from age 2 years 3 months. Over the years, her seizure pattern included a feeling that she was about to have a seizure, followed by deviation of the head and eyes to the right, cursive seizures in which she walked to the right, and occasional generalized tonic-clonic convulsions. She is a candidate for surgery to remove a left posterior mesotemporal lobe lesion identified on MRI.

Her mother brought her to see Dr. Lee because she expressed death wishes. She first said she wanted to die at age 7.5 years when she was placed in a special education class because of poor learning and socialization skills. At that time, the parents attributed this to difficulties Pauline had adjusting to a new schoolteacher. Now, however, they are unaware of any other possible trigger factors for the child's death wishes.

The developmentally based dialogue below between Dr. Lee and Pauline reveals that she is experiencing auditory, olfactory, and visual hallucinations. These are associated with significant distress and poor reality testing. Although she told her parents about these experiences, they told her it was just her imagination. Pauline's death wishes express that she feels there is no other way to rid herself of the hallucinations.

Epilepsy, Hallucinations, and Death Wishes

DR. LEE: *Pauline, who did you bring with you today?*
PAULINE: *My favorite doll.*
DR. LEE: *What's her name?*
PAULINE: *Angel.*
DR. LEE: *Is she a good angel?*
PAULINE: *She looks after me when I sleep.*
DR. LEE: *What can happen to you when you are asleep?*
PAULINE: *Dreams.*
DR. LEE: *Oh, so she can help you if you have bad dreams.*
PAULINE: *If she's with me, no bad dreams.*
DR. LEE: *What does she do in the daytime?*
PAULINE: *Sleep.*
DR. LEE: *I see. So in the daytime you feel safe.*
PAULINE: *My mom looks after me.*
DR. LEE: *I get it. At night your mom sleeps, so Angel takes care of you.*
Pauline nods and hugs her doll.
DR. LEE: *What bad things happen in the daytime?*
PAULINE: *Talking.*
DR. LEE: *Who is talking?*
PAULINE: *My brain.*
DR. LEE: *What is your brain saying?*

PAULINE: *Bad stuff.*

DR. LEE: *Like what?*

PAULINE: *This side (pointing to the left side of her head) says I am stupid.*

DR. LEE: *Oh, that is not nice. Who does it say it to?*

PAULINE: *This side (pointing to the right side of her head)*

DR. LEE: *And then what?*

PAULINE: *They say I am stupid and laugh at me.*

DR. LEE: *I am sorry to hear they are so mean. What do you do when they talk about you?*

PAULINE: *I do this (putting her fingers in her ears).*

DR. LEE: *How does that help?*

PAULINE: *It doesn't. They just go blah, blah, blah.*

DR. LEE: *And then what do you do?*

PAULINE: *I tell my mom I want to die.*

DR. LEE: *Does she know that they are talking about you?*

PAULINE: *She said I am just imagining.*

DR. LEE: *Oh, I see. What makes them say such bad things about you?*

PAULINE: *I don't know. But they don't go away.*

DR. LEE: *Can you see who is saying this?*

PAULINE: *No, I can't see in my brain!*

DR. LEE: *Do your eyes play tricks on you and sometimes you can see things no one else can see?*

PAULINE: *No, but there is a horrible smell, like throw up.*

DR. LEE: *That's not fun. Who else in your family smells the throw up?*

PAULINE: *No one. They say it's my imagination.*

DR. LEE: *How does that make you feel?*

PAULINE: *They think I am "cuckoo" in the head.*

DR. LEE: *Oh wow, your brain makes fun of you, there's a bad smell in your nose, and your family think you are "cuckoo."*

PAULINE: *If I die, no more talking.*

DR. LEE: *It all really makes you feel so bad you want to die.*

Pauline suddenly looks very scared and is staring at the corner of the room.

DR. LEE: *What's wrong Pauline?*

PAULINE: *There she is.*

DR. LEE: *Who?*

PAULINE: *The witch.*

DR. LEE: *Who brought her here?*

PAULINE: *She did this.*

DR. LEE: *What did she do?*

PAULINE: *A spell.*

DR. LEE: *She put a spell on you.*

Pauline puts her fingers in her ears and starts crying.

DR. LEE: *Are the voices bothering you again?*

Pauline nods yes.

DR. LEE: *Pauline, there is medicine that can make all these horrible things stop bothering you.*

Pauline (taking her fingers out her ears): *There is?*

DR. LEE: *Yes.*

PAULINE: *For me?*

DR. LEE: *But first I will have to talk with your parents and explain to them all the things you told me.*

PAULINE: *Okay.*

DR. LEE: *I have one more thing I want to understand so I can make sure I can help you.*

PAULINE: *Okay.*

DR. LEE: *When you say you want to die, is it because of the talking, the smell, and the witch, or also something else?*

PAULINE: *Nothing else.*

DR. LEE: *Do you think about how you would make yourself die?*

PAULINE: *No.*

DR. LEE: *So you say you want to die, but not do something to make you die?*

PAULINE: *Yes.*

Dr. Lee applied several developmental guidelines in this interview. She spoke about the child's death wishes only after she had established good rapport with Pauline. From Pauline's responses to "What" questions, Dr. Lee understood that Pauline was scared at night, but less so in the day when she could be with her mother. Dr. Lee expressed empathy and checked with Pauline to make sure she correctly understood the child's negative experiences. She gave Pauline positive feedback for being a good talker and asked for her permission to repeat some questions about her death wishes. Pauline's answers to these questions helped Dr. Lee understand that Pauline had no active suicidal plan.

SUMMARY

- Hallucinations are rare in children under age 7 years.
- Children are the best source of information on hallucinations.
- The interviewer can help young children talk about hallucinations using:
  - Concrete language
  - "What" questions
  - Examples from other children
  - Empathy
  - And by avoiding words that imply the child is abnormal, weird, strange, crazy, and the like.

DELUSIONS

Delusions are erroneous beliefs that are held despite evidence to the contrary. Similar to hallucinations, delusions are rare in children under age 7. They typically present as fears or cosmic threats (invading aliens, end of the world) rather than as the systematized persecutory delusions focused on one topic ("The FBI is trying to get me.") found in older individuals.

Although parents might be aware of their children's delusional thoughts, they might consider them to be age-appropriate fears and fantasies, or just creative imagination as in the following example. An 8-year-old boy believed that evil spirits were about to take over the world. To protect himself, he wore a leather dagger attached to his belt at all times, slept with a night light, and surrounded his bed with shields. He constantly made detailed plans of how he would vanquish the evil sprits with the help of figurines that he knew were really drones with brains.

His parents thought he had a vivid imagination and age-appropriate fears. However, his cosmic fears were rigid delusions that were not open to rational explanations by others. He was preoccupied with them all the time, and acted on them by arming himself and making war plans. The boy also had delusions of grandeur (able to vanquish the evil spirits) as well as visual illusions (misperceived plastic figurines as drones with brains).

Unlike age-appropriate fears, delusions that involve fears are pervasive, associated with poor reality testing, and the child will act on them. In contrast, children with "normal" fears, fantasies, and creative imagination have good reality testing and insight regarding the imaginary quality of these phenomena. See chapter 3 on how to interview young children about their fears.

Table 7–1 lists different types of delusions and suggested interview questions to identify, confirm, or rule out delusions in young children. A child with *ideas of reference* refers the actions of other people to herself and is convinced that their intentions are malevolent and derogatory toward her. For example, a 9-year-old girl thinks everyone at a mall is looking at her and that some people are talking about her. When asked, "What do they say?" she answers, "That I am ugly." When asked how she knows that people think she is ugly, she responds with, "By the way they look at me, I know they think I am ugly." Her answer demonstrates that she assigns negative meaning to behavior that has nothing to do with her, and it supports that she has a delusion.

Persecutory delusions (Table 7–1) are fixed ideas that others are trying to harm the child. Follow-up questions of a child's claim that others are being mean toward the child are essential because this might be true. The interviewer should find out what these children do, and whether they also do this to other children. After collecting this information, inquiring how the child knows that he is the target of other children's "mean" behavior helps the interviewer decide if the child's "persecutory" concern is reality-based or a delusion.

More specifically, if the child justifies the "malevolent" intentions of others based on incidents of arguments and fights, there probably is no underlying persecutory delusion. However, answers such as "in order to watch me, they always sit in the same seat behind me on the school bus," "they stand behind me in line every morning at school," or "they go to my church," could support a persecutory delusion.

Table 7–1. TYPES OF DELUSIONS AND INTERVIEW QUESTIONS

Delusion Type	Interview Questions
Reference	When you walk in the street (cross the playground at school), do kids look at you and talk about you? What do they say? How do you know?

Table 7–1. (CONTINUED)

Delusion Type	Interview Questions
Persecution	Are there people who do bad or mean things to you or to your family? What do they do? How do you know?
Guilt	If you do something wrong or bad, how does that make you feel? Do you forget about it or think about it again and again? If something bad happens to someone you know, even though you did nothing to them, do you feel you made that happen? How do you know?
Nihilism	Do you sometimes think that the world is coming to an end? How do you know?
Grandiosity	Have you got special powers? What special powers? Who else has these powers? Can you do things that no one else can do? Like what? Who else can do that? How did you get to be so special?
Somatic	When you look at yourself in the mirror, is there any part of you that looks strange or different? Did someone say that or is that what you think? How about inside your body, is everything in there okay? How do you know?
Thought broadcasting	Do people on TV, YouTube, or the Internet talk about what you are thinking? What do they say? How do you know? Who are they?
Thought insertion	Can people put thoughts into your head and make you think what they want you to think? How do you know? Who are they? What do they want you to think?
Thought withdrawal	Can they take thoughts out of your head and not let you think what you want to think? How do you know? Who are they? What do they want from you?
Thought control	Can people know what you are thinking? Do you know what other people are thinking? How do you do it?
Message	Does people on TV, YouTube, or the Internet say things especially for you? What do they say? How do you know?
Motor control	Do you sometimes feel like someone else, not you, is in your body and makes it work? Who/What is it? What does it/the person want you to do? How do you know?

In contrast to delusions of reference and persecution, follow-up questions on *grandiosity* (Table 7–1) usually reveal positive content, as in the following example of Patrick, a 9-year-old boy with acute lymphoblastic leukemia, who developed delusions of grandeur several weeks after he began treatment with prednisone and intrathecal methotrexate.

Delusions of Grandeur

DR. JONES: *Hi, Patrick. How are you feeling today?*
PATRICK: *Great.*
DR. JONES: *What did mom and dad bring you in for today?*
PATRICK: *To check if I am okay.*
DR. JONES: *So you are feeling great. What's been good for you?*
PATRICK: *Will you tell my mom and dad?*
DR. JONES: *You tell me; do you want me to tell them or not?*
PATRICK: *If you tell them, they will get mad.*
DR. JONES: *Mad at what?*
PATRICK: *They don't like it if I say I have special powers.*
DR. JONES: *You have special powers? What can you do with them?*
PATRICK: *Everything. I can get anything I want.*
DR. JONES: *What else?*
PATRICK: *I am smarter than all the kids in my class.*
DR. JONES: *That is really something. How did you find this out?*
PATRICK: *Don't tell my parents; they will get mad. God.*
DR. JONES: *What did God do?*
PATRICK: *He told me.*
DR. JONES: *He spoke with you?*
PATRICK: *Yep.*
DR. JONES: *What did he say?*
PATRICK: *That I have special powers and am the best at everything.*
DR. JONES: *Is it okay for me to tell your parents not to get mad about this?*
PATRICK: *Only if they won't be mad.*

In this interview Dr. Jones asked "What" and "How" questions, expressed empathy for the child's problems, and was respectful and not judgmental of the child. Dr. Jones's good rapport with the child encouraged Patrick to talk about experiences he was scared to share with his parents.

Patrick's acknowledgment of both delusions of grandeur and auditory hallucinations is evidence that he lacks insight, has impaired reality testing, and is psychotic. The chronology of the development of these symptoms suggests that the psychosis is steroid-induced. By asking Patrick how he found out that he had special powers, Dr. Jones obtained information on his auditory hallucination. This emphasizes the importance of follow-up questions to validate or confirm symptoms under inquiry. In addition to assuaging the child's fear, ending the interview by requesting the child's permission to tell his parents helps consolidate the child's trust and rapport with Dr. Jones.

Although rare in young children, *nihilism* (a pervasive thought that the end of the world is about to happen) can occur in children with psychotic depression or mania (see chapter 3) and in those with schizophrenia. For examples of questions to probe for nihilism, see Table 7–1. The section on differential diagnosis provides more details on how to differentiate nihilism and other delusions in children with mood disorders and psychosis from those in children with schizophrenia.

Children might also have *somatic delusions* that involve pervasive thoughts that something is wrong with their body (external appearance or internal organs). As evident from the follow-up question on somatic delusions in Table 7–1, the interviewer should ascertain if the child's thoughts are his own product (come from within) or derive from comments made by others. In the latter case, this would not be regarded as a delusion, because body image can be influenced by comments made by family and peers even in young children. Similarly, the goal of the follow-up questions on delusions involving *thought control, messages, and motor control* is to prevent misdiagnosis of one of these delusions. This is important because young children think that their parents control their thoughts and actions and might answer, "Yes" to these questions.

SUMMARY
- Delusions are rare in children under age 7 years.
- They usually take the form of cosmic fears and need to be differentiated from age-related "normal" fears.
- The assessment of delusions involves the use of concrete language and follow-up questions to confirm or rule out the delusional content of the child's thoughts.

THOUGHT DISORDER

Thought disorder involves impaired formulation and organization of thoughts and represents abnormalities in the form of language rather than in its content, as in delusions. Signs of thought disorder include illogical thinking (impaired reasoning) and loose associations (unpredicted change in the topic of conversation). From the clinical perspective, the listener has difficulty following the reasoning (illogical thinking) of the child with thought disorder, as well as the changes in the topic of conversation (loose association), and what the child is talking about (Caplan et al. 1996; Caplan et al. 2000).

As discussed in chapter 1, children's communication skills mature with age. The ability to talk coherently and cohesively develops from the toddler period through adolescence and involves basic and higher-level linguistic (discourse) and cognitive skills (see review in Caplan 1996). Although the term thought disorder has been used synonymously with schizophrenia, a wide range of disorders other than schizophrenia impact the development of a child's basic linguistic, discourse, and/or cognitive skills, including language disorders (Caplan 2011), intellectual disability (Caplan 2011), ADHD (Caplan et al. 2001), high functioning autism (van der Gaag et al. 2005), epilepsy (Caplan et al. 2006), and traumatic brain injury (Babikian et al. 2011).

When faced with a child with difficult-to-understand or disorganized speech, interviewers should consider the previously listed common disorders in their differential diagnosis, rather than the more infrequent psychotic disorders (schizophrenia, mood disorder and psychosis). It is particularly important that the interviewer obtain speech samples of adequate length—mini-paragraphs of one to two sentences rather than "Yes/No" answers—to assess thought disorder. If the interviewer applies the developmental guidelines but nevertheless continues to have difficulty making sense of what the child is saying, referral to a speech and language therapist could help determine if the child has a language disorder.

Three clinical examples of thought disorder follow. In addition to helping the reader identify thought disorder, these examples demonstrate how application of the developmental guidelines can help the interviewer make sense of the child's speech and clarify the underlying diagnosis

Tara, a 10-year-old girl with systemic lupus erythematosus, was brought to Dr. Spence because of weight loss, sleep problems, irritability, and anger. She is treated with corticosteroids and has had no medication changes in the past six months.

Thought Disorder and Hallucinations

DR. SPENCE: *Come in, Tara. It's been a while since I saw you last. What brings you here today?*

TARA (looking toward the door): *You can ask <u>her</u>.*

DR. SPENCE: *Looks like you have lost some weight.*

TARA: *<u>She</u> bugs me about food.*

DR. SPENCE: *Your mom does?*

TARA (looking angry): ***It's always like that when she talks to me.***

DR. SPENCE: *What is like that when she talks to you?*

TARA (raising her voice and looking around the room): ***Can't you see how mean she is?***

DR. SPENCE: *Tara, who is being so mean?*

TARA: *<u>She</u> is a witch.*

DR. SPENCE: *Who is?*

TARA (looking toward the door): *My mother.*

DR. SPENCE: *How do you know?*

TARA (again looking around the room): **Because she puts potions in the food**.

DR. SPENCE: *You mean your mother puts potions in the food?*

TARA (looking to the corner of the room): *Yes, <u>she</u> is saying that right now.*

DR. SPENCE: *So there is woman over there, and she tells you that your mother is putting potion in your food?*

TARA: **Because I am stupid.**

DR. SPENCE: *What does that woman look like?*

TARA: *Mean and ugly just like a witch.*

Dr. Spence is having difficulty following who and what Tara is talking about, because she makes unclear references by using the pronouns "her" and "she" without indicating beforehand whom she is talking about (indicated by underline). Dr. Spence also has difficulty following the topic of conversation, because the child makes unpredicted topic changes, as in loose associations (indicated by bold italics), without preparing the listener for the topic change. Dr. Spence also does not understand the child's reasoning due to her illogical thinking (indicated by bold highlight).

Through concrete "What" and "How" questions, Dr. Spence confirmed that, in addition to thought disorder, Tara is experiencing both auditory and visual hallucinations. She also has poor reality testing. Her weight loss is probably the result of not eating due to her fear that the mother is poisoning her food. However, additional questions are needed to confirm this delusion.

Hal is a 5-year-old boy with sickle cell anemia whose most recent blood transfusion was about six months ago. The parents told Dr. Raj that his kindergarten teacher says he is inattentive, does not follow instructions, and acts aggressively toward peers. The teacher told Hal's parents to take him to the doctor to find out if he has ADHD. His parents' reported that when they talk with him at home he often seems to be thinking about something else. Similar to his behavior at school, he frequently does not do what his parents ask of him. When they remind him, he begins to cry.

Thought Disorder or Language Disorder

DR. RAJ: *Hi, Hal. I think you must be already in kindergarten.*
Hal smiles.
DR. RAJ: *What do you like to do at school?*
HAL: *Go home.*
DR. RAJ: *What don't you like to do at school?*
HAL: *School.*
DR. RAJ: *What work at school don't you like?*
HAL: *Work.* **My dog is Scott.**
DR. RAJ: *What work is hard at school?*
HAL: **We play.**
DR. RAJ: *With the kids at school?*
HAL: *Scott.*
DR. RAJ: *What do you like to play with Scott?*
HAL: *Play.*
DR. RAJ: *When your teacher talks, is it difficult or easy to understand?*
HAL: *She yells.*
DR. RAJ: *At you?*
Hal nods yes.
DR. RAJ: *That must make you angry?*
HAL: They *laugh.*
DR. RAJ: *Who laughs?*
HAL: *Kids.*
DR. RAJ: *At you?*
Hal nods yes.
DR. RAJ: *That's not nice.*
Hal nods yes.
DR. RAJ: *So the work is hard.*
Hal nods yes.
DR. RAJ: *And your teacher yells at you.*
Hal nods yes and his eyes begin to tear.
DR. RAJ: *And the kids are mean and laugh.*
HAL CRIES.
DR. RAJ: *What do mom and dad say?*
HAL: Not listening.
DR. RAJ: *Who is not listening?*

HAL: *Me.*
DR. RAJ: *You mean they say you are not listening to them.*
Hal sobs.

This interview illustrates that concrete language, "What" questions, empathy, and acting as the child's communication assistant are how Dr. Raj made sense of the speech of this young child with language problems. This example is particularly important because, to the uninformed interviewer, Hal might appear to have thought disorder. His answers to Dr. Raj's questions about "work" were off topic as in loose association (indicated by italics and bold). Dr. Raj also needed to use several "Who" questions to clarify who Hal was talking about, because the boy used the pronoun they without previously specifying to whom they refers (indicated by underline). However, Hal's one to two word sentences (including a grammatically incomplete sentence indicated by a broken underline) and the difficulties he appeared to have with "work" at school suggested a need for comprehensive testing of language to determine if he has a language disorder and related learning difficulties. Although labeled as ADHD by his teacher and parents (see chapter 5), throughout this interview Hal focused on the concrete questions Dr. Raj asked and sat without fidgeting.

Pablo is a 12-year-old boy who underwent hemispherectomy at age 3 years for intractable seizures and Rasmussen syndrome treated by surgical removal of the left side of his brain. Language development was delayed until after his surgery and his mental age is that of a normally developing 8-year-old child. His parents divorced following his surgery and he lives with his mother and spends weekends with his father. Dr. Hill is seeing him today because of recent aggressive behavior both at school and toward his father.

Thought Disorder, Hallucinations, and Delusions
DR. HILL: *Hi, Pablo. Who did you bring with you today to my office?*
PABLO (showing Dr. Hill his stuffed animal): *James. The others didn't come. He is mad. They are laughing. But they listen to me. Stop laughing you guys.*
DR. HILL: *Who is making James mad?*
PABLO: **Hey, knock it off you guys. She wouldn't let me bring them in.**
DR. HILL: *Oh, you mean other stuffed animals?*
PABLO: *I'm their boss.*
DR. HILL: *What do they do when you go to school?*
PABLO: *Get mad because they're at home. But I cheer them up so they won't be lonely.*
DR. HILL: *How do they hear you?*
PABLO: *The wires in my head from surgery.*
DR. HILL: *What wires?*
PABLO: *In my head. Stop fighting you guys. You'll get time out when I'm in the car.*

As evident from this example, Pablo's conversation is difficult to follow because his answers are unrelated to the topic of conversation as in loose association (indicated italics and bold) and he uses pronouns without identifying who he is talking about (indicated by underline). In addition, he has auditory hallucinations and grandiose delusions. Dr. Hill uses short concrete "What," "Who," and "How" questions rather than "Yes/No" questions to try to understand what Pablo is communicating.

SUMMARY

- A listener's difficulties in understanding the logic of a child's conversation, following the topic changes, and who and what the child is talking about could reflect:
  - Developmental immaturity
  - A language disorder
  - Intellectual disability
  - Psychotic disorders and other psychiatric disorders
  - Neurological disorders associated with language and cognitive deficits
- To assess thought disorder, the interviewer needs to encourage the child to speak in mini-paragraphs of one to two sentences because "Yes/No" questions yield one-word answers.
- The interviewer's use of developmental guidelines to elicit speech and make sense of the child's communication are essential tools to identify hallucinations, delusions, and thought disorder, as well as the underlying diagnosis.

DIFFERENTIAL DIAGNOSIS OF PSYCHOTIC SYMPTOMS IN YOUNG CHILDREN

Psychotic symptoms, such as hallucinations, delusions, and thought disorder, are rare in young children. Yet, how young children communicate about their feelings, particularly negative feelings (sadness, anger, poor self-esteem), is often misunderstood by adults. Rather than using verbal communication, young children tend to act out their feelings. As a result, their behavior at times of stress might mistakenly be described as "psychotic" because it appears to be disorganized, strange, or regressed.

Hallucinations, delusions, and thought disorder occur in psychosis due to psychiatric, neurological, medical disorders, and adverse effects of different medications (Table 7–2). (The reader can find a detailed discussion of how to differentiate between these conditions in Caplan 2011.) In this section, we first briefly summarize how to differentiate between schizophrenia and mood disorders with psychosis, because mood disorders are frequent in children with medical and neurological illnesses. It then describes how to determine when symptoms of the comorbidities of medical and neurological disorders (mood disorders, anxiety disorders, ADHD) might, in fact, be symptoms of psychosis in young ill children.

The distinguishing features in the differential diagnosis between schizophrenia and mood disorders associated with psychosis are that the content of hallucinations and delusions is bizarre in schizophrenia but mood-congruent in the psychosis

Table 7–2. DISORDERS ASSOCIATED WITH PSYCHOTIC SYMPTOMS

Schizophrenia
Mood disorders (depression, mania, bipolar)
Dissociative disorder
Medical disorders
Neurological disorders
Iatrogenic disorders (caused by medications or medical procedures)

found in mood disorders. Thus, whereas a child who is both depressed and psychotic would think he is to blame for the end of the world (nihilism and delusion of guilt), a child with mania might think he has the powers to bring about this end (grandiose delusion). A child with schizophrenia, however, might attribute the upcoming end of the world to an evil ruling force or power (bizarre delusion). Thus in contrast to the bizarre content in the delusions of children with schizophrenia, the content of delusion in children with a mood disorder and psychosis matches the sad negative or euphoric grandiose mood of the underlying disorder.

Similarly, the suicidal ideation of children with schizophrenia is based on hallucinations and delusions with bizarre content, whereas in children with psychosis and a mood disorder, the suicidal ideation is congruent with the child's mood. For example, a child with schizophrenia might want to kill herself because there is an electronic device in her abdomen that transmits messages to her indicating that the devil wants her to come down to hell. A depressed child who is psychotic might have auditory hallucinations telling her that she is so bad that she deserves to die.

In terms of the comorbidities of neurological and medical illness, interviewers should be aware that psychosis in young children can present with fears; with symptoms of anxiety disorders, including separation anxiety, generalized anxiety, obsessions, and posttraumatic stress symptoms; with mood disorder symptoms, such as depressed mood, social withdrawal, anger, irritability, suicidal or self-harm behavior, insomnia and sleep disturbances, including nightmares, a change in appetite and eating behaviors; with inattention; and with aggression. When children confirm any of the above symptoms, the interviewer should always determine if these symptoms are associated with hallucinations or delusions.

Thus, the earlier example in the Delusions section of the child who wore a dagger because he feared that evil spirits will take over the world highlighted that, in contrast to fears, delusions are pervasive, reflect poor reality testing, and are acted upon by the child. The following example illustrates that hallucinations might also present as fears and/or symptoms akin to those of a separation anxiety disorder.

Ben, aged 7, began having crying or screaming episodes in which he would cling to one of his parents. The frequency of the episodes increased, he refused to go to school, slept with his parents, and would not separate from them throughout the day. His nurse practitioner, Ms. Cooper, spoke to Ben together with his mother.

Hallucinations vs. Fears and Separation Anxiety Symptoms

MS. COOPER: *Ben, I haven't seen you for a long time. What did your mother bring you in for today?*

BEN: *I don't know.*

MS. COOPER: *Did you come here straight from school?*

BEN: *I didn't go to school.*

MS. COOPER: *Oh, were you sick?*

BEN: *I don't want to go to school.*

MS. COOPER: *What's happening at school that isn't good?*

BEN: *Nothing.*

MS. COOPER: *Some kids don't like school because they get scared.*

BEN: *Of what?*

MS. COOPER: *Not being with their parents.*

BEN: *Me too.*

MS. COOPER: *What can happen if you are not with them?*
BEN: *I don't know.*
MS. COOPER: *Are you scared something might happen to you or to your parents?*
BEN: *Me.*
MS. COOPER: *What might happen to you?*
Ben becomes tearful.
MS. COOPER: *It looks like it is scary for you even to talk about it.*
Ben starts crying.
MS. COOPER: *Is it easier for you to draw what is making you scared?*
Ben draws a monster-type figure.
MS. COOPER: *What does that scary thing in your picture do to you?*
Ben starts to sob and clings to his mother who tries to console him.
MS. COOPER: *Is it easier for you to draw or to tell me what it's doing?*
BEN (shouting): *It wants to kill me.*
MS. COOPER: *Does it say that or does it look like it wants to hurt you?*
BEN: *Both.*

Ms. Cooper carefully and indirectly approached the topic of Ben's school refusal by asking him if he had just come from school. She then asked if he had not gone to school because he was sick. The child then told her that he did not want to go to school. Using examples from other children who are scared to go to school, "What" questions, and Ben's drawing, she found out that he was scared of a monster that he saw and heard.

Although Ben's presenting problem appeared to be separation anxiety disorder symptoms, Ms. Cooper's careful developmentally based questions revealed that the child experiences both auditory and visual hallucinations. The child's significant distress and clinging behavior suggest that his reality testing is impaired and that these experiences are very real for him. Additional questions, as well as a physical and neurological exam, are needed to determine the underlying diagnosis.

Similarly, delusions might underlie the worries of a child with generalized anxiety disorder or the obsessions or compulsions of a child with obsessive-compulsive disorder. Misdiagnosis might occur if an interviewer asks a child about these symptoms without follow-up validation questions which help clarify the source of the worries or the thought processes associated with what appear to be obsessions or compulsions, as in the two examples that follow.

Carol is a 10-year-old girl seen by Dr. Mills because of headaches that began about a month ago. Dr. Mills's interview thus far has revealed that Carol's headaches occur mainly in the morning before she goes to school and on afternoons when she goes to the Girl Scouts. In addition, Carol has been feeling quite sad recently but she was unable to talk with Dr. Mills about what makes her sad. However, she confirmed having worries.

Psychotic vs. Generalized Anxiety Disorder Symptoms

DR. MILLS: *Carol, what things do you worry about?*
CAROL: *Different things.*
DR. MILLS: *Would you like me to tell you what other kids worry about and see if any of those are like your worries?*
CAROL: *Okay.*

DR. MILLS: *Kids your age often tell me they worry about what other kids think of them.*

CAROL: *They do?*

DR. MILLS: *Yes.*

CAROL: *What else?*

DR. MILLS: *They also worry that the kids might be talking about them?*

CAROL: *I know that they are. I see how they look at me and then laugh.*

DR. MILLS: *Carol, do they do that to other kids or only to you?*

CAROL (SADLY): *Only to me.*

DR. MILLS: *What do you think they are thinking or saying?*

CAROL: *I don't think it. I know it!*

DR. MILLS: *I wasn't sure about that. Thanks for correcting me. So what are they thinking and saying?*

CAROL: *Bad stuff.*

DR. MILLS: *Like what?*

CAROL: *I don't want to say.*

DR. MILLS: *When you are not at school or scouts, are they talking about you?*

CAROL: *Yes.*

DR. MILLS: *How do you know?*

CAROL: *I hear them.*

DR. MILLS: *How does that make you feel?*

CAROL: *Sad.*

DR. MILLS: *Before you said you get sad, but you didn't want to say what was making you sad. How does seeing and hearing the kids talk bad stuff about you make you feel?*

CAROL: *Sad.*

The techniques Dr. Mills used in this interview included asking "What" and "How" questions, giving Carol examples of what makes other children scared, and apologizing for saying that Carol thinks the kids are laughing at her rather than saying that Carol knows this. When Carol did not want to answer what bad stuff kids were saying about her, Dr. Mills did not repeat the question and changed the topic of conversation.

As evident from this interview, ideas of reference and auditory hallucinations underlie Carol's worries and sadness. If Dr. Mills would not have clarified the nature of these symptoms, she might have misdiagnosed Carol with an anxiety or mood disorder. As in the previous example, comprehensive psychiatric, medical, and neurological examinations are indicated to determine the child's underlying diagnosis.

"AJ" is an 8-year-old boy who began a ritual when going to bed after his most recent emergency room visit because of a severe attack of asthma. He folds his bedding, checks under the bed, makes sure his windows are closed, and then asks his parents to come into his room, and go through these same actions. A medical social worker on the asthma team, Mr. Sparks, had the following conversation with AJ.

Delusions vs. Compulsions vs. Medical Trauma Symptoms

MR. SPARKS: *AJ, you are breathing much better than when I saw you last at the emergency room.*

AJ: *I never want to go there again.*

MR. SPARKS: *Did something bad happen in the ER?*

AJ: *I don't want any more asthma.*

MR. SPARKS: *It is scary when you feel you can't breathe.*

AJ: *I don't want any more attacks.*

MR. SPARKS: *I understand that this last time made you very scared.*

AJ averts eye contact and nods.

MR. SPARKS: *What were you scared might happen?*

AJ: *I can't say.*

MR. SPARKS: *Some kids get scared that the asthma might make them die. Does that happen to you?*

AJ: *No.*

MR. SPARKS: *How about when you go to sleep at night—what makes you scared?*

AJ: *I'm not scared. I close the windows and check under my bed.*

MR. SPARKS: *What can come in through your windows?*

AJ: *The ghosts.*

MR. SPARKS: *Which ones?*

AJ: *From the haunted house next to our house.*

MR. SPARKS: *How do you know it is haunted?*

AJ: *Because the lady died.*

MR. SPARKS: *Oh that is scary. Did you tell your mom and dad?*

AJ: *They said there is not such thing as ghosts and haunted houses.*

MR. SPARKS: *Who told you about the lady and the house?*

AJ: *No one.*

MR. SPARKS: *So how do you know?*

AJ: *One was under my bed.*

MR. SPARKS: *Oh, so you saw one there?*

AJ: *Yes, but then it was gone.*

MR. SPARKS: *Did it come back?*

AJ: *Not if I close my windows.*

MR. SPARKS: *What does it want to do in your room?*

AJ: *Scare me.*

MR. SPARKS: *Does it also do that to other kids?*

AJ: *I don't know. They don't live next to a haunted house.*

MR. SPARKS: *Oh, so the ghost comes from there.*

In this example, the child appeared to have a ritual prior to going to sleep. As evident from the dialogue above, AJ's thinking and the associated ritual before going to sleep were unrelated to his recent asthma attack and reflected his fear of a ghost from the neighboring haunted house. From a cultural perspective, some people believe in haunted houses and ghosts. However, Mr. Sparks established that this was neither a family belief nor ideas he heard from his friends. In fact, his parents tried unsuccessfully to convince him that the house was not haunted. Since AJ believed that he could see the ghost (visual hallucination) and that it wanted to scare him (delusion), this was not an obsession.

Mr. Sparks's interview demonstrates the importance of not talking about the child's main problem until rapport is established and the child is comfortable talking with the interviewer. Mr. Sparks uses questions about asthma and asthma-related fears to talk to AJ about sleep and the child's bedtime rituals. Use of "What" and "How" questions and action-based concrete language help Mr. Sparks encourage the child to talk about his hallucinations.

SUMMARY

- The differential diagnosis of psychosis in young children should include psychiatric, neurological, and medical disorders.
- The content of hallucinations and delusions is mood congruent in children with mood disorders and bizarre or unusual in children with schizophrenia.
- Use of the developmental guidelines help the interviewer ask young children about hallucinations and delusions.
- Follow-up validating questions assess the child's insight, reality testing, and judgment for these symptoms.
- Hallucinations and delusions might also present as mood, anger, irritability fear, anxiety, attention, and aggression symptoms.

INSIGHT, JUDGMENT, AND REALITY TESTING IN YOUNG ILL CHILDREN

Neurological disorders (epilepsy, delirium/encephalopathy, degenerative disorders) (Caplan et al. 1991; Bursch and Stuber 2004; Caplan et al. 2004) and medical disorders (systemic lupus erythematosus) (Sibbitt et al. 2002) cause psychotic symptoms with impaired insight, judgment, and reality testing. More commonly, young ill children present with delirium (see review in Bursch and Stuber 2004), posterior reversible encephalopathy (see review in Ishikura et al. 2011), and epilepsy related encephalopathy (Wirrell et al. 2005). Chapters 10–12 discuss epilepsy in detail. In this section, we briefly highlight the main signs and symptoms of delirium and how to differentiate between psychosis due to psychiatric disorders and delirium. A clinical example then illustrates these diagnostic difficulties.

Delirium is defined as sudden, severe confusion and rapid changes in brain function. It is most often caused by physical or mental illness and is usually temporary and reversible. Young ill children who have preexisting brain damage, sleep deprivation, or sensory overload are at higher risk to develop delirium. Essential information to obtain from caregivers include the presence of a fluctuating mental status (waxing and waning of orientation, cognition, and language skill) and changeable levels of awareness, as well as the behaviors listed in Box 7–1, Signs and Symptoms of Delirium. Some children with delirium hallucinate and have disorganized thinking (thought disorder).

Several features help differentiate delirium from psychosis found in psychiatric disorders. First, psychosis is unlikely if the child has a primary medical illness known to be associated with delirium (Table 7–3). Second, disorientation, together with waxing and waning of awareness usually does not occur in a psychosis associated with psychiatric disorders. Third, fluctuating impairment of both receptive and expressive language with disorganized, disjointed, or incoherent speech and, in severe cases, loss of speech, suggest delirium rather than psychosis. Fourth, visual hallucinations without auditory hallucinations can be seen in delirium but not in psychosis due to other psychiatric and neurological disorders. Talking to oneself

---

Box 7–1.

SIGNS AND SYMPTOMS OF DELIRIUM

- Visual hallucinations
- Pulling at lines, picking, grabbing air
- Waxing and waning mental status
- Delusional thoughts and/or paranoia
- Disorganized thinking and speech
- Cessation of spontaneous speech
- Sleep–wake disturbance; extreme fatigue
- Impaired attention, disorientation
- Irritability, agitation, anxiety, affective lability
- Confusion, impaired memory, depressed mood, apathy

---

or a focused look associated with mumbling, picking, fear, or laughter might suggest that a child with delirium has auditory hallucinations. However, a reliable and valid assessment of hallucinations can be done only if a child is speaking and can confirm the hallucinatory experience.

As can be seen in the next case example, it is not uncommon for children with delirium to have visual hallucinations of bugs and/or delusions of persecution. Amy is an 8-year-old girl who was hospitalized for a heart transplant. Her transplant was uneventful, however she remained intubated (on a ventilator) for three days. Once she was no longer intubated, Amy's parents noted bizarre behavior. Amy reported that she felt a spider crawling on her body and a fly on her face. In addition to these tactile hallucinations (involving sensations on her skin), she also had a visual illusion in which she saw a shadow out of the corner of her eye that seemed like a scary person.

Notably, an incident was documented by her medical team members in which Amy appeared to have experienced hallucinations in response to pain medication. At that time, she was intubated and did not verbalize what she was seeing, however she appeared to see something in the room that greatly frightened her. Although that medication was discontinued, her perceptual disturbances persisted. Amy and her father denied any previous history of hallucinations or poor reality testing.

Amy also described a sense of dread that a vague entity she could not describe was trying to kill her. In addition, she reported having feelings that the hospital doctors were trying to kill her when they gave her medications. She also had dreams in which doctors were attempting to kill her with knives. Amy reported a frequent state of fear and exhibited withdrawn behavior.

Delirium, Hallucinations, and Delusions

DR. GIBSON: *Hi, Amy. I hear you have been having some worries. Can you tell me about it?*

Amy does not answer.

Table 7–3. DELIRIUM/ENCEPHALOPATHY AND INTERMITTENT CHANGE IN
CONSCIOUSNESS: RELATED MEDICAL CONDITIONS AND MEDICATIONS

CNS DISTURBANCES
• Seizure
• Migraine
• Head trauma
• Brain tumor
• Infection—meningitis or encephalitis
• Vascular
METABOLIC/ENDOCRINOPATHIES
• Electrolyte abnormalities
• Fluid abnormalities
• Diabetes (hypoglycemia, hyperglycemia, insulin resistance)
• Adrenal abnormality
• Thyroid abnormality
• Parathyroid abnormality
• Hyperammonemia
SYSTEMIC ILLNESSES
• Cardiac, such as failure, arrhythmia, myocardial infarction, assist device, surgery
• Pulmonary, including hypoxia, SIADH,* acid base disturbance
• Hematological, such as anemia, leukemia, transplant, blood transfusions
• Neoplasms
• Renal failure or uremia
• Hepatic disorders
• Infections, including enterovirus, pneumonia, aspergillosis, Lyme disease, syphilis
• Autoimmune disorders, including systemic lupus erythematosus
• Other: Nutritional deficiency, sleep deprivation, surgery
MEDICATIONS AND TOXINS
• Over the counter medications, including antihistamines, decongestants, analgesics
• Herbals such as jimsonweed, oleander, foxglove, hemlock
• Heavy metals such as mercury, lead, arsenic, aluminum
• Prescription medications, including pain medication, anesthesia, cardiac medications, antihypertensives, steroids, antibiotics, antivirals, antifungals, sedative-hypnotics, histamine H2 antagonist, antineoplastics, anticholinergics, antituberculous medications, antispasmotics, ephedrine, lithium, contrast, colchicine, indomethacin, levodopa
• Neuroleptic malignant syndrome
• Serotonin syndrome
• Abuse of stimulants, opiates, sedatives, or organic molecules (pesticides, insecticides, solvents, gasoline, glue, ethylene glycol

* Syndrome of inappropriate antidiuretic hormone hypersecretion

DR. GIBSON: *I am hoping that if I understand what is happening, I might be able to help you.*

AMY: *Bad dreams.*

DR. GIBSON: *You are having bad dreams?*

AMY: *Yeah.*

DR. GIBSON: *What else?*

AMY: *Bugs.*

DR. GIBSON: *What about bugs?*

AMY: *They keep crawling on me. And, they are giving me poison.*

DR. GIBSON: *Who is giving you poison?*

AMY: *The doctors and nurses. They want to kill me.*

DR. GIBSON: *That sounds scary. What makes you think they want to kill you?*

Amy starts rubbing her face.

DR. GIBSON: *Amy, what are you doing?*

AMY: *Get rid of the bugs!*

DR. GIBSON: *Do you feel bugs?*

AMY (crying out): *Get rid of them.*

In the dialogue above, Dr. Gibson encouraged the child to speak by being explicit about the desire to help her, by asking very brief "What" questions, by being empathic about the experiences being frightening, and by not challenging the reality of her experiences. The interviewer was able to obtain evidence for tactile hallucinations and delusions of persecution (poisoning). It is not clear from this brief conversation if the child's "bad dreams" are nightmares or if they are related to her fluctuating awareness and scary thoughts. Given her lack of a psychiatric history and her current medical condition, these symptoms are most consistent with delirium.

SUMMARY

- Psychosis occurs in medical and neurological disorders.
- Delirium should be considered in children who undergo a marked change in behavior, fluctuation of awareness, waxing and waning of cognitive, linguistic, and perceptual abnormalities (visual and tactile hallucinations).

IMPAIRED INSIGHT, JUDGMENT, AND REALITY TESTING: CONCLUSIONS

A comprehensive evaluation of the young, medically ill child includes the assessment of insight, judgment, and reality testing to rule in or out psychotic symptoms including hallucinations, delusions, and thought disorder. Psychosis is rare in young children. What might appear to be psychotic symptoms, therefore, needs to be differentiated from normal developmental phenomena and from mood, anxiety, and attention deficit/hyperactivity disorders, as well as language disorders and intellectual disability. This can be achieved by conducting a developmentally based interview.

The possibility of delirium should be considered in young children with regressive, withdrawn, or agitated behavior who have a medical or neurological in behavior, and fluctuations in level of awareness associated with abnormalities in behavior, cognition, language, and perception.

REFERENCES

Babikian T, Satz P, Zaucha K, Light R, Lewis RS, and Asarnow RF (2011). The UCLA longitudinal study of neurocognitive outcomes following mild pediatric traumatic brain injury. *J Int Neuropsychol Soc* 17: 886–895.

Bursch B and Stuber M (2004). Pediatrics. In: *Textbook of Psychosomatic Medicine*, JL Levenson (ed.). Arlington, VA: American Psychiatric Publishing, Inc.

Caplan R (1996). Discourse deficits in children with schizophrenia spectrum disorder. In: *Language, Learning, and Behavior Disorders*, JH Beichtman, N Cohen, M Konstantareas, and R Tannock (eds.). Cambridge, UK: Cambridge University Press: 156–177.

Caplan R (2011). Childhood schizophrenia: Diagnostic and treatment challenges. *Cutting Edge Psychiatry in Practice* 1: 55–64.

Caplan R, Guthrie D, and Komo S (1996). Conversational repair in schizophrenic and normal children. *J Am Acad Child Adolesc Psychiatry* 35: 950–958.

Caplan R, Guthrie D, Komo S, Tang B, and Asarnow R (2000). Thought disorder in childhood schizophrenia: Replication and update of concept. *J Am Acad Child Adolesc Psychiatry* 39: 771–778.

Caplan R, Guthrie D, Tang B, Nuechterlein KH, and Asarnow RE (2001). Thought disorder in attention-deficit hyperactivity disorder. *J Am Acad Child Adolesc Psychiatry* 40: 965–972.

Caplan R, Shields WD, Mori L, and Yudovin S (1991). Middle childhood onset of interictal psychosis. *J Am Acad Child Adolesc Psychiatry* 30: 893–896.

Caplan R, Siddarth P, Bailey CE, Lanphier EK, Gurbani S, Shields WD, and Sankar R (2006). Thought disorder: A developmental disability in pediatric epilepsy. *Epilepsy Behav* 8: 726–735.

Caplan R, Siddarth P, Gurbani S, Ott D, Sankar R, and Shields WD (2004). Psychopathology and pediatric complex partial seizures: Seizure-related, cognitive, and linguistic variables. *Epilepsia* 45: 1273–1286.

Correll CU and Kratochvil CJ (2008). Antipsychotic use in children and adolescents: Minimizing adverse effects to maximize outcomes. *J Am Child Adolesc Psychiatry* 47: 9–20.

Fiorentini A, Volonteri LS, Dragogna F, Rovera C, Maffini M, Mauri MC, and Altamura CA (2011). Substance-induced psychoses: A critical review of the literature. *Curr Drug Abuse Rev* 4: 226–240.

Hornstein NL and Putnam FW (1992). Clinical phenomenology of child and adolescent dissociative disorders. *J Am Acad Child Adolesc Psychiatry* 1077–85.

Ishikura K, Hamasaki Y, Sakai T, Hataya H, Mak R, and Honda M (2012). Posterior reversible encephalopathy syndrome in children with kidney diseases. *Pediatr Nephrol* 27: 375–384.

Sibbitt WL, Brandt JR, Johnson CR, Maldonado ME, Patel SR, Ford CC, Bankhurst AD, and Brooks WM (2002). The incidence and prevalence of neuropsychiatric syndromes in pediatric onset systemic lupus erythematosus. *J Rheumatol* 29: 1536–1542.

Tillman R, Geller B, Klages T, Corrigan M, Bolhofner K, and Zimerman B (2008). Psychotic phenomena in 257 young children and adolescents with bipolar I disorder: Delusions and hallucinations (benign and pathological). *Bipolar Disorders* 10: 45–55.

Ulloa RE, Birmaher B, Axelson D, Williamson DE, Brent DA, Ryan ND, Bridge J, and Baugher M (2000). Psychosis in a pediatric mood and anxiety disorders clinic: Phenomenology and correlates. *J Am Acad Child Adolesc Psychiatry* 39: 337–45.

van der Gaag RJ, Caplan R, van Engeland H, Loman F, and Buitelaar JK (2005). A controlled study of formal thought disorder in children with autism and multiple complex developmental disorders. *J Child Adolesc Psychopharmacol* 15: 465–476.

Wirrell E, Farrell K, and Whiting S (2005). The epileptic encephalopathies of infancy and childhood. *Can J Neurol Sci* 32: 409–418.

Somatization

Somatization is defined as the process whereby physical symptoms are experienced in response to stress (Lipowski 1988). Examples include a tension headache or a gastrointestinal symptom (such as abdominal pain, nausea, or diarrhea) that is triggered or exacerbated by a stressful event (such as a school test or a family argument). The most frequently reported symptoms experienced via somatization are pain, gastrointestinal and/or neurological. It is important to recognize that an underlying illness or injury can itself be a significant stressor that triggers or exacerbates somatization. For example, a child with epilepsy might also have non-epileptic seizures, or a child with cancer might get nauseated in anticipation of a hospital admission for chemotherapy.

Somatization is not intentional; it is an automatic or habitual physical and behavioral response to stress. While it is possible with training and practice to gain some control over one's symptoms, somatization is not equivalent to falsifying symptoms (as one might see in malingering or a factitious disorder). Therefore, to simply suggest that one cease somatizing is not helpful.

Likewise, it is inaccurate to conclude that "nothing is wrong" when a somatizing individual seeks assistance for symptoms and medical testing fails to reveal an underlying medical condition. A child or parent may feel disbelieved or discounted unless the symptom is adequately explained. Additionally, parents are more likely to accept treatment recommendations if they feel the clinician has a good understanding of the child's symptoms. The clinician who concludes "there is nothing wrong" or that the symptom is "stress-related" (without explaining how that is possible) can inadvertently increase distress, anxiety, and somatizing in the child and the family.

While everyone responds physically to stress, some individuals are more prone to somatization than others, and some are more distressed and/or disabled than others by somatic (physical) symptoms. For example, behaviorally inhibited (reserved, avoidant, anxious) children appear to be at higher risk for somatization (Biederman et al. 1993; Boyce et al. 1992; Kagan et al. 1988; Manassis et al. 1995). Stuart and Noyes (1999) have hypothesized that somatizing behavior is a response that is conditioned (learned) within the family system and reinforced by the positive caregiving responses of others (such as increased positive attention and assistance with daily activities by the parent), or by the successful avoidance of aversive experiences (such as bullying at school or abuse at home).

Increased levels of psychopathology (especially anxiety and depression), family dysfunction, poor school performance and attendance, perceived health impairment, and more frequent use of health and mental health services are observed in families with somatizing children (Campo et al. 1999; Tamminen et al. 1991). Although anxiety disorders are the most common psychiatric comorbidity, somatization can occur in the absence of a psychiatric condition (Andresen et al. 2011; Smith et al. 2005; Torgersen 1986).

Individuals who have medically unexplained physical symptoms and who are inexplicably distressed or disabled by symptoms that appear to be in excess of what would be expected from the history, physical examination, and/or laboratory findings, are defined by the DSM-IV as having a Somatoform Disorder. In the DSM-5, these disorders are reconceptualized and referred to as Somatic Symptom Disorders. Due to the unreliability of assessments of "medically unexplained symptoms," this aspect of the diagnoses is no longer a key feature. Instead, the Somatic Symptom Disorder diagnoses are defined by physical symptoms and excessive maladaptive illness-related cognitions and behaviors (such as high health anxiety, excessive concern about the seriousness of one's symptoms, and/or devotion of excessive time and energy to one's health concerns).

One way symptom-associated disability develops is when a recognized or unrecognized significant life event, physical stressor, or developmental challenge surpasses the "at-risk" child's coping abilities. The child's inefficacious coping results in a physiological stress response, rendering the child vulnerable to the development of somatic symptoms. A child in this vulnerable state, who does perceive a physical symptom, may retreat to a dependent role and/or take steps to avoid the stressor. Because retreat from the stressor prohibits mastery over the challenge and strengthens the child's belief that the child cannot effectively cope with the

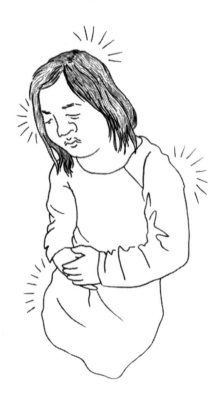

stressor, a progressively declining course follows, with decreasing functioning, as well as increasing distress and vulnerability to emotional and physical impairment. Well-meaning and concerned parents and clinicians may perpetuate this downward spiral of symptoms and disability by fostering the dependent role and/or by contributing to the stress of the child.

COMMUNICATION

The manner in which the clinician communicates with the somatizing child and family plays a significant role in the accuracy of the evaluation and in the willingness of the family to accept treatment recommendations. Due to the physical presentation of the symptoms and the complex nature of somatization, many parents question the validity of a behavioral or psychiatric diagnosis and treatment plan, especially if they feel blamed for the disorder. When each clinician working with the child and family uses the same words to describe the problem and the treatment plan, confusion is minimized.

An explanation that includes how the body physiologically responds to physical or psychosocial stress may help the family better understand the biopsychosocial model (which posits that illness and disability are best explained by a combination of biological, psychological, and social factors rather than purely in biological terms). Additionally, it is important to explicitly state that neither the child nor the family are to blame for the symptoms and disability, but that there are things they can learn to do to reverse the downward disabling spiral. Even if the child or parent does not understand or remember the details of how the mind and body interact, the physiological explanation can be sustaining for them throughout the assessment and treatment of the child. The child and parent need to understand that while it is not always possible to identify specific stressful triggers, somatization is a valid problem that requires treatment. It is also important to inform the child and parent that, fortunately, this diagnosis is not life-threatening and progress has been made in understanding how to best treat such symptoms.

Because young children have little ability for introspection and are not always aware of their emotional states, they may be more aware of and able to discuss their somatic distress. Therefore, in order to prevent excessive medical intervention and to increase accurate assessment, it is important for the clinician to understand how to assess and interpret symptoms and triggers of somatization.

ASSESSMENT

By far, the most researched form of pediatric somatization is pain. Because pain is discussed in chapter 14, in this chapter, we will focus on general topics related to somatization and our examples will emphasize gastrointestinal and neurological complaints. Consequently, it is recommended that the reader who is evaluating a somatizing child utilize the information presented in both the present chapter as well as the pediatric pain chapter. Generally, the biopsychosocial framework and assessment approach provided in the chapter on pediatric pain can also be applied to children who experience other forms of somatization.

The most productive information to obtain from the somatizing child is information about his or her somatic symptoms; life stressors, and health-related behaviors, beliefs, and emotions used by the child and parent to cope. Not only do these domains of inquiry best assist the clinician in identifying somatization, such information also allows the evaluator to implement or recommend specific interventions designed to alter the salient stressors, improve the child's coping, and/or better manage the child's symptoms.

SYMPTOMS

Physical Symptoms

The number, frequency, and severity of physical symptoms can be considered a measure of somatization and its severity. This can be evaluated through a clinical interview or with a questionnaire (such as the Childhood Somatization Inventory, Walker et al. 2009). Although the somatizing child may spontaneously complain of one somatic symptom (typically the most distressing symptom), it is not uncommon for additional physical symptoms to be identified during a thorough assessment. It is helpful to ask both the child and a parent about the child's physical symptoms. Parents may be unaware of symptoms unless the child has complained about them. Because children have poor perception of chronology and time, however, parents are typically better equipped than children to report frequency of known symptoms. Table 8–1 presents a list of symptoms for use during an interview.

Non-epileptic seizures (NES) is the term used to describe seizure-like phenomena that does not have an established medical cause and that appears to be psychologically mediated (Plioplys et al. 2007). Children who are significantly disabled and/or distressed by NES are defined by the DSM as having a Conversion Disorder or a Functional Neurological Disorder. A diagnosis of NES is confirmed in children presenting with seizures by a videotaped electroencephalogram (EEG). Videotape of the child's behavior and electrodes placed on the scalp will indicate if behaviors thought to be seizures caused by epilepsy are associated with epileptiform activity on the EEG. The typical psychological profile of these children is that they, like children with other somatization disorders, speak about their seizures as the main problem and typically initially deny any other problems when interviewed by clinicians.

The following dialogue is an example of an interview with a young girl about her physical symptoms. Notice that the interviewer uses the words that the girl uses to describe her symptoms. The interviewer also learns about the girl's abdominal pain by asking her specifically about it rather than refraining from further pain questions when the girl indicates that she generally does not have any pain.

Physical Symptoms
INTERVIEWER: *Hi, Margi. How are you feeling today?*
CHILD: *Good.*
INTERVIEWER: *What happened at school this morning?*
CHILD: *I had a fit.*
INTERVIEWER: *I see. What happens when you have a fit?*
CHILD: *My legs shake and I can't walk.*

Table 8–1. SOMATIC SYMPTOMS

Pain symptoms	*Neurological symptoms*
• abdomen • back • chest • head • joints • limbs • rectum *Gastrointestinal/Urinary symptoms* • bloating • cramping • diarrhea • encopresis (voluntary or involuntary passage of stools in a child over 4 years old who has been toilet trained, and which causes the soiling of clothes) • enuresis (involuntary urination in a child over 6 years old, and which causes the soiling of clothes) • food intolerance • nausea • urinary retention • vomiting • weight changes	• seizures • coordination problems • dizziness or fainting • fatigue or decreased energy • impaired balance • numbness or tingling • paralysis • difficulties with memory • sensory disturbances (for example, blurred or double vision) • speech problems or aphonia (inability to speak) • tremor *Other symptoms* • dry mouth • hot or cold spells • lump in throat • rapid heartbeat • sweating • trouble breathing (shortness of breath or hyperventilating) • trouble sleeping (falling asleep, staying asleep, nightmares)

INTERVIEWER: *Wow. Did that ever happen to you before?*

CHILD: *Yeah.*

INTERVIEWER: *Do you get scared when that happens?*

CHILD: *No. It doesn't hurt.*

INTERVIEWER: *I see. I am glad it doesn't hurt. What else happens when you have a fit?*

CHILD: *I don't know. Nothing.*

INTERVIEWER: *Do you stay at school when you have a fit or do you go home?*

CHILD: *I just wait and it goes away.*

INTERVIEWER: *I see. You said that it doesn't hurt?*

CHILD: *Hmm. No.*

INTERVIEWER: *Does any part of your body hurt at other times?*

CHILD: *No.*

INTERVIEWER: *What about your tummy? Do you ever get pain in your stomach?*

CHILD: *Yeah. But, my tummy only hurts in the morning.*

INTERVIEWER: *I see. What else happens in the morning when your tummy hurts?*

CHILD: *Sometimes I throw up.*

INTERVIEWER: *And, then what happens?*

CHILD: *That's all.*

INTERVIEWER: *Do you go to school?*

CHILD: *If I have a temperature, no. If I don't have a temperature, yes.*

INTERVIEWER: *I see. Do you ever have pain in your head?*

CHILD: *No.*

INTERVIEWER: *What about your arms or legs?*

CHILD: *No.*

INTERVIEWER: *Does any part of your body hurt at other times?*

CHILD: *No.*

INTERVIEWER: *You said earlier that your tummy sometimes hurts and then you throw up. Do you have any other trouble with your tummy?*

CHILD: *Only in the morning, like I said before.*

INTERVIEWER: *I see. Do you ever have any trouble with peeing or pooping?*

CHILD: *No.*

INTERVIEWER: *Do you ever have trouble sleeping?*

CHILD: *No.*

INTERVIEWER: *Eating?*

CHILD: *No.*

INTERVIEWER: *Walking or running?*

CHILD: *Only when I have a fit.*

INTERVIEWER: *Okay. What about problems talking or thinking?*

CHILD: *No!*

INTERVIEWER: *Okay. Do you ever have trouble seeing or hearing?*

CHILD: *Hmm. No.*

INTERVIEWER: *What about trouble breathing?*

CHILD: *If I get a cold.*

INTERVIEWER: *Okay. Does your body ever feel funny in any other way or give you any other kind of trouble?*

CHILD: *No.*

INTERVIEWER: *So, let me see if I got it right. You have fits that make your legs shake and you can't walk, but you wait until it goes away, and sometimes you have pain in your tummy in the morning and throw up. Is that right?*

CHILD: *Right.*

INTERVIEWER: *Thank you for telling me all that. You did a great job.*

Psychological Symptoms

The assessment of psychological symptoms in somatizing children is sometimes hindered by alexithymia (greater than developmentally expected difficulty identifying and/or expressing one's emotional state). Therefore, it is especially important in somatizing children to assess alexithymia before asking questions related to the child's emotional functioning as demonstrated in the example below. If alexithymia is endorsed, the child may have an easier time identifying the physical symptoms associated with their emotional state (such as rapid heartbeat and sweaty hands when anxious). Children with alexithymia may indicate that their emotions are hard to distinguish from each other (most commonly stating that anxiety, anger, and sadness are all perceived as general distress), or they might deny experiencing emotions. If alexithymia is not endorsed, the interviewing techniques described in the other chapters of this book may be used. The following example demonstrates how to ask young children if they have alexithymia.

Alexithymia—Example 1

INTERVIEWER: *For some kids, it is easy for them to figure if they are feeling mad, sad, scared, or happy. Other kids know they are having feelings, but have a hard time figuring out which one, like their feelings all get jumbled together. What type of kid are you? Is it easy or hard for you to figure out how you are feeling?*

CHILD: *Easy! That is silly.*

The next example demonstrates how a child with alexithymia might respond to the same question. Notice that this child looks for external cues to determine an internal feeling state.

Alexithymia—Example 2

INTERVIEWER: *For some kids, it is easy for them to figure if they are feeling mad, sad, scared, or happy. Other kids know they are having feelings, but have a hard time figuring out which one, like their feelings all get jumbled together. What type of kid are you? Is it easy or hard for you to figure out how you are feeling?*

CHILD: *I don't have any feelings.*

INTERVIEWER: *That is interesting. How do you know if you are sad?*

CHILD: *Maybe I cry?*

INTERVIEWER: *That sounds right. How do you know if you are mad?*

CHILD: *I think I yell or maybe I hit my sister.*

INTERVIEWER: *I see. How do you know if you are scared?*

CHILD: *Well, when I walk by the mean dog on my street, sometimes I feel my heart go boom-boom-boom.*

INTERVIEWER: *Okay. That does sound scary. How do you know if you are happy?*

CHILD: *Hmm. I act silly and run around more.*

INTERVIEWER: *That is a very good way to explain it. What did you feel like when everyone left your birthday party yesterday?*

CHILD: *Like I was shrinking!*

INTERVIEWER: *Oh my. That is interesting. What feeling do you think that was? Do you think you were sad or mad or some other feeling?*

CHILD: *I don't know. It was bad though.*

STRESSORS

Stressors come in many forms; they can be catastrophic for the child (such as a rape, a strong earthquake, the death of a grandparent or pet, or a move to a new city), chronic (such as marital discord between the parents, a learning difficulty that is interfering with school success, separation anxiety, or encountering a bully at school), developmental (such as starting preschool, experiencing a significant growth spurt, or learning to swim), or related to a medical disorder (such as acute gastroenteritis or a recent diagnosis of diabetes).

The young child is unlikely to understand the word "stressor" (an abstract concept) or to recognize any of the stressful events described above as related to his or her physical symptoms. Likewise, the parents of the somatizing child are often unaware of factors causing stress to the child, and they are also unlikely to link known stressors to physical symptoms. Because the symptom(s) can persist after the stressor has resolved, the child and family may have great difficulty with the very concept of somatization. Additionally, significant concerns about a possible undiagnosed medical disorder or the worsening of a chronic medical condition can make it difficult for them to accept the possibility of somatization. Furthermore, children and their parents might not discuss certain family stressors with the interviewer due to embarrassment and the genuine belief that such information is not relevant to the child's physical symptoms. Consequently, it can be a significant challenge for the clinician to obtain a good understanding of the various stressors that are potentially contributing to somatization in a child. Table 8–2 includes a partial list of potential stressors for use during an interview.

Table 8–2. POTENTIAL STRESSORS

Abuse or neglect by parent, sibling, peer, or stranger, including: • emotional • verbal • physical • sexual • exposure to domestic violence • medical
A problem with or changes in an important life domain, such as: • family constellation or functioning • health • independence or responsibilities • living arrangement • recreational activities • school • social life
Developmental milestones and achievements, such as: • starting school • potty training • learning to swim • growth spurt • accepting an award at school
Natural disaster, including: • tornado • hurricane • floods • fire • earthquake
Other major events, such as: • Car accident or other frightening accident or event • Family member with significant psychopathology or behavioral disturbance • Illness, injury, or death in a close friend, family member, or pet • Parent or other family member deployed in the military • Personal illness, injury, learning problem, communication or psychiatric disorder, surgery, or medical procedure

The following dialogue is an example of stressors acknowledged by an 8-year-old boy with chronic vomiting and no other medical disorder. With excellent grades at school, good friends, and a close and supportive family, the source of his primary worry was not readily apparent or fully appreciated by his parents until this interview.

Stressors

INTERVIEWER: *Jimmy, I am wondering if you can tell me a little about your life.*
CHILD: *Like what?*
INTERVIEWER: *Well, let's see, what is your favorite thing to do?*
CHILD: *Play with my dog.*
INTERVIEWER: *Oh, that sounds fun. What do you do with your dog?*
CHILD: *Well, I try to teach him tricks, and sometimes we go to the park and pretend that we live in a cave. His name is Leo.*
INTERVIEWER: *That sounds fun. Leo is a lucky dog. What else do you do for fun?*
CHILD: *Hmm. I don't know.*
INTERVIEWER: *Do you ever play with your sister or with other kids?*
CHILD: *Oh yeah. Not my sister, she's too little, but I play videogames with friends from school. They come over when I am not throwing up.*
INTERVIEWER: *I see. And, how is school for you?*
CHILD: *Fine. I am good at math.*
INTERVIEWER: *Wow. That is great. What is your hardest topic?*
CHILD: *I don't know; I like them all.*
INTERVIEWER: *I see. Do you have any problems at school?*
CHILD: *Hmm. No.*
INTERVIEWER: *How is it at home, with your parents and your little sister?*
CHILD: *Okay.*
INTERVIEWER: *Do you have any problems at home?*
CHILD: *Hmm. No.*
INTERVIEWER: *What about your parents and your sister, do they have any problems?*
CHILD: *Just me.*
INTERVIEWER: *You? What makes you a problem?*
CHILD: *Throwing up all the time.*
INTERVIEWER: *I see. What makes that a problem?*
CHILD: *My dad misses work to take me to doctors and my mom cries.*
INTERVIEWER: *What do you think about your dad missing work?*
CHILD: *I wish he would stay at work.*
INTERVIEWER: *What would be better if he stayed at work?*
CHILD: *Then, he could have weekends off, like he used to, but now he is either going to the doctor or working all the time, even at nights and on weekends. We can never go to the park anymore.*
INTERVIEWER: *I see. No time for fun. What about your mom? What do you think about your mom crying?*
CHILD: *She just cried one time. She was sad because I was throwing up.*
INTERVIEWER: *I see. Does she also go to the doctors with you?*
CHILD: *Yeah. Me, my mom, and my dad go to the doctors. My sister stays with grandma.*

INTERVIEWER: *I see. What would you say is the worst thing that ever happened to you?*

CHILD: *Throwing up all the time.*

INTERVIEWER: *It must be pretty bad. What makes throwing up all the time the worst thing that ever happened to you?*

CHILD: *My dad might die.*

INTERVIEWER: *Oh my. What would make your dad die?*

CHILD: *From working too much.*

INTERVIEWER: *I see. What makes you think he might die from working too much?*

CHILD: *My grandpa died from working too much.*

INTERVIEWER: *Oh, that is sad. Have you told your dad that you think he might die from working too much?*

CHILD: *Yes, all the time. He just says don't worry.*

INTERVIEWER: *Does that help make you feel better?*

CHILD: *No.*

INTERVIEWER: *Hmm. Do you want me to help you explain to your dad how much this bothers you?*

CHILD: *Yes!*

In the above example, Jimmy had previously informed his parents that he was worried that his father would die from working too much, but his parents did not realize *how much* this was bothering Jimmy. The family agreed that they could use a number scale, from 1 to 5, to help them understand how strongly they each felt. Jimmy explained to his parents that his frequent vomiting bothered him about a "3" (with "5" being the strongest worry and "1" being no worry). However, when they asked him to rate his worry about his dad dying, he gave a rating of "10."

With this increased insight, Jimmy's father immediately stopped joining them at doctor appointments and cut back on his overtime. Additionally, the family learned that when Jimmy is sharing his emotions, he does not change his facial expression or use other nonverbal communication (such as hand gestures) to indicate how strongly he is feeling. The number scale also greatly improved the family communication related to other emotionally charged topics, such as when Jimmy wanted his family to understand how he felt about going to sleep-over camp.

COPING: HEALTH-RELATED BEHAVIORS, BELIEFS, AND EMOTIONS

Infants cope with stressors by regulating their physiological arousal, behavior, and emotions with automatic, biologically based processes (including attempts to engage the caregiver by looking cute or by crying). Repeated patterns of interaction between parent and child have long-term effects on the child's central nervous system, including how the child physiologically responds to stress. Over time, the growing child develops an increasing capacity for conscious coping that has been shaped by brain development and by his or her early experiences (Compas and Boyer 2001).

Cognitive capacities that develop as the child matures and that impact coping efficacy include the emergence of intentionality (differentiating the intentions of others), representational thinking (imagining someone or something not present), language, meta-cognition (thoughts about thoughts), and the capacity for delay of gratification. Specific skills that contribute to helpful coping include the capacity for reframing a problem (thinking about it a different way), cognitively representing absent caregivers (imagining what they might say or do if they were present), using self-talk to calm negative emotions, and generating various solutions to problems (Compas and Boyer 2001). So, for example, it is very helpful for a hospitalized child to understand that his mother loves him even though she had to go to work, to successfully imagine how she might soothe him, and to use that information to develop a way to self-soothe. Conversely, a young child who is unable to use these more advanced cognitions may simply feel devastated and helpless because his mother left him alone in the hospital.

To assess for maladaptive coping, the child and the parents should be interviewed separately to learn about the health-related behaviors, beliefs, and emotions of the child and the parents. The goals are to determine if the child and/or parent demonstrate excessive maladaptive illness-related cognitions and behaviors, including high health anxiety, anxiety sensitivity (defined as a tendency to interpret bodily sensations or physical symptoms as dangerous), and devotion of excessive time and energy to health concerns.

Parental behaviors that may contribute to excessive somatization in the child include excessive sympathy and attention for symptoms, external help-seeking (seeking medical assistance rather than self-management of symptoms), strong parental distress responses to the child's physical symptoms, parent modeling of symptoms and/or illness behaviors (exhibiting symptoms or illness behaviors), and parental support and/or encouragement for the child's efforts at task avoidance. Table 8–3 includes a list of potential health-related behaviors, beliefs and emotions for use during an interview with the child and parent.

The following dialogue between a clinician and a child with NES illustrates the complete sense of helplessness that many somatizing children report. One is able to discern from this short exchange that the parent also feels a sense of fear, urgency, and helplessness when her child experiences symptoms.

Efficacy of Coping
INTERVIEWER: *So, what kinds of things do you do to try to help yourself when you have seizures?*
CHILD: *Go to the hospital.*
INTERVIEWER: *And, what happens at the hospital?*
CHILD: *We wait and wait and then they check me and tell us nothing is wrong. Then, my mom gets mad and we leave.*
INTERVIEWER: *And, what is making your mom mad?*
CHILD: *Because they don't fix me. It just keeps happening. So, she gets mad.*
INTERVIEWER: *I see. Okay, and, what else do you do?*
CHILD: *Stay home from school and lie down so I won't fall.*
INTERVIEWER: *Is there anything you do that helps the seizures?*
CHILD: *No. I can't do anything. They just happen.*
INTERVIEWER: *Oh, I see. Does anything make them worse?*

CHILD: *I don't know.*
INTERVIEWER: *What does your mom do when you have seizures?*
CHILD: *She calls 911 emergency and gives me medicine.*

SUMMARY

- Somatization is as the process whereby somatic (physical) symptoms are experienced in response to physical or psychosocial stress.
- Somatization is not intentional; it is an automatic or habitual physical and behavioral response to stress.
- Somatization can become a focus of clinical attention when associated with significant health-related distress or disability.

Table 8–3. HEALTH-RELATED BEHAVIORS, BELIEFS, AND EMOTIONS

TOPICS FOR CHILD

• Impact of symptoms on daily life
  ▪ Child
  ▪ Family
• Child's thoughts, emotions, and behaviors associated with the symptoms
  ▪ Beliefs about the seriousness of the symptoms
  ▪ General health anxiety (distress related to somatic symptoms)
  ▪ Beliefs about what will and will not help symptoms
  ▪ Coping responses; ability to tolerate the symptoms
• How others react to the symptoms
  ▪ Parents
  ▪ Teachers
  ▪ Others

TOPICS FOR PARENT

• Impact of symptoms on daily life
  ▪ Child, including school history and number of school days missed
  ▪ Family, including the number of work days missed by parent(s)
• Parent's thoughts, emotions, and behaviors associated with the child's symptoms
  ▪ Beliefs about the seriousness of the symptoms
  ▪ General health anxiety (distress related to somatic symptoms)
  ▪ Beliefs about what will and will not help symptoms
  ▪ Coping responses; ability to tolerate the symptoms
• How others react to symptoms
  ▪ Child
  ▪ Parents
  ▪ Teachers
  ▪ Others
• Parent concerns about the child's health, behavior, or emotional well-being.
• Medical history of the child and other family members: Illnesses, hospitalizations, surgeries, injuries, ER visits, including other family members who have chronic and recurrent symptoms and dysfunction in the primary areas of life (family, peers, work, and school).
• Parents' emotional functioning, marital stress, and coping skills

- Somatization is best explained by the biopsychosocial model. Maintaining an organic versus nonorganic etiology of symptoms dichotomy is misleading and can be harmful, potentially leading to excessive medical intervention and/or to a lack of empathy for the child with physical symptoms.
- Increased levels of psychopathology (especially anxiety and depression), family dysfunction, poor school performance and attendance, perceived health impairment, and more frequent use of health and mental health services are observed in families with disabled somatizing children.

REFERENCES

Andresen JM, Woolfolk RL, Allen LA, Fragoso MA, Youngerman NL, Patrick-Miller TJ, and Gara MA (2011). Physical symptoms and psychosocial correlates of somatization in pediatric primary care. *Clin Pediatr (Phila)* 50(10): 904–909.

Biederman J, Rosenbaum JF, Bolduc-Murphy EA, Faraone SV, Chaloff J, Hirshfeld DR, and Kagan J (1993). Behavioral inhibition as a temperamental risk factor for anxiety disorders. *Child Adolesc Psychiatr Clin N Am* 2: 667–683

Boyce W, Barr R, and Zeltzer L (1992). Temperament and the psychobiology of childhood stress. *Pediatrics* 90: 483–486

Campo JV, Jansen-McWilliams L, Comer DM, and Kelleher KJ (1999). Somatization in pediatric primary care: Association with psychopathology, functional impairment and use of services. *J Am Acad Child Adolesc Psychiatry* 38:1093–1101.

Compas BE and Boyer MC (2001). Coping and attention: Implications for children's health and pediatric conditions. *J Dev Behav Pediatr* 22: 1–11.

Kagan J, Reznick J, and Snidman N (1988). Biological bases of childhood shyness. *Science* 40: 167–171.

Lipowski ZJ (1988). Somatization: The concept and its clinical application. *Am J Psychiatry* 145(11): 1358–1368.

Manassis K, Bradley S, Goldberg S, Hood J, and Price-Swinson R (1995). Behavioural inhibition, attachment and anxiety in children of mothers with anxiety disorders. *Can J Psychiatry*, 40:87–92.

Plioplys S, Asato M, Bursch B, Salpekar J, Shaw R, and Caplan R (2007) Multidisciplinary management of pediatric nonepileptic seizures. *J Am Acad Child Adolesc Psychiatry* 46(11): 1491–1495.

Smith RC, Gardiner JC, Lyles JS, Sirbu C, Dwamena FC, Hodges A, Collins C, Lein C, Given CW, Given B, and Goddeeris J (2005). Exploration of DSM-IV criteria in primary care patients with medically unexplained symptoms. *Psychosom Med* 67(1): 123–129.

Stuart S and Noyes R (1999). Attachment and interpersonal communication in somatization. *Psychosomatics* 40: 34–43.

Tamminen TM, Bredenberg P, Escartin T, Kaukonen P, Puura K, Rutanen M, Suominen I, Leijala H, and Salmelin R (1991). Psychosomatic symptoms in preadolescent children. *Psychother Psychosom* 56(1–2):70–77.

Torgersen S (1986). Genetics of somatoform disorders. *Arch Gen Psychiatry* 43(5): 502–505.

Walker LS, Beck JE, Garber J, and Lambert W (2009). Children's Somatization Inventory: Psychometric properties of the revised form (CSI-24). *J Pediatr Psychol* 34: 430–440.

Symptoms Associated with Autism Spectrum

Children with autism spectrum disorders (ASDs) are significantly more likely than those without autism to have co-occurring medical and psychiatric conditions, high health-care utilization (including frequent physician visits for preventive care, nonemergency and hospital emergency care) and high medication usage (Gurney et al. 2006; Peacock et al. 2012). Additionally, children with ASDs have symptoms and deficits that impact how they experience illnesses, injuries, and interactions with health-care professionals. With prevalence estimated to be 1 in 88 births in the United States and almost 1 in 54 boys (ADDM 2008), clinicians can expect to assess children with ASDs (as well as children of adults with ASDs).

ASDs are neurodevelopmental disorders that occur in all ethnic and socioeconomic groups and affect every age group. Impairments are observed in reciprocal social communication and social interaction, and affected individuals demonstrate stereotyped behavior, interests, and activities. An ASD is best diagnosed with a comprehensive evaluation conducted by a multidisciplinary team of clinicians, including a pediatrician, pediatric neurologist or child psychiatrist, a psychologist, a speech and language pathologist, and an occupational therapist.

The goal of this chapter is to review the specific challenges one might face when interviewing a medically ill child with an ASD. The specific objectives are to give a brief overview of common symptoms and deficits one might encounter with medically ill children on the autism spectrum and to provide suggestions for interviewing such children. Consistent with the other chapters in this book, we will focus on children with ASD symptoms or features who fall within the average or higher level of intellectual functioning.

SYMPTOMS AND DEFICITS ASSOCIATED WITH AUTISM SPECTRUM

Core Features

ASDs impact each person in a different way, ranging in severity from very mild to severe. Individuals with milder ASDs might have social challenges, unusual

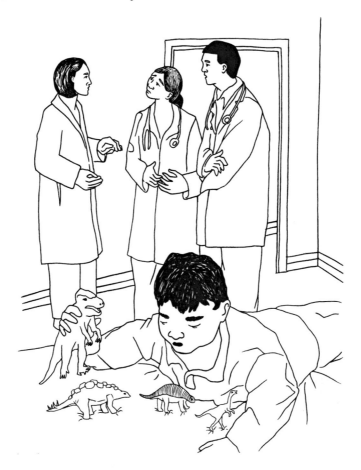

behaviors, and specific interests, but no problems with language or intellectual disability. Those with more severe ASDs might be nonverbal and have severe cognitive impairment. Clinical indicators of a possible ASD can be found in Table 9–1.

To meet diagnostic criteria for an ASD, the individual must have persistent deficits in social communication and social interaction across contexts, including deficits in social-emotional reciprocity; in nonverbal communicative behaviors used for social interaction; and in developing and maintaining relationships that are developmentally appropriate (other than relationships with caregivers). Additionally, the affected individual must exhibit two of the following four traits: stereotyped or repetitive speech, movements, or use of objects; excessive adherence to routines or rituals; excessive resistance to change; unusual sensory processing evidenced by hyper-or hypo-reactivity to sensory input or unusual interest in sensory aspects of environment.

Co-occurring Diagnoses

Children identified with an ASD have high frequencies of one or more co-occurring non-ASD developmental, psychiatric, neurological, and possibly causative medical diagnoses. ASDs occur more often than expected among those who have Fragile

Table 9–1. INDICATORS OF POSSIBLE AUTISM SPECTRUM DISORDER

Early indicators:
• no babbling or pointing by age 1
• no single words by 16 months or no two-word phrases by age 2
• no response to hearing name
• loss of language or social skills
• poor eye contact
• excessive lining up of toys or objects
• no smiling or social responsiveness
Later indicators:
• impaired ability to make friends with peers
• impaired ability to initiate or sustain a conversation with others
• absence or impairment of imaginative and social play
• stereotyped, repetitive, or unusual use of language
• restricted patterns of interest that are abnormal in intensity or focus
• preoccupation with certain objects or subjects
• inflexible adherence to specific routines or rituals

X syndrome, tuberous sclerosis, congenital rubella syndrome, and untreated phenylketonuria (APA 2000). These disorders are usually associated with intellectual disability. Thalidomide taken during pregnancy has also been linked with a higher risk of autism (APA 2000). In terms of other co-occurring diagnoses, recent population surveillance suggests that the most common co-occurring conditions among children with an ASD are attention deficit/hyperactivity disorder (ADHD) (21.3%), intellectual disability (18.3%), and epilepsy (15.5%) (Levy et al. 2010). Other common psychiatric co-occurring diagnoses include anxiety disorders, mood disorders, and tic disorders (Mukaddes et al. 2010).

Associated Features/Traits That Impact the Medically Ill Child

Medically ill children with ASDs can face numerous challenges, some that clinicians may never consider. Descriptions of associated features and traits that are particularly important for the clinician to consider when assessing a medically ill child with an ASD are presented next. Some of these associated features or traits are considered core features (as described above) and others are commonly seen, but not considered core features.

SENSORY ABNORMALITIES
Due to sensory and communication abnormalities, some individuals with an ASD have great difficulty knowing when they are ill and even greater difficulty describing their symptoms. Many have confused internal senses and may use atypical words to describe symptoms, such as saying they feel "weak" when others might say they feel "pain." Likewise, it can be difficult for such individuals to locate pain or other symptoms. Not having a good sense of what is considered normal, it can be confusing to someone with an ASD to simply be asked, "Do you feel sick?"

As indicated above, individuals with ASDs may experience hyper- or hyporeactivity to sensory input, such as indifference to pain, heat or cold that most others would find distressing, or distress to specific sounds, smells or textures that most others would find benign. Children with sensory hypersensitivities might not like getting their hands dirty with sand or finger paint, might be highly distressed when groomed or unexpectedly touched, or might not be able to tolerate tags in clothing. Nader and colleagues (2004) found that autistic children undergoing venipuncture showed a larger behavioral pain response and appeared to be more pain sensitive then a group of age-matched children without autism. For sensory sensitive children, medical settings can be a source of significant sensory overload. This can cause them great emotional and/or physical distress. By contrast, children with hyposensitivities may be at an increased risk for illness or injury due to reduced pain reactivity and inattention to stimuli indicating potential danger.

THEORY OF MIND DEFICITS

Some individuals with an ASD suffer from "Theory of Mind" deficits, such as difficulty determining the intentions of others, impaired understanding of how their behavior affects others, and difficulty with social reciprocity. They may expect others to perceive, think, feel, sense, and behave exactly like they do. It may, therefore, be difficult for them to understand how others could disagree with them, leading to an incorrect conclusion that the other person is being malevolent or irrational. With limited ability to use past and current experiences to determine the motivations and intentions of others, it is easy for such individuals to develop a protective, suspicious stance toward others. Consequently, interpersonal conflicts and misunderstandings are not uncommon. Children with ASD may conclude that clinicians who cause them pain (such as nurses and physical therapists) are intentionally harming them.

Deficits in pragmatic language (the practical ability to use language in a social setting; knowing what is appropriate to say, and where and when to say it) and concrete thinking are related to deficits in "Theory of Mind." For example, a young child who just moved to town sees his new pediatrician for the first time. When the doctor asks him where he comes from, the child responds: "From home." This child's concrete answer is precise, but he misses the meaning of the question and does not realize this is an effort by the doctor to initiate a longer conversation. Consequently, seemingly benign comments made by a clinician, such as, "We need to see what's going on inside your brain," can be quite terrifying to a child with an ASD who might concretely think that the doctor plans to open up his brain to look inside. Finally, attempts at jokes, especially sarcasm, are likely to be missed. A clinician who, in an attempt to establish rapport, sarcastically says to a child just admitted to the hospital on her birthday, "This must be just how you wanted to spend your birthday" may be met with confusion. Not understanding the humor, the child with an ASD might respond with a serious explanation of what she had hoped to do on her birthday.

RIGIDITY

Many individuals with an ASD demonstrate resistance to change and excessive adherence to routines and/or rules. For example, they may eat the very same food every day or have rituals they must follow to remain calm. New diagnoses, changes in treatment plans, unexpected complications, or unpredictable health-care contacts can be highly distressing. This rigidity might be problematic for medical adherence, or quite helpful depending on the decision of the affected individual to accept or reject a medical recommendation. Finally, some rigid behaviors can cause medical problems or injuries to the child. For example, a child who will only eat meat might develop nutritional or gastrointestinal problems.

DIFFICULTY WITH FACIAL RECOGNITION
Some children with an ASD have severely impaired facial identity recognition skills (Wilson et al. 2011). This can place the child at risk for harm if he cannot tell who is a friend and who is not a friend. In a medical setting, these children might find it extremely difficult to be separated from a parent, identify their clinicians, and/or cope with multiple clinicians who come into the exam or hospital room in groups.

DIFFICULTY WITH EMOTIONAL FUNCTIONING AND COPING
Children with ASDs are at increased risk for ADHD, anxiety disorders, mood disorders, tic disorders, and other behavioral/emotional disturbance (Levy et al. 2010; Mukaddes et al. 2010). Problems in the regulation of attentional focus, inflexible cognitive coping strategies, language and communication deficits, and chronic high arousal can make it exceptionally difficult for individuals with an ASD to cope and function with stressors. It is not uncommon for individuals with ASDs to have periods of aggressiveness, self-injurious behaviors, and/or temper tantrums. It may be difficult to understand the emotional reactions of individuals with ASDs, as they might be fearful of harmless objects, lack fear in dangerous situations, appear not to be emotionally distressed in response to upsetting information, or laugh for no apparent reason. These difficulties with emotional functioning and coping add another layer of challenges for the medically ill child with an ASD.

MOTOR DYSFUNCTION
Motor dysfunction, including deficits in gait, coordination, and the performance of skilled movements (praxis) has been documented in children with ASDs (Fournier et al. 2010; Van Waelvelde et al. 2010). Such motor dysfunction can impact other areas of development, including speech clarity, social interactions, and self-confidence. Children with motor difficulties are also at higher risk for injury and, thus, are more likely to have encounters with medical professionals.

EXAMPLES OF CLINICAL PRESENTATIONS

The specific traits of individuals with ASDs can increase the likelihood of presentation to a medical facility. For example, general pediatricians or pediatric gastroenterologists might see a child with an ASD for complaints of weight loss, obesity, nausea, vomiting, constipation, or diarrhea due to unusual eating habits, abnormal sensory signaling or underlying gastrointestinal problems. Children with ASDs might be seen in the emergency department for injuries caused by self-injurious behavior, sensory signaling problems (such as not feeling pain when they pick up a hot iron), physical altercations due to social misunderstandings, or accidents caused by lack of fear, inattentiveness, or clumsiness. Due to the abnormalities in sensory processing, clinicians might encounter children on the spectrum with chronic pain disorders or other somatic symptoms. Mental health clinicians or developmental specialists might be consulted for psychiatric symptoms or for general difficulty with coping.

PARENTS WITH ASDS

Parents with ASDs are also vulnerable in the same ways as children with ASDs. For example, due to "Theory of Mind" deficits, some adults with ASDs have limited empathic responses to distress cues. This can be problematic when parenting an ill or otherwise distressed child. Parents with ASDs might be suspicious of the intentions of health-care providers and may reject medical recommendations for reasons that are confusing to health-care providers. They might also appear extremely rigid and have difficulty distinguishing important from unimportant details. For example, a parent with an ASD might have great difficulty understanding that some abnormal laboratory tests are highly concerning while other abnormal laboratory tests are essentially ignored or discounted by clinicians. Likewise, a parent with an ASD might not be able to tolerate medical recommendations to do nothing for a benign abnormality (such as a functional heart murmur or benign mole) and might, consequently, insist on treatment for the condition or removal of the abnormality.

CLINICAL ASSESSMENT

ASDs typically become evident during the first three years of life, but might not be diagnosed in those mildly affected until much later. Consequently, the family will not always be aware that the child has an ASD. Likewise, a child with an ASD who is high functioning may or may not appear unusual to medical providers when they first encounter the child. However, clinicians might become aware of the child's communication limitations, seemingly unusual emotional reactions, unusual interests or routines, concrete thinking, sensitivity to sounds or smells in the exam or hospital room, and/or difficulty adapting to new information or treatment plans.

Assessment of a child with traits or symptoms of an ASD requires that the interviewer learn the best way to develop rapport and communicate with the particular child. Generally speaking, most children with an ASD will respond well to the interviewer's efforts to be consistent, maintain a predictable schedule, share their interests and communication style, reinforce their efforts with praise or other rewards, respect their sensory sensitivities, understand their challenges, and utilize the developmental guidelines described in this book.

DEVELOPING RAPPORT

The importance of rapport development cannot be overstated when assessing a child with an ASD. Although there may be common traits among children with ASDs, the clinical approach should be based on understanding how each specific child engages their world. This requires the clinician to gather information. The parent may be able to provide guidance about the child's preferred topics of conversation and manner of communication. In addition to obtaining information from the parent, it is helpful to spend at least 10 minutes simply observing the child, without overwhelming the child with premature conversation. During this observational period, the clinician should notice what the child does to communicate with others, what he or she talks about, plays with, is startled by, pays attention to, and thinks is funny. Even a rigid, controlling, defiant child can become more flexible and adherent to medical recommendations once he trusts and invites the clinician into his world. When changes are gradual enough, significant progress can be achieved. When interventions are adapted to the interests and worldview of the child, it is less frightening and he might even become more trusting of new relationships.

As illustrated in the following example, information about the child's interests can be used to reinforce skills and motivate him to participate in treatment.

Developing Rapport—Example 1

Gavin is a 6-year-old boy with ASD traits who was recently diagnosed with leukemia. Adjustment to the new diagnosis has been a challenge for Gavin and his family due to Gavin's extreme fear of needles. Clinicians in the pediatrician's office found that their usual teaching methods were not effective, so they referred Gavin to a mental health clinician.

The mental health clinician found that she was able to develop rapport with Gavin by listening to him talk about his primary interest, koala bears. The therapist then adapted a cognitive-behavioral therapy intervention (skills training that helps children recognize anxious feelings and more effectively cope with anxiety-provoking situations) to include koala bears in the examples. Photographs of koala bears were used during the sessions to demonstrate what it looks like to be "relaxed" and to reward Gavin for paying attention in the therapy sessions. His parents agreed to arrange for a trip to the zoo to see live koala bears upon graduating from the psychotherapy, which he called "needle school."

When he gained mastery over his needle anxiety, the therapist gave him a certificate of completion with a koala bear on it and a stuffed koala bear from his oncologist. Gavin then brought his stuffed koala bear to appointments to help him remember his new techniques.

In the next example, the interviewer uses information about the child's communication style to engage the child.

Developing Rapport—Example 2

James is a 9-year-old boy with an ASD who was referred to a weight management clinic. Although he learned to read at a very young age, James is mostly nonverbal. With few other interests, he loves to read computer manuals and to work on his computer. Initial efforts by the clinicians to engage James in a discussion regarding the need for him to track what he eats and increase his physical activity were completely ineffective, with James simply ignoring them. James's mother also tried to get him to engage, but she was unsuccessful. She told the clinicians that she and her husband are at their wits' ends due to their inability to increase his willingness to verbalize.

Finally, the dietician brought her laptop into the exam room, typed "What did you eat for breakfast?" and handed the computer to James. James then typed, "Pancakes" and handed it back. Once they discovered his willingness to communicate via computer, they were able to set him up with a computerized food diary to track what he ate and also with a schedule for increased physical activity, which was rewarded with increased computer time. They were able to use this modality to teach him about food groups and calories as well. He became fascinated with this topic and ended up doing very well with his weight and nutrition goals, even preparing grocery lists for his mother without prompting.

In the following example, the medical team came to suspect an ASD diagnosis was warranted after a concerted effort to better understand the child's nonadherence to medical recommendations and his seemingly defiant and immature behavior with medical staff.

Developing Rapport—Example 3

Jermaine is a 10-year-old boy with a history of diabetes mellitus and a diagnosis of anxiety. There has been a history of concern that Jermaine's mother has difficulty managing his diet and insulin. He has recently been exhibiting aggressive behaviors during outpatient medical appointments and often refused to follow medical recommendations. He was admitted to the hospital for acute management of his diabetes after he was seen in clinic with an HbA1C of 9.7 (which indicates chronically very high blood glucose). A multidisciplinary team worked closely with Jermaine while he was an inpatient to better understand his challenges.

According to school records, the team learned that Jermaine has average cognitive functioning. However, it became apparent that he often became nonverbal or would have a crying tantrum in certain situations, such as when clinicians attempted to increase his independent functioning or during morning medical rounds. Jermaine would spontaneously speak when engaged in something of interest to him (e.g., video games), but his eye contact was poor. He was often seen as noncompliant when asked to take medication, drink water, order food, and undertake other tasks that the team felt a 10-year-old would normally be able to complete.

Over time, clinicians began to suspect that Jermaine had an ASD. When this was understood, further discussion with him revealed that Jermaine felt overwhelmed during morning medical rounds because so many people were in the room. He was very excited when it was suggested he make a sign that asks the medical teams to limit their visits to three people at a time and to speak one at a time. Additionally, it was discovered that Jermaine was scared to order his meals because he did not feel confident he could answer questions, such as how he wanted his eggs cooked.

However, once he was able to practice ahead of time, he took great pride in being able to order his own meals. Jermaine responded well to consistency, routines, and calm limit-setting, with a time limit for him to make his decision or complete his task. Jermaine was taught relaxation skills, which he liked very much. Jermaine and the medical team learned that when he starts to become upset or agitated, he can be reminded by his mother or another trusted adult to count to 10 or to take deep breaths and to be given some time alone to calm himself. Based on this hospital admission, Jermaine was referred for formal evaluation of possible ASD and to appropriate additional services.

SYMPTOM ASSESSMENT

Due to impairments in social reasoning and deficits in vocabulary and idioms, many individuals with ASDs interpret language very concretely. Consequently, they may have difficulty understanding certain words used in a new context and may not do well when asked open-ended questions. Careful use of the developmental guidelines will assist communication. Additionally, many children with ASDs have greater than expected difficulty identifying or describing their emotional experiences (alexythmia). Therefore, it is important to assess alexithymia in a child with an ASD before asking questions related to emotional functioning. With this information, the interviewer may be able to discern what words the child uses to describe emotional experiences and use those words to shape future discussions. If alexithymia is not endorsed, the interviewing techniques described in the other chapters of this book may be more directly used to assess symptoms related to emotional functioning.

The example below demonstrates how a child with an ASD and significant alexithymia might respond to being asking about alexithymia. It is clear from this exchange that this child has great difficulty identifying and communicating about emotions.

Alexithymia

INTERVIEWER: *For some kids, it is easy for them to figure out if they are feeling mad, sad, scared, or happy. Other kids know they are having feelings, but have a hard time figuring out which feeling, like their feelings all get jumbled together. What type of kid are you? Is it easy or hard for you to figure out how you are feeling?*

CHILD: *I don't have feelings.*

INTERVIEWER: *Hmm. How do you know if you are sad?*

CHILD: *My mom or my dad tells me.*

INTERVIEWER: *I see. I know your cat died two weeks ago. Do you remember what happened when you found out your cat died?*

CHILD: *We buried him in the backyard.*

INTERVIEWER: *How was that for you?*

CHILD: *Easy, we have soft dirt in the backyard. I helped.*

INTERVIEWER: *What about your feelings? How did you feel when he died?*

CHILD: *I was used to him sleeping on my bed and now he isn't there. My mom says maybe we will get another cat. I want a black cat.*

INTERVIEWER: *I see. What else has been different since your cat died?*

CHILD: *My mom has to sleep in my room.*

INTERVIEWER: *Oh? What makes her have to sleep in your room?*

CHILD: *I already told you! Because my cat isn't there!*

INTERVIEWER: *What happens if you sleep by yourself?*

CHILD: *I don't sleep by myself!*

In the dialogue above, the child did not readily understand that the clinician wanted to know if it was *emotionally* hard for him when his cat died or how to answer that question once he understood it. It is likely that this child would have great difficulty directly answering any questions about his emotional experiences.

Nevertheless, using concrete action-based questions, the interviewer identified how difficult it has been for the child since the death of his cat.

The next example demonstrates how an interviewer might adapt to the language used by a child with an ASD to describe her symptoms. With careful questioning, the interviewer learns a great deal about a symptom even though the child uses an unusual word to describe it.

Language and Symptom Assessment
INTERVIEWER: *Hi, Sumiko. How are you doing today?*
CHILD: *Fine.*
INTERVIEWER: *It has been two weeks since we started you on your new medication. Have you noticed a change since you started it?*
CHILD: *It makes me fragile.*
INTERVIEWER: *Fragile?*
CHILD: *Yes.*
INTERVIEWER: *What does fragile feel like to you?*
CHILD: *Like something is wrong.*
INTERVIEWER: *I see. Can you tell me more?*
CHILD: *No. I just feel fragile.*
INTERVIEWER: *That's okay. You are doing a good job trying to help me understand. What makes you think it is the new medication that is making you feel fragile?*
CHILD: *I feel fragile after I take it.*
INTERVIEWER: *Okay, that makes sense. Does anything else happen when you feel fragile?*
CHILD: *Sometimes I throw up.*
INTERVIEWER: *Do you feel better after you throw up?*
CHILD: *Yes.*
INTERVIEWER: *That is very helpful. Does anything else help you feel better and not fragile?*
CHILD: *If I eat something when I take my medicine.*
INTERVIEWER: *If you eat something with your medicine, then you do not feel fragile afterwards?*
CHILD: *Right.*
INTERVIEWER: *And, does anything make it worse?*
CHILD: *If I don't eat.*
INTERVIEWER: *It is really good you figured that out. Does feeling fragile make you not want to take the medication or do you think you will be able to keep taking it?*
CHILD: *If I eat something, I can take it.*

SUMMARY
- Children with ASDs are more likely than those without autism to have co-occurring medical and psychiatric conditions, high health-care utilization, and high medication usage.
- Children with ASDs have symptoms and deficits that can impact how they experience illnesses, injuries, and interactions with health-care professionals.
- Due to the specific traits of those with ASDs, it is important to spend time developing rapport based on the child's interests and preferred modes of communication.

- The developmental guidelines presented in this book are applicable to the medically ill child with an ASD. However, the interviewer may find that they need to be even more concrete, specific, and creative when evaluating a young child with an ASD.

REFERENCES

American Psychiatric Association. (2000). *Diagnostic and statistical manual of mental disorders* (4th ed., text revision). Washington, DC: American Psychiatric Association.

Autism and Developmental Disabilities Monitoring (ADDM) Network Surveillance Year 2008 Principal Investigators, and Centers for Disease Control and Prevention (CDC) (2012). Autism and Developmental Disabilities Monitoring Network, United States, 2008. *MMWR Surveill Summ* 60 (SS03): 1–19.

Fournier KA, Hass CJ, Naik SK, Lodha N, and Cauraugh JH (2010). Motor coordination in autism spectrum disorders: A synthesis and meta-analysis. *J Autism Dev Disord* 40: 1227–1240.

Gurney JG, McPheeters ML, and Davis MM (2006). Parental report of health conditions and health care use among children with and without autism. *Arch Pediatr Adolesc Med* 160: 825–830.

Levy SE, Giarelli E, Lee LC, Schieve LA, Kirby RS, Cunniff C, Nicholas J, Reaven J, and Rice CE (2010). Autism spectrum disorder and co-occurring developmental, psychiatric, and medical conditions among children in multiple populations of the United States. *J Dev Behav Pediatr* 31: 267–275.

Mukaddes NM, Hergüner S, and Tanidir C (2010). Psychiatric disorders in individuals with high-functioning autism and Asperger's disorder: Similarities and differences. *World J Biol Psychiatry* 11(8): 964–971.

Nader R, Oberlander T, Chambers C, and Craig K (2004). The expression of pain in children with autism. *Clin J Pain* 20(2): 88–97.

Peacock G, Amendah D, Ouyang L, and Grosse SD (2012). Autism Spectrum Disorders and Health Care Expenditures: The Effects of Co-occurring Conditions. *J Dev Behav Pediatr* 33(1): 2–8.

Van Waelvelde H, Oostra A, Dewitte G, Van Den Broeck C, and Jongmans MJ (2010). Stability of motor problems in young children with or at risk of autism spectrum disorders, ADHD, and or developmental coordination disorder. *Dev Med Child Neurol* 52:e174–e178.

Wilson CE, Palermo R, Burton AM, and Brock J (2011). Recognition of own- and other-race faces in autism spectrum disorders. *J Exp Psychol* (Hove) 64(10): 1939–1954.

Application of the Developmental Guidelines

A Comprehensive Assessment of Pediatric Epilepsy

Overview to Part III

WHAT THE READER NOW KNOWS

The reader is now equipped with the developmental guidelines and clinical examples that demonstrate techniques on how to interview young children about their emotions and behavior and understand what they are communicating. The clinical examples have also highlighted how the interviewer patiently and methodically works at making sense of what the child is saying in order to obtain the needed information. These skills are the building blocks that enable the interviewer to comprehensively evaluate symptoms and the impact of illness on children's emotions, behavior, and functioning.

WHERE TO NOW?

In the next two chapters, the reader will learn how to use these building blocks to conduct a developmentally sensitive comprehensive interview of young children with epilepsy. Pediatric epilepsy is a good model for demonstrating how to apply the developmental guidelines to comprehensively assess the emotions and behavior of a young ill child for the following reasons.

First, like many other pediatric chronic illnesses, epilepsy is a complex biopsychosocial disorder. While historically equated with seizures, research over the past two decades has demonstrated involvement of brain development (both structural and functional) with related problem behavior, emotions, cognition, language, and social skills in children with epilepsy with average intelligence who have no neurological handicaps other than seizures. The biology of epilepsy underlies both the neurological (e.g., seizures) and neurobehavioral symptoms (also known as the comorbidities) of the disorder. The seizures and the comorbidities, in turn, engender psychosocial responses by the child and the parents (see reviews in Caplan 2010 and in Austin and Caplan 2007).

Likewise, as an example, in addition to pulmonary-related asthma symptoms, children with asthma are at risk for a broad range of symptoms, such as rhinosinusitis (inflammation of the tissues of the nose and the sinuses), gastroesophageal reflux disease (a condition in which food or liquid leak backwards from the

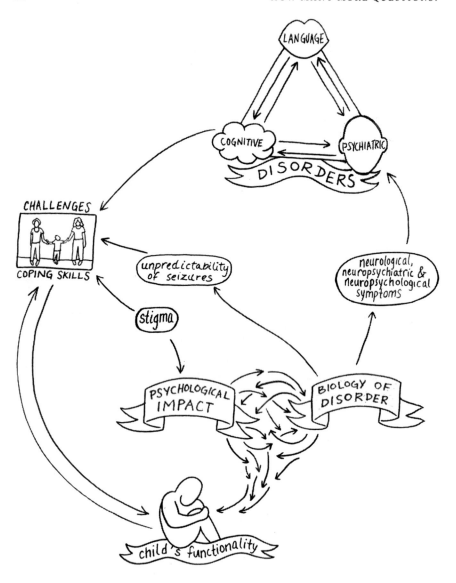

stomach into the esophagus), vocal cord dysfunction (an abnormal adduction of the vocal cords during the breathing cycle), obesity, bone loss, anxiety, and sleep apnea. As in pediatric epilepsy, the stressful and impairing nature of these co-occurring disorders serves to further challenge the coping ability of the child and family. Therefore, a comprehensive evaluation of a child presenting with asthma symptoms also requires a careful review of potentially co-occurring medical and psychiatric symptoms.

Second, similar to other pediatric chronic illnesses, epilepsy is both an acute and a chronic disorder. Seizures are acute events that are recurrent and sometimes intractable (resistant to treatment). Epilepsy is also a chronic disorder, requiring daily medication, emotional coping, and behavioral adaptation. As an acute, chronic, and sometimes intractable disorder, the illness taxes the coping skills of children and their parents, in a manner similar to medical disorders. Other examples of pediatric chronic illnesses that are both acute and chronic in nature include diabetes, asthma, cancer, sickle cell anemia, Crohn's disease, lupus, cystic fibrosis, and chronic heart conditions.

Third, as found in a number of other pediatric illnesses, the stigma and perception of epilepsy among different cultural groups make additional coping demands on children and their families. Examples of other pediatric illnesses that often carry significant social stigma include HIV, sickle cell anemia, cancer, tuberculosis, chronic pain, and mental illness.

Therefore, knowledge on how to conduct a comprehensive interview of children with epilepsy that teases out the biological and psychosocial components and their effects on the child's functioning serves as an excellent model for other neurological disorders and for medical disorders that do not involve the brain. Applying the developmental guidelines, each of the chapters on epilepsy focuses on interview techniques that aid in identifying the multiple factors that might influence the clinical presentation of children with this disorder.

These include obtaining information from children on the specific neurological features of the underlying disorder; associated problems with behavior, emotions, cognition, language, and social skills; side effects of medications; illness-related fears; the psychosocial impact on the child, parents, siblings, and family functioning; and the stigma of epilepsy. Individuals who master the skills required for such complex clinical interviewing can easily apply their knowledge and skills to other patient populations.

DEFINITION AND CLASSIFICATION OF SEIZURES

The Commission on Classification of the International League Against Epilepsy uses the definition of seizures proposed by Fisher et al. (2005) as "a transient occurrence of signs and/or symptoms due to abnormal excessive or synchronous neuronal activity in the brain" and has proposed a new classification of the epilepsies (Berg et al. 2010). To familiarize the reader with terms used in the next two chapters, Table 10–1 summarizes the clinical manifestations, EEG findings, and treatment of some of the more common epilepsy syndromes and the types of seizures found in children with average intelligence.

Interested readers can find detailed reviews of the neurology (Pellock et al. 2007), neuropsychology (MacAllister and Schaffer 2007), neuropsychiatry (Hamiwka et al. 2011), and family functioning (Rodenburg et al. 2011) of pediatric epilepsy. Understanding how to use knowledge about the biological aspects of the disorder—the neurology, neuropsychiatry, and neuropsychology—and the psychosocial impact of pediatric epilepsy is key to the comprehensive evaluation of young children with epilepsy. Application of this knowledge and use of the developmental guidelines and techniques, as shown in the next two chapters on epilepsy, serve as a model to assess the impact of illness on young children.

Table 10–1. Features of Epilepsy Syndromes and Types of Seizures Found in Children with Average Intelligence

Classification[1]	Names	Symptoms	EEG	Most Commonly Used Generic (Brand) AEDs[2,3]
GENERALIZED				
Tonic-clonic (GTCS)	Grand mal, primary generalized epilepsy	Eye rolling, loss of consciousness, body becomes rigid followed by rhythmic contractions and relaxation of the trunk and extremities and subsequent sleep, tiredness, confusion	Normal or spikes; sharp waves; spike, sharp and slow wave complexes (SWC) over all EEG leads	Levetiracetam (keppra, LEV), topiramate (topamax, TPM) lamotrigine (lamictal, LTG), valproate (depakote, VPA), carbamazepine (tergretol, CBZ), oxcarbamazepine (trileptal, OXC), phenobarbital (PB), phenylhydantoin (dilantin PHT)
ABSENCE				
Typical	Petit mal, child-hood absence epilepsy	Brief, sudden change in state of consciousness, eyelid fluttering, lip twitching, unchanged tone, no sleep, tiredness, confusion	Normal background, hyper-ventilation induces SWC at 3 per second (Hz)	VPA, ethosuximide (zarontin), LTG
Myoclonic	Childhood/Juvenile mycolonic epilepsy	Jerks of arms, shoulders, legs in early morning, sometimes followed by GTCS with sleep, tiredness, confusion	Interictal 3.5–6 Hz SWC; ictal rapid spike followed by irregular slow waves, often in response to flashing lights	VPA, LTG, LEV, TPM
FOCAL				
No impairment of consciousness/ awareness				
Motor	Simple partial seizure	Localized motor activity (jerk) involving a group of muscles, no sleep, tired-ness, confusion	Spikes, sharp waves in motor area of the frontal lobe (Broca's area)	CBZ, OXC, LTG, LEV, VPA

Autonomic	Panayiotopoulos syndrome	Pallor, cyanosis, nausea, retching, vomiting, widening/narrowing of pupils, tachycardia, loss of bladder control no sleep, tiredness, confusion	Shifting and/or multiple spikes with occipital predominance	CBZ, VPA only if seizures are frequent. If prolonged, benzodiazepine (e.g., valium)
Subjective sensory or psychic phenomena	Aura	Distinct motor, sensory (hallucination, illusion), or psychological perception (fear with epigastric discomfort, déja phenomena, forced thinking) around the time of a CPS or GTCS before loss of consciousness	Spikes, sharp waves, or SWC in right or left temporal lobe leads	See AEDs for GTCS or CPS
Impairment of consciousness/ awareness	Complex partial seizures (CPS)	Blank stare, chewing clumsy meaningless random movements followed by sleep, tiredness, confusion	Spikes, sharp waves in temporal or other brain regions	CBZ, OXC, LTG, LEV, zonisamide (zonegran), TPM, clobazapam, lacosamide
Evolving to bilateral convulsive seizures	Secondary generalized seizures			As for CPS and GTCS
Unknown cause	Benign Rolandic epilepsy, benign epilepsy with centrotemporal spikes	Typically during sleep, twitching of face or cheek, tingling numbness, or unusual sensations in tongue, drooling, difficulty speaking, consciousness preserved, not followed by tiredness or confusions	Centrotemporal (Rolandic area) interictal spikes (occur between seizures)	If frequent, daytime, or secondarily generalized, sulthiame, gabapentin[4]

[1] Based in part on ILAE revised terminology and concepts (Berg et al. 2010). [2] AEDS = Antiepileptic drugs most commonly used. [3] Based on review in Hussain and Sankar 2011. [4] See Shields and Snead 2009.

REFERENCES

Austin K and Caplan R (2007). Behavioral and psychiatric comorbidities in pediatric epilepsy: Toward an integrative model. *Epilepsia* 48: 1639–1651.

Berg AT, Berkovic SF, Brodie MJ, Buchhalter J, Cross JH, Van Emde Boas W, Engel J, French J, Glauser TA, Mathern GW, Moshé SL, Nordli D, Plouin P, and Scheffer IE (2010). Revised terminology and concepts for organization of seizures and epilepsies: Report of the ILAE Commission on Classification and Terminology, 2005–2009. *Epilepsia* 51: 676–685.

Caplan R (2010). Pediatric epilepsy: A developmental neuropsychiatric disorder. In: *Epilepsy: Mechanisms, Models, and Translational Perspectives*, J Rho, R Sankar, and J Cavazos J. Boca Raton, FL: RC Press—Taylor & Francis Group, 535–549.

Fisher RS, Boas WvE, Blume W, Elger C, Genton P, Lee P, and Engel J (2005). Epileptic seizures and epilepsy: Definitions proposed by the International League Against Epilepsy (ILAE) and the International Bureau for Epilepsy (IBE). *Epilepsia* 46: 470–472.

Hamiwka L, Jones JE, Salpekar J, and Caplan R (2011). Child psychiatry: Special edition on the future of clinical epilepsy research. *Epilepsy Behav* 22: 38–46.

Hussain S and Sankar R (2011). Pharmacologic treatment of intractable epilepsy in children: A syndrome-based approach. *Semin Pediat Neurol* 18: 171–178.

MacAllister W and Schaffer SG (2007). Neuropsychological deficits in childhood epilepsy syndromes. *Neuropsychol Rev* 17: 427–444.

Pellock J, Bourgeois B, Dodson E, Nordli D, and Sankar R (2007). *Pediatric Epilepsy: Diagnosis and Therapy*. New York: Demos Medical Pub.

Rodenburg R, Wagner JL, Austin JK, Kerr M, and Dunn DW (2011). Psychosocial issues for children with epilepsy. *Epilepsy Behav* 22: 47–54.

Shields WD and Snead C (2009). Benign epilepsy with centrotemporal spikes. *Epilepsia* 50: 10–15.

Biological Aspects
of Pediatric Epilepsy

In this chapter, we apply the developmental guidelines described in chapter 1 to the assessment of young children with epilepsy. The evaluation of children with epilepsy, similar to other central nervous disorders, such as traumatic brain injury and brain tumor, is complex and challenging because it involves teasing out if the child's symptoms reflect biological and/or psychosocial aspects of the disorder.

To help the reader meet this challenge, we summarize main aspects of the biological impact of the disorder, describe their relevance to the interview of the young child, and present clinical examples that demonstrate how to interview children about these aspects of the disorder using the developmental guidelines. A brief review of the relevant research is included for readers interested in the knowledge base for this clinical information. The two main biological aspects discussed in this chapter are the direct effects of epilepsy on brain functions, including behavior/emotions, cognition, language, and social skills (also known as the comorbidities of epilepsy) and the adverse cognitive and behavioral/emotional effects of antiepileptic drugs. We also briefly discuss seizure manifestations that might be misdiagnosed as psychiatric symptoms and psychiatric symptoms that may be incorrectly labeled as seizures.

THE COMORBIDITIES

Overview

Given this book's focus on the clinical interview, the description of the comorbidities focuses on children with epilepsy whose average cognitive and language skills (or mild deficits) enable them to be interviewed. We will reintroduce the reader to the concept presented in the previous chapter that, like seizures, the psychiatric, behavioral, cognitive, linguistic, and social functioning difficulties found in pediatric epilepsy are integral components of epilepsy. Based on this premise, the National Institute of Neurological Disorders and Stroke designated the study of these comorbidities as an institute benchmark to ensure that research on the comorbidities will improve the understanding and treatment of all aspects of the disease. Given the

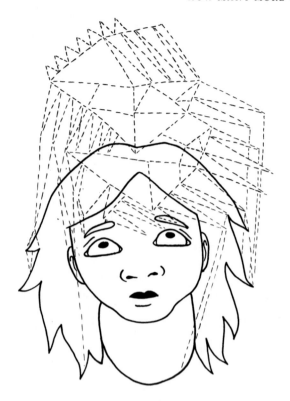

impact of these comorbidities on the quality of life of children with epilepsy and their families (Baca et al. 2011), the assessment of these comorbidities should be part of the comprehensive evaluation of every child with epilepsy.

PSYCHOPATHOLOGY

What We Know

- Children with epilepsy with average intelligence have prevalent psychopathology (psychiatric diagnoses, behavior problems).
- They have a wide range of psychiatric diagnoses including attention deficit/hyperactivity disorder (ADHD), anxiety disorders, depression, combinations of these diagnoses, psychosis, and autism.
- In most children with epilepsy, these disorders are undiagnosed and untreated.
- Children are essential informants about their symptoms and problem behaviors and emotions.
- Developmentally based assessment of psychopathology early in the course of the illness might therefore:
  - Reduce the unmet mental health needs of these children
  - Prevent the poor long-term psychopathology outcome in adults with childhood onset epilepsy

Relevance for the Interview of Young Children with Epilepsy

The findings of numerous studies suggest that children with new onset and chronic epilepsy with average intelligence have a wide range of psychiatric diagnoses, internalizing behavior problems (depressed, anxious, physical complaints, withdrawn behavior), and suicidal ideation that are related to structural abnormalities in the brain rather than direct effects of ongoing seizures (see review in Caplan 2010). The clinical examples provided in this and the following chapter on the psychosocial impact of pediatric epilepsy demonstrate that identifying the behavior and emotional problems of children with epilepsy—their association with cognitive, linguistic, and academic problems, as well as with coping difficulties in the parents—is essential for the comprehensive assessment of children with epilepsy and other similar pediatric disorders.

The importance of a comprehensive interview for these children is further emphasized by the high rate of unmet mental health needs in these children. About two-thirds of the children with epilepsy who also have psychiatric diagnoses, behavior/ emotional problems, and suicidal ideation are undiagnosed and untreated (Ott et al. 2003; Caplan et al. 2008b; Hanssen-Bauer et al. 2010). Yet, the need for diagnosis and treatment of mental health problems in these children is underscored by the poor long-term social, educational, vocational, and psychiatric outcome in adults with childhood onset epilepsy even when seizures are controlled (Sillanpää et al. 2004; Camfield and Camfield 2009).

Of relevance to the interviewer, several factors might contribute to this high rate of unmet mental health needs. First, treating physicians and parents focus primarily on the child's seizures. Second, parents might incorrectly perceive their child's inattention (Ott et al. 2003) and somatic symptoms of anxiety (Caplan et al. 2008b) as seizures (Oostrom et al. 2001). Third, young children aware of their parents concern about their epilepsy might not want to add to their parents' burden by sharing their emotional difficulties with them. Fourth, as previously described in chapters 3 and 4 on mood and anxiety disorders, respectively, young children might act out their emotions and be inaccurately labeled as misbehaving rather than depressed and anxious. Fifth, due to lack of knowledge about the comorbidities of epilepsy (Wu et al. 2008), parents might misinterpret their child's resistance to doing homework as laziness or "bad" behavior rather than possible problems with attention or subtle cognitive and linguistic difficulties. Finally, the need to deal with the double stigma of epilepsy and mental illness might deter parents from telling physicians about their children's behavior and emotional problems (Wu et al. 2008).

Providing clinicians with the developmental guidelines and interviewing techniques included in this book, together with the background information needed to conduct a comprehensive evaluation of children with epilepsy, can help address the unmet mental health needs of these children. The clinical examples below highlight the importance of recognizing that young children with epilepsy are the essential informants regarding the problems they might have with their behavior and emotions. These examples will also illustrate the need for clinicians to formulate developmentally appropriate questions, understand children's concrete use of language, and use validation questions to clarify the children's exact communication intent.

Clinical Examples

Separation Anxiety Disorder: Anne, an 8-year-old only daughter to older parents, was diagnosed with epilepsy two months ago after being taken to the emergency room because her parents were unable to rouse her from sleep in the morning. Other than an EEG with focal epileptic activity in the right temporal lobe, she had no abnormal findings on her physical and neurological exams, and her blood work and an MRI were also normal. On the assumption that she had complex partial seizures originating in the temporal lobe (temporal lobe epilepsy) (Table 11–1) and experienced a seizure during her sleep, she was given an antiepileptic drug.

Her parents brought her to see a pediatric clinical psychologist because she has had frequent temper tantrums over the last month during which she sometimes hit her mother. They are concerned that the seizure might have done something to her brain and changed her because she was never a behavior problem for them. As far as they are concerned, her outbursts of anger and aggression have been unprovoked. They usually occur when the mother picks her up from school, so they think that the medicine for her seizures might make her tired by the end of the school day.

Separation Anxiety Disorder

INTERVIEWER: *How is third grade going for you, Anne?*
ANNE: *Good.*
INTERVIEWER: *What is your favorite subject?*
ANNE: *Everything.*
INTERVIEWER: *Sounds like you like school.*
ANNE: *But sometimes my mom doesn't pick me up after school.*
INTERVIEWER: *When she doesn't pick you up, who does?*
ANNE: *I wait for her and my teacher gets mad.*
INTERVIEWER: *Do you mean that your mom sometimes comes late to pick you up?*
ANNE: *A lot.*
INTERVIEWER: *So while you wait for her, what do you think about?*
ANNE: *That she had an accident.*
INTERVIEWER: *That's scary. What other things do you think about?*
ANNE: *That the teacher will be mad and leave me there by myself.*
INTERVIEWER: *And then what could happen?*
ANNE: *I could get kidnapped.*
INTERVIEWER: *That is really scary. Does you mother know about all these scary thoughts?*
ANNE: *I cried one day. She said 8-year-olds don't cry because their mothers come a little late.*
INTERVIEWER: *How did that make you feel?*
Anne's eyes fill with tears.
INTERVIEWER: *Looks like it made you sad. Is it easy or difficult for you when your mom and dad go out?*
ANNE: *It's okay.*
INTERVIEWER: *Who stays with you?*
ANNE: *My grandmother babysits me because I had a seizure.*
INTERVIEWER: *When she babysits you, do you worry something bad might happen to them or to you?*

Table 11-1. FEATURES OF COMMON SEIZURES

GENERALIZED TONIC-CLONIC SEIZURES (GTCS)
• Eye rolling
• Loss of consciousness
• Body becomes rigid
• Rhythmic contractions and relaxation of trunk and extremities
• Sleep, tiredness, confusion follows
COMPLEX PARTIAL SEIZURES (CPS)[1]
• Blank stare
• Chewing
• Clumsy meaningless random movements
• Sleep, tiredness, or confusion follows
SIMPLE PARTIAL SEIZURE (AURA)
• Occurs around the time of a CPS or GTCS before loss of consciousness
• Distinct motor, sensory (hallucination, illusion, déjà phenomena), autonomic, or psychological perception (fear with epigastric discomfort)
• Forced thinking
• Not followed by sleep, tiredness, confusion
CHILDHOOD ABSENCE EPILEPSY
• Brief, sudden change in state of consciousness
• Eyelid fluttering
• Lip twitching
• Unchanged tone
• Sleep, tiredness, or confusion do not follow
BENIGN ROLANDIC EPILEPSY
• Typically occurs during sleep
• Twitching of face or cheek
• Tingling numbness, or unusual sensations in tongue
• Drooling
• Difficulty speaking
• Preservation of consciousness
• No tiredness or confusion
FRONTAL LOBE EPILEPSY
• Prominent motor symptoms
• Occurs during sleep
• Brief
• Rapid secondary generalization
• Complex automatisms

[1] Commonly originate in temporal lobe and called temporal lobe epilepsy

ANNE: *A little.*
INTERVIEWER: *Not like when you are waiting at school for your mom?*
Anne nods yes.
INTERVIEWER: *When you were in second grade, did this also happen?*
ANNE: *My mom would drive the morning car pool and Carrie's mom picked us up.*
INTERVIEWER: *Did you have the same scary thoughts when you waited for her after school?*

ANNE: *She was always waiting in front of school.*
INTERVIEWER: *Anne, what things make you angry?*
ANNE: *When she calls me a baby.*
INTERVIEWER: *Who does?*
ANNE: *My mom.*
INTERVIEWER: *What do you do when you get mad?*
Anne starts crying.
INTERVIEWER: *I see it is difficult for you to talk about this.*
Anne continues to cry.
INTERVIEWER: *Some kids get sad when they are mad. How about you?*
Anne nods yes.
INTERVIEWER: *Some shout and scream.*
Anne nods yes.
INTERVIEWER: *And some hit.*
Anne nods yes.
INTERVIEWER: *Looks like these scary thoughts and being told you are a baby are really making things difficult for you.*
Anne cries even more.
INTERVIEWER: *How about we explain to your mom about all these scary thoughts and bad feelings?*
ANNE: *She says I am bad and hit.*
INTERVIEWER: *Maybe she needs to understand that you are scared something bad might happen to her or to you while you wait for her after school.*
ANNE: *Okay.*

The psychologist's developmental approach helped Anne talk about her separation anxiety. The interviewer achieved this goal by beginning the conversation with a question about school rather than the behavior problems reported by the mother. Using "How" and "What" questions, working on understanding the emotions underlying the child's action-based communication, checking if this was what Anne meant, and expressing empathy for Anne's difficulties encouraged the child to talk.

In this case, as in many cases of pediatric epilepsy, parents blame the seizures and the medicine for changes in their children's behavior. Although the parents previously said that Anne had no prior behavior problems, after interviewing the child, the psychologist asked them if in the past Anne had difficulties separating from them. They said that she had from the toddler period until about second grade. They thought it was normal for young children to have these difficulties and that she had outgrown them.

The psychologist told the parents that Anne had separation anxiety disorder and that separation fears can continue through middle childhood. They asked the psychologist if Anne's seizure induced the separation fears. The psychologist explained that the child had separation anxiety disorder from an early age and that the onset of seizures might have exacerbated her separation fears. She counseled them on how to prevent triggering the fears unnecessarily. She also recommended that if Anne continues to have these symptoms, they should consider treatment for her separation anxiety disorder.

Depression: The parents of Jonathan, aged 10 years, have brought him for a follow-up evaluation by a child psychiatrist. Jonathan has left frontal lobe epilepsy

(Table 11–1) with what appear to be well-controlled seizures since he began taking an antiepileptic drug. From the beginning of the current school year, the parents reported increasingly "bad" behavior, including talking back, anger, temper tantrums, oppositional behavior, and threats to run away. He has also become a picky eater and wakes up frequently at night. Although the children in the neighborhood want to play with him, he says none of them are his friends. There have been no complaints from school about his behavior. The parents had read that "bad" behavior can occur in children with frontal lobe epilepsy and were concerned that he might be having seizures of which they were unaware.

Depression

INTERVIEWER: *Jonathan, how have you been feeling since I saw you during your summer vacation?*

JONATHAN: *Fine*

INTERVIEWER: *What's going fine for you and what's not so fine?*

JONATHAN: *School is fine.*

INTERVIEWER: *What's not fine?*

JONATHAN: *Nothing.*

INTERVIEWER: *How about your mood? Are you happy, sad, or in-between?*

JONATHAN: *Happy.*

INTERVIEWER: *What about getting angry? Who bugs you these days?*

JONATHAN: *Everyone.*

INTERVIEWER: *Who bugs you the most?*

JONATHAN: *My parents.*

INTERVIEWER: *What are they doing that makes you angry?*

JONATHAN: *They just bug me.*

INTERVIEWER: *Is it things they say or ask you to do?*

JONATHAN: *They don't let me watch TV.*

INTERVIEWER: *What else don't they want you to do?*

JONATHAN: *Play video games.*

INTERVIEWER: *Anything else?*

JONATHAN: *Be in my room.*

INTERVIEWER: *And what's the reason they don't let you do all these things?*

JONATHAN: *My seizures.*

INTERVIEWER: *What do these things do to your seizures?*

JONATHAN: *They can make me have a seizure.*

INTERVIEWER: *So if you watch TV, play video games, or be by yourself in your room you might have a seizure?*

JONATHAN: *Ask them.*

INTERVIEWER: *Looks like my questions are also bugging you.*

Jonathan looks down and nods yes.

INTERVIEWER: *Sorry about that. Maybe you can help me to understand what else bothers you because you look kind of mad and sad to me.*

JONATHAN: *No one likes me.*

INTERVIEWER: *Your family or friends?*

JONATHAN: *All of them.*

INTERVIEWER: *That's not a good feeling. What about you don't they like?*

JONATHAN (shrugging his shoulders): *Everything.*

INTERVIEWER: *Jonathan, in the summer time, did you also think that no one liked you?*

Jonathan shakes his head no.

INTERVIEWER: *What is making them not like you?*

JONATHAN (starting to cry): *I just want to go home.*

INTERVIEWER: *I know it is difficult for you to talk about this. Can we talk for a few minutes longer so I can figure out how to help you?*

JONATHAN: *No one can.*

INTERVIEWER: *Do you mean you think nothing will get better for you?*

Jonathan nods yes.

INTERVIEWER: *That's a really sad thought.*

Jonathan nods yes.

INTERVIEWER: *Do you sometimes feel it would be better if you were dead?*

JONATHAN: *I ran away to do it, but they caught me.*

INTERVIEWER: *What were you going to do?*

JONATHAN: *I don't remember.*

INTERVIEWER: *Does that mean you don't want to talk about it?*

Jonathan nods yes.

INTERVIEWER: *Let me ask you this, do you still want to hurt or kill yourself?*

Jonathan nods yes.

INTERVIEWER: *Do you think you will try again?*

Jonathan nods yes.

INTERVIEWER: *Do your mom and dad know how bad you feel about yourself and everything?*

Jonathan shrugs his shoulders.

INTERVIEWER: *And that you want to die.*

JONATHAN: *No.*

INTERVIEWER: *Would you like to feel how you were feeling in the summer?*

Jonathan makes eye contact with the psychiatrist, nods his head yes, and cries.

Rather than the "bad" behavior described by the parents, this child's irritability, hopelessness, feelings of social isolation, and suicidality are symptoms of major depressive disorder. The severity of his symptoms and his intentions to kill himself are indications for treatment in an inpatient child psychiatry unit to ensure his safety. The interviewer obtained this information from Jonathan through "How," "What," and "Who" questions and nonbiased questions with positive and negative options (fine/not fine, happy, sad, or in-between). The psychiatrist checked with the child to make sure he correctly understood what Jonathan was saying. He expressed empathy for how bad Jonathan felt, apologized for questions that irritated the child, and was sensitive to cues indicative of the child's difficulty talking about feeling rejected by others and his suicidal plans.

ADHD: Tommy, a 10-year-old boy, had his first seizure at age 4 years and a subsequent EEG that demonstrated left centrotemporal interictal spikes typical of benign Rolandic epilepsy (Table 11–1). He has had a total of three seizures since age 4, and is on no antiepileptic drugs. His mother brought him to a pediatrician because he underwent neuropsychological testing due to school difficulties and the testing revealed that he was inattentive and distractible. The child's past history provides no evidence of hyperactivity, impulsivity, and prior behavior problems in preschool or elementary school. The mother noted that her husband had been treated for ADHD when he was in elementary school and outgrew it. While the pediatrician spoke to the mother, Tommy could not separate from his mother and played games on her cell phone.

ADHD (Inattentive Type)

INTERVIEWER: *Tommy, I am not sure if you could hear what your mom told me about your testing while you were playing games on her phone.*

Tommy shakes his head no.

INTERVIEWER: *Did you like or not like the testing?*

TOMMY: *I liked it. But some things were hard.*

INTERVIEWER: *What was the hardest for you?*

TOMMY: *When I had to remember and draw the picture of the shapes.*

INTERVIEWER: *How about at school, what is easy and what is hard for you to do?*

TOMMY: *The kids are easy.*

INTERVIEWER: *Oh, so you have a lot of friends?*

Tommy nods yes.

INTERVIEWER: *What is hard to do at school?*

TOMMY: *Listening.*

INTERVIEWER: *That's important for me to understand. Can you help me understand?*

Tommy nods yes.

INTERVIEWER: *When you say that it is hard to listen, do you mean that when the teacher speaks you are thinking of other things?*

Tommy nods yes.

INTERVIEWER: *What kind of things?*

Tommy shrugs his shoulders.

INTERVIEWER: *Does that mean that you think about different things and not only one thing?*

TOMMY: *I guess so.*

INTERVIEWER: *So you don't remember what they are, but you know that you think about other things, not what the teacher is talking about?*

Tommy nods yes.

INTERVIEWER: *Does not listening also mean that when other kids are talking, you listen to them and not to the teacher?*

Tommy smiles and nods yes.

INTERVIEWER: *Is what they are talking about more interesting than what the teacher is saying?*

Tommy smiles and nods yes.

INTERVIEWER: *Sometimes do you not listen to the teacher because you don't understand what she is teaching?*

TOMMY: *No.*

INTERVIEWER: *Thank you that is all very helpful for me. Now when you have to do homework, are you thinking about all kinds of other things?*

TOMMY: *Yes.*

INTERVIEWER: *And when you play video games?*

Tommy smiles and shakes his head.

INTERVIEWER: *Does your teacher ever say you make mistakes on work you know well?*

TOMMY: *Yes.*

INTERVIEWER: *What about your desk at school and your backpack? Are they neat or messy?*

TOMMY: *A big mess.*

INTERVIEWER: *Oh really, and how about your room at home?*

TOMMY: *Makes my mom real angry.*

INTERVIEWER: *So your things are in a bit of a mess?*

TOMMY: *A big mess.*

INTERVIEWER: *Are you the type of kid who loses stuff or not?*

TOMMY: *Loses stuff.*

INTERVIEWER: *How easy is it for you to wait your turn in line?*

TOMMY: *Hard.*

INTERVIEWER: *Are you a kid who does things and then thinks about them or are you the type of kid who first thinks and then does them?*

TOMMY: *The first.*

INTERVIEWER: *Of all the different things you told me about, what would you like help with?*

TOMMY: *Listening.*

INTERVIEWER: *Well, thank you. You really helped me understand what is difficult and what is easy for you, and how we can fix it.*

TOMMY: *Don't mention it.*

The pediatrician established rapport with Tommy at the beginning of the interview by asking him if he heard what his mother was saying about him. Rather than talking about inattention and distractibility, the mother's presenting complaint about the child, the interviewer asked him how the testing went. Based on Tommy's answers to unbiased "What" and "How" questions about attention and learning, and on evidence for problems with attention in neuropsychological testing, the pediatrician diagnosed Tommy with ADHD inattentive type.

Similar to other types of pediatric epilepsy, benign Rolandic epilepsy is also associated with the inattentive type of ADHD (see review in Kavros et al. 2008). Other than the problems with attention, the interview and test results did not confirm a learning disorder. The pediatrician recommended treatment with a stimulant, given recent evidence that stimulants do not appear to increase seizure frequency (Gonzalez-Heydrich et al. 2010).

Psychosis: Juan is a 9-year-old boy with a lesion in the right posterior temporal lobe secondary to a neonatal hemorrhage, and with relatively well-controlled complex partial seizures (Table 11-1) that began at age 3 years. A pediatric neuropsychiatrist first saw him at age 5 years when he was expelled from a summer day camp because of aggression toward other children. She diagnosed him with Asperger's disorder due to circumscribed preoccupations with the gardening of vegetables, fruit, and other plants, together with impaired social and pragmatic skills. His aggression toward children at the summer camp occurred because they encroached on his body boundaries, and he was unable to tolerate their intrusion into his space. He presents today at the physician's office because he has been spitting repeatedly.

Schizophrenia-like Psychosis Associated with Epilepsy

INTERVIEWER: *Hi, Juan. You are holding a tissue on your tongue. Is something in your mouth bothering you?*

JUAN (spitting into the tissue): *It feels gross.*

INTERVIEWER: *So sorry to hear this. Is the gross feeling on your tongue or in your mouth?*

JUAN: *Both.*

INTERVIEWER: *What does it feel like?*

JUAN (averting eye contact): *A snail.*

INTERVIEWER: *Do you mean that it is wet like a snail or there is a snail moving in your mouth?*

JUAN: *In my mouth.*

INTERVIEWER: *How did it get there?*

JUAN (spitting into the tissue again): *That's what I want to know.*

INTERVIEWER: *Did someone put it there?*

JUAN: *Not sure.*

INTERVIEWER: *Who would do a thing like that?*

JUAN: *My sister—she's pretty sneaky, you know.*

INTERVIEWER: *How did you realize that it was a snail?*

JUAN: *The mirror.*

INTERVIEWER: *Oh, I see. I should have thought of that.*

JUAN: *Yes, that was a stupid question.*

INTERVIEWER: *It must have scared you when you saw it?*

JUAN: *It first started in the back of my throat and then came to my mouth.*

INTERVIEWER: *I can imagine how uncomfortable it is.*

JUAN: *That's why I spit.*

INTERVIEWER: *Now I understand. Did you tell you parents about the snail?*

JUAN: *They don't believe me. They said snails are in my vegetable and fruit tree garden, not in my mouth.*

INTERVIEWER: *Did you also tell them that you thought your sister was making this happen?*

JUAN: *No, 'cause they won't believe me.*

INTERVIEWER: *So we need to figure out a way to get rid of this snail.*

JUAN: *Can you?*

INTERVIEWER: *Let me first talk with your parents and then come up with a plan to help you.*

Empathy for Juan's unpleasant symptoms and asking "What," "How," and "Who" questions helped the pediatric neuropsychiatrist determine that Juan has both gustatory (taste) and visual hallucinations that are multimodal (involve more than one sensory system) and changing (from throat to the mouth) rather than fixed and stereotyped (see Differential Diagnosis of Psychotic Symptoms in chapter 7). He also has a persecutory delusion in that he is convinced that his sister put the snail in his mouth. He has poor reality testing, insight, and judgment but no formal thought disorder. His hallucinations and delusions are not followed by the tiredness, confusion, or memory loss that is experienced after complex partial seizures. With psychotic symptoms occurring between seizures (during the interictal period), Juan meets criteria for an interictal schizophrenia-like psychosis associated with temporal lobe epilepsy.

Brief Literature Review

As previously mentioned, in contrast to the historical focus on seizures, clinicians and researchers are now well aware of the importance of the comorbidities of pediatric epilepsy. The prevalence of psychiatric diagnoses in children with epilepsy with average intelligence is significantly higher than in children with other chronic illnesses with rates of about 60% in community studies and 37% in epidemiological studies (see review in Caplan 2010). Children with epilepsy have a wide range of psychiatric diagnoses including ADHD in 12%–39% (mainly the inattentive type), anxiety disorders in 11%–40%, depression in 16%–36%, and both ADHD and anxiety/affective disorders in about 18% (see review in Caplan 2010). A schizophrenia-like psychosis is rare in children with epilepsy (Caplan et al. 2004). Similar to the high rate of autism (De Bildt et al. 2005) and ADHD (Baker et al. 2010) among children with intellectual disability, autism (Steffenburg et al. 1996; Berry-Kravis et al. 2010) and ADHD, mainly the combined or hyperactive type (Sherman et al. 2007), are the most frequent psychiatric diagnoses in children with both epilepsy and intellectual disability.

In addition to formal psychiatric diagnoses, child self-report of depression and anxiety symptoms (see review in Caplan in press), as well as parent reports of internalizing problem behaviors (depressed, anxious, physical complaints, withdrawn behavior) (see review in Rodenburg et al. 2005) are consistently found in children with epilepsy. Similar to children with other chronic illnesses (Barnes et al. 2010) and physical disabilities (Scott et al. 2010), about 20% of children with epilepsy have suicidal symptoms, mainly suicidal ideation/thoughts (Caplan et al. 2005b). These are associated with both depression/anxiety and ADHD diagnoses. Parents' reports of behavior problems that differentiate children with epilepsy from those with chronic illness include inattention, thought problems, and social problems (see review in Rodenburg et al. 2005).

It is important to note that the psychopathology found in cross-sectional studies of children with epilepsy with average intelligence is unrelated to seizure variables, such as seizure frequency and control, antiepileptic drugs, EEG findings, duration of illness, past history of febrile or prolonged seizures (see review in Caplan 2010). In fact, from both the perspective of children and their parents, poor quality of life in a large sample of children with epilepsy is related to the presence of psychiatric diagnoses in the children rather than to continued uncontrolled seizures or having complicated epilepsy (Baca et al. 2011).

Furthermore, some children with new or recent onset epilepsy have psychiatric diagnoses and parent-reported behavior problems *prior* to their first seizure (see review in Caplan 2010). In addition, follow-up studies of psychiatric diagnoses among children with chronic epilepsy reveal no change in the prevalence of psychiatric diagnoses over a 2-year period (Jones et al. 2010. Thus, evidence for behavior and emotional problems prior to the onset of seizures (Austin et al. 2002; Oostrom et al. 2003; Jones et al. 2007), together with structural cortical and subcortical abnormalities in children with epilepsy who have a psychiatric diagnosis and in those with suicidal ideation, imply a possible role for the neuropathology underlying the disorder (see review in Caplan 2010).

Recent findings also suggest that genetic aspects of both epilepsy and psychopathology play a role in determining which children with epilepsy are at risk for psychopathology (Caplan 2010; Hesdorffer et al. 2012). Supporting the role of familial psychopathology, maternal depression is related to both the behavior problems (Shore et al. 2002) and poor quality of life (Ferro et al. 2011) in children with epilepsy. This is particularly relevant since from one-third (Shore et al. 2002) to half of the mothers of children with epilepsy (Ferro and Speechley 2009) are depressed. In chapter 12, Psychosocial Impact of Pediataric Epilepsy, we discuss the implications of these findings on the child's functioning in more detail.

Although the prevalence of psychiatric diagnoses does not appear to change over time, a recent large 3-year follow-up study of parent reports of child internalizing behavior problems (depressed, anxious, physical complaints, withdrawn behavior) demonstrated a significant improvement over time. However, those children with continued problems three years later had uncontrolled seizures (Austin et al. 2011), as well as poor self-esteem, depression, and poor academic performance (Dunn et al. 2010). Poor academic achievement is related to anxiety and depression in children in the general population (Corapci et al. 2006; Voci et al. 2006; Lundy et al. 2010) and ongoing seizures impact children's cognition and language (as described in the next section under Cognition and Language). Thus, poor academic performance (and associated cognitive and linguistic difficulties) might underlie the internalizing behavior problems that children with epilepsy and uncontrolled seizures continue to experience over time.

Summary

- Psychiatric diagnoses, behavior, and emotional problems are often undiagnosed and untreated in young children with epilepsy.
- The presence of psychopathology rather than seizures is associated with poor quality of life in children with epilepsy.
- The wide range of psychiatric diagnoses and behavior/emotional symptoms underscore the need to evaluate mood, anger, and irritability; fear and anxiety; attention; aggression; insight, judgment, and reality testing; somatization; and symptoms associated with autistic spectrum in children with epilepsy.
- A developmentally sensitive interview of young children is essential to obtain information on these symptoms.

COGNITION

What We Know

- Some children with epilepsy have cognitive and learning deficits despite average range intelligence.
- Ongoing seizures, underlying neuropathology, family dysfunction, parent anxiety, and child psychopathology play a role in these cognitive and learning deficits.
- The association of cognition and school performance with seizure control highlights the importance of early detection of cognitive/learning problems in children with uncontrolled seizures.

- It is important to rule out cognitive difficulties and poor academic achievement in children with epilepsy who have poor self-esteem and symptoms of depression.

Relevance for the Interview of Young Children with Epilepsy

The presence of cognitive/academic difficulties prior to the onset of seizures; the association with seizure variables; stable cognitive trajectories; and cognition-related structural and functional brain abnormalities suggest that cognitive/academic functioning reflects a combined effect of having epilepsy (the underlying pathology) and ongoing seizures in children with epilepsy (see review in Caplan 2010). Yet young children might not be cognizant of their cognitive deficits. In addition, when they are aware of their learning problems, they might not share them with their parents.

In some cases, parents might not understand or accept what their children are saying when they tell their parents about these difficulties. Parents might misinterpret the children's behaviors associated with frustrations related to learning difficulties as "bad" behavior. Sometimes they perceive the child's requests for help or complaints that the work is too hard as laziness or immature unwillingness to apply his/herself to the task at hand. Often children are too embarrassed to tell their parents (and their teachers) that they are having learning difficulties, particularly when they have siblings who do well at school.

Therefore, the comprehensive assessment of each child with epilepsy should always include questions about school performance. Some children might deny difficulties even when they have them because they are embarrassed and do not want to be perceived as "stupid." The clinical examples below demonstrate how the clinician can help young children talk about these difficulties.

Clinical Examples

Childhood Absence Epilepsy, ADHD, or Cognitive Deficits: Candice is an 8-year-old girl in third grade with childhood absence epilepsy that initially presented as attention problems when she was in second grade. Her neurologist identified 3Hz spike and wave epileptic activity on the EEG (see Table 10–1 in chapter 10), diagnosed childhood absence epilepsy, and treated her with valproate. However, the mother was unable to describe what the child's seizures look like and was uncertain if Candice ever had or was having seizures. Candice continued to do poorly at school and her neurologist then changed her valproate to ethosuximide and subsequently prescribed lamotrigine instead of the ethosuximide due to the mother's complaints that Candice continued to have learning problems.

At home, the mother would plead with Candice to do her homework. She would do some work if the mother sat with her but she found many reasons why she had to stop and do other things. The teacher suggested to the mother that Candice has ADHD. However, the mother thought that Candace, an only child to a single mother, was spoiled and immature and preferred to play with her artwork rather than do school work. The mother decided to get a second opinion from another pediatric neurologist about her daughter's epilepsy and Candice having possible ADHD.

Childhood Absence Epilepsy, ADHD, or Cognitive Deficits?

INTERVIEWER: *I see you brought an art kit with you. Show me what you did in the waiting room?*

CANDICE: *I drew pretty flowers.*

INTERVIEWER: *Wow, you are a really good artist. I love those colors. Besides flowers, what else do you like to draw?*

CANDICE: *Lots of things.*

INTERVIEWER: *Do you draw at home and at school?*

CANDICE: *My art teacher says I am a real artist.*

INTERVIEWER: *So you get to draw in your art classes at school. And at home?*

CANDICE: *My mom doesn't let me until I finish my homework.*

INTERVIEWER: *And is it easy or difficult to do the homework?*

CANDICE: *Difficult.*

INTERVIEWER: *Is that because you are thinking about your artwork or because the work is hard?*

CANDICE: *Both.*

INTERVIEWER: *Well how about at school—is it easy or hard for you to pay attention to the teacher?*

CANDICE: *Hard.*

INTERVIEWER: *Is it easy or hard to understand what she is teaching?*

CANDICE: *Hard.*

INTERVIEWER: *How about in art class, is it easy or hard to pay attention?*

CANDICE: *Easy.*

INTERVIEWER: *So when you say it is hard to understand what the teacher is saying, what do you do?*

CANDICE: *I think about what I want to draw when I will be in art class or get home.*

INTERVIEWER: *Are you the type of kid who thinks about how hard the work is a lot or a little?*

CANDICE: *Not really.*

INTERVIEWER: *How about what your teacher will say if you don't finish your homework?*

CANDICE: *No, only that my mom gets mad at me.*

INTERVIEWER: *So we need to figure out what is making it hard for you to understand your teacher and the homework.*

CANDICE: *My mom thinks I am just being a big baby.*

INTERVIEWER: *How does that make you feel?*

CANDICE: *I cry when she says that.*

INTERVIEWER: *Let's try and see what we can do to help with all this.*

CANDICE: *Look! I just made a picture for your office.*

INTERVIEWER: *Oh, how beautiful. You are both a good artist and a good talker. You really helped me understand how to help you.*

The neurologist established rapport with the child through questions about her art kit and drawing skills. The physician then indirectly approached the child's homework problem by asking if the child gets to do her artwork at home after school. This case demonstrates the importance of obtaining information from the child using a developmental approach to differentiate inattentiveness due to ongoing seizures from the inattentive type of ADHD that is interictal (between seizures) in children with absence epilepsy (Caplan et al. 2008b; Killory et al. 2011).

In the absence of a clear description of absence seizures by the mother, however, the pediatric neurologist recommended that Candice have an EEG with hyperventilation after gradually stopping her current antiepileptic drug, lamotrigine. The information the pediatric neurologist obtained from the child during the interview suggested that Candice might have a learning disorder and not ADHD. To determine if she has a primary learning disorder with inattentiveness secondary to learning difficulties, the inattentive type of ADHD, or both, the physician referred Candice for neuropsychological testing.

Depression, Seizures, or Impaired Cognition: Sami is an 8-year-old boy with complex partial seizures (Table 11–1) who was brought to see the social worker at the outpatient pediatric clinic by his mother because of her concerns that he was depressed. She described crying in the morning and resistance to going to school, poor appetite, lack of interest in his sisters, who he loves dearly, loss of his sense of humor, and increased tiredness and sleepiness. When asked to do his homework, he would cry. She felt she had lost her son whose personality had changed from what she described as a previously happy and related child.

Depression, Seizures, or Impaired Cognition
Sami slowly walked into the room and sat down without facial expression.
INTERVIEWER: *Hi, Sami. I just heard from your mother that you have three older sisters and they call you their baby brother.*
Sami slowly nods yes.
INTERVIEWER: *Are they nice or mean sisters?*
SAMI (slowly): *Nice.*
INTERVIEWER: *What nice things do they do for you?*
SAMI (after hesitation): *Buy me presents.*
INTERVIEWER: *That is nice. What mean things do they do to you?*
SAMI: *Nothing.*
INTERVIEWER: *So they sound like nice sisters. What do you like about your teacher?*
SAMI: *Sheeee* (voice trails off)
INTERVIEWER: *She what?*
Sami gets a brief fixed look in his eyes.
INTERVIEWER: *Sami, remind me who were we talking about?*
Sami looks through the interviewer.
INTERVIEWER: *Now I remember; it was about your teacher.*
SAMI (slowly): *My teacher.*
INTERVIEWER: *Yes, what do you like about her?*
SAMI (slowly): *Who?*
INTERVIEWER: *Your teacher.*
SAMI (slowly): *She's nice.*
INTERVIEWER: *Is the work at school easy or hard?*
SAMI: *It is* (voice trails off)
INTERVIEWER: *Sami*
Sami looks through the interviewer.

INTERVIEWER: *Sami, what were we talking about?*
Sami bursts out crying.

Despite the developmental approach used by the social worker in this interview, the child's one word answers, short sentences, inattention, repetition of the interviewer's last word of a sentence, voice trailing off, and recurrent fixed stare suggested he was experiencing seizures during the interview. The social worker then asked the mother to join her and Sami. The child continued to cry. She told the mother that Sami had been zoning in and zoning out and asked the mother if this has also been happening at home and at school.

The mother then told the social worker that the school had called her many times to come take him home from school because he was crying. She thought the teacher of his regular education class did not want him in the class because of his epilepsy. So she was engaged in a battle with the school administration to stop sending him home from school. She told the social worker that she felt the school's behavior had made her child depressed.

The social worker explained to the mother that he appeared to be having many seizures which she would discuss with Sami's neurologist to find out if the boy needed to have a video-EEG to clarify the nature of his seizures. Although Sami appeared to be depressed (lack of affect, slow speech and motor movements, crying) based on how adults perceive depression, these behaviors were probably the effects of having many seizures close to each other. The social worker also told the mother that Sami's academic skills needed assessment because he had been zoning in and out of what was being taught in class for an indeterminate period due to these frequent unnoticed seizures.

A video-EEG confirmed that Sami was, in fact, having ongoing seizures. Educational testing, done once he had better seizure control on a new antiepileptic drug combination, identified a broad range of difficulties involving attention, executive function, language, and slowed processing time. He was authorized to receive special education resources. This case, therefore, again underscores the importance of the individual interview of the child and that parents should not be the sole informants about their children's problem behaviors and emotions.

ADHD, Oppositional Defiant Disorder, or Cognitive Difficulties: The parents of Dwayne, a 10-year-old boy, were told by his teacher to have him checked out for ADHD because he was not paying attention in class and his grades had deteriorated. He had a past history of nocturnal motor seizures from age 5 years and enjoyed complete seizure control for the past four years. He had immigrated to the United States three years ago and spoke fluent English. Both parents were professionals and the grandparents, who lived with the nuclear family, played a major role in the boy's upbringing.

Although Dwayne had been a good student in a regular class, during the past few months, he began avoiding doing homework and his grades began to drop at school. His parents were very concerned about his poor performance at school. When they or the grandparents tried to make him do his homework, he would have a temper tantrum and, more recently, throw things.

While the parents described the child's condition to the pediatric epilepsy nurse practitioner, Dwayne was in the waiting room with his grandparents. However, all four adults brought the unwilling boy in to see the nurse practitioner. Since Dwayne refused to see the nurse practitioner alone, the mother stayed with him. He sat on her lap and began to playfully tap/hit her. The mother told him to stop but he smiled at her and continued to hit her.

ADHD, Oppositional Defiant Disorder, or Cognitive Difficulties

INTERVIEWER: *Dwayne, what has your mom done that you are hitting her?*

DWAYNE (smiling): *She knows.*

INTERVIEWER: *Well, I know that you did not want to come in here to speak with me.*

DWAYNE: *What do you want to talk about?*

INTERVIEWER: *About your school, friends, family, and your epilepsy.*

DWAYNE: *Why?*

INTERVIEWER: *To find out if things are going okay for you.*

DWAYNE: *Ask her. She knows.*

INTERVIEWER: *Oh, that's a good idea. When I ask a question that you think your mom should answer, just tell me.*

DWAYNE: *You're weird. What do you want to talk about?*

INTERVIEWER: *What you like to do at school?*

DWAYNE: *Nothing.*

INTERVIEWER: *What schoolwork would you say is hard and what is easy?*

DWAYNE: *That's stupid.*

Dwayne turns to his mother and tries to pull her toward the door.

INTERVIEWER: *Thanks for telling me, Dwayne. I will try not say stupid things.*

Dwayne laughs.

INTERVIEWER: *How about your teacher? Is she nice or not so nice?*

DWAYNE: *Stupid like you.*

INTERVIEWER: *What stupid things does she do?*

DWAYNE: *Work.*

INTERVIEWER: *Okay, now I get it. You don't like the schoolwork.*

DWAYNE: *It's stupid.*

INTERVIEWER: *What do you do with your friends at school?*

DWAYNE: *You know.*

INTERVIEWER: *So who lives with you at home?*

DWAYNE: *You know that.*

INTERVIEWER: *What do you like to do for fun?*

DWAYNE: *Basketball. Do you play?*

INTERVIEWER: *What do you think?*

DWAYNE: *Do you know how?*

INTERVIEWER: *No.*

DWAYNE: *I play.*

INTERVIEWER: *What position?*

DWAYNE (turns to mother): *Talk.*

MOTHER: *Defense.*

INTERVIEWER: *Which team is your favorite?*

DWAYNE (pulling his mother's elbow): *You say.*

MOTHER: *You know who you like, the Lakers.*

DWAYNE: *You like them, right?*

In contrast to the previous clinical example, there were no overt signs that this child was having seizures. If the nurse practitioner had focused on Dwayne's disinhibited behavior (hitting mother, talking back, calling the nurse practitioner stupid), she would have missed the cognitive gaps that became apparent during the dialogue between her and the child. The clue to these cognitive difficulties was that Dwayne repeatedly said, "You know" or told the nurse practitioner to ask his mother not him. Dwayne also made efforts to cover up his cognitive gaps through what might be interpreted as impertinent, funny, or disrespectful behavior. His anxiety about how he would fare during the interview is also probably why Dwayne wanted the mother in the room together with him and was hitting her.

The nurse practitioner applied the twelfth developmental guideline, *work to understand* (see chapter 1), to make sense of what the child was, in fact, communicating to her. She assumed that Dwayne's aggressive statements about her being stupid and weird were due to his fear about how well he would do during the interview. Her response to his statement about her being stupid was to thank him and that she would try to change her behavior. This positive approach, together with her neutral response to his name-calling, helped establish rapport with the child.

From the diagnostic perspective, an overnight video-EEG showed electrical status epilepticus during sleep (sleep activated epileptic discharges) (see reviews in Nickels and Wirrell 2008 and Akman 2011) without overt seizures. Treatment with valium resulted in severe disinhibition. However, subsequent gammaglobulin (blood plasma protein that includes antibodies) treatments lead to gradual improvement in the child's sleep EEG, his cognition, and his behavior. He was then able to cooperate and undergo neuropsychological testing, which revealed a wide range of deficits in attention, executive function, memory, and language.

Brief Literature Review

Standardized cognitive testing of children with epilepsy demonstrates values that range from high intelligence to intellectual disability (see review in Caplan 2010). Children with generalized and focal epilepsy (Table 11–1) usually have intelligence in the normal range. In contrast, children with epilepsy syndromes associated with symptomatic etiology (identified causes in the brain) and early onset are more likely to have intellectual disability (Hoie et al. 2005; Berg et al. 2008). As previously described, this chapter focuses on children with epilepsy who have average intelligence.

Seizure variables, such as age of onset, seizure frequency, number and type of antiepileptic drugs, and history of prolonged seizures are related to cognition in both children with new onset (Fastenau et al. 2009) and chronic epilepsy (Caplan et al. 2004; Oostrom et al. 2005; Caplan et al. 2008b). However, cognitive deficits are also reported prior to onset of seizures (Oostrom et al. 2003) in children with new (within the past three months) (Fastenau et al. 2009) and recent onset (within the past six months) seizures (Hermann et al. 2006; Hermann et al. 2008). Yet, the findings of prospective studies demonstrate stable trajectories of cognitive functioning in children with epilepsy (Aldenkamp et al. 1990; Oostrom et al. 2005; Hermann et al. 2008; Jones et al. 2010).

Although the findings of the cross-sectional and prospective studies seem to be contradictory, they suggest that children with uncontrolled seizures and/or related high doses of antiepileptic drug polytherapy (more than one antiepileptic drug), and who have associated cognitive impairment, continue on that same trajectory over time in terms of both their seizures and cognition. Similarly, children without cognitive impairment before or shortly after onset of the disorder who have easy-to-control seizures keep on their normal developmental trajectory (Hermann et al. 2008).

Regarding the type of cognitive deficits, children with new onset epilepsy (Hermann et al. 2006; Fastenau et al. 2009) and chronic epilepsy (Schoenfeld et al. 1999) have a broad range of deficits including attention/executive/construction, verbal memory and learning, and language. Despite similar intelligence (IQ) scores and performance on tests of attention/executive/construction in both children with complex partial seizures and in those with childhood absence epilepsy (Caplan et al. 2004; Caplan et al. 2008b; Fastenau et al. 2009), they differ from each other in tests for memory (Fastenau et al. 2009). Children with complex partial seizures perform significantly worse on delayed word list memory and delayed story memory tasks (Kernan et al. 2011), as well as on verbal memory and learning tests (Fastenau et al. 2009). Those with absence epilepsy show deficits in immediate and delayed story memory. Youth with juvenile myoclonic epilepsy have executive function deficits involving skills necessary for purposeful, goal-directed activity that enable an individual to synthesize information, plan an appropriate strategy, and execute that strategy (Pulsipher et al. 2009).

Seizure variables associated with these cognitive profiles also vary across these different types of epilepsy. Thus, longer duration of the illness and antiepileptic drug treatment are related to cognition and attention in childhood absence epilepsy (Caplan et al. 2008b; Glauser et al. 2010). But, age of onset, more years with active seizures, higher seizure frequency, antiepileptic drug polytherapy, and a history of prolonged seizures and/or febrile convulsions are associated with IQ in children with complex partial seizures (Schoenfeld et al. 1999; Caplan et al. 2004). Inconsistent findings for the association of cognitive function with EEG findings and other seizure variables in benign Rolandic epilepsy might reflect the small sample sizes and heterogeneity of subjects included in these studies (see review in Kavros et al. 2008).

In addition to effects of ongoing seizures and seizure severity, structural (Hermann et al. 2006; Daley et al. 2007; Pulsipher et al. 2009; Tosun et al. 2010; Tosun et al. 2011) and functional imaging studies (Killory et al. 2011) provide evidence for involvement of brain structure and function in the overall intelligence, attention, and neuropsychological deficits of children with epilepsy. Thus, the presence of cognitive difficulties prior to onset of seizures; the association of cognition and cognitive profiles with seizure variables; stable cognitive trajectories over time; and cognition-related structural and functional brain abnormalities together suggest that cognitive functioning reflects a combined effect of having epilepsy (the underlying neuropathology) and ongoing seizures in children with epilepsy with average intelligence.

From the clinical perspective, these findings emphasize the need to test intelligence and specific areas of cognitive functioning soon after a child is diagnosed with epilepsy to determine if the child has cognitive deficits. Early detection and intervention are important because of the association of deficits in cognitive functioning with both problem behavior and poor academic performance. Thus, both cross-sectional and prospective studies have shown that, similar to the findings for cognition, some children have learning difficulties prior to onset of seizures (Oostrom et al. 2005; Hermann et al. 2008; Berg et al. 2011), others develop them over time (Berg et al. 2011), and/or they worsen in association with the severity of seizures (Dunn et al. 2010).

Identified learning difficulties include problems with reading, writing, and math, and are related to cognitive deficits revealed by neuropsychological test findings (Dunn et al. 2010). Aldenkamp et al. (2005) have shown that IQ mediates the role of epilepsy syndrome (focal epilepsy and symptomatic generalized epilepsy) on educational underachievement in children with epilepsy. Both at the baseline and at follow-up, slow processing speed predicts learning difficulties (Dunn et al. 2010; Berg et al. 2011). Over a 36-month period, the increase in learning problems in children with epilepsy is associated with a decrease in language and verbal learning scores (Dunn et al. 2010). This finding emphasizes the importance of language skill (discussed in the next section) in the academic performance of children with epilepsy

However, standardized testing alone does not appear to identify which children with epilepsy receive special education services compared to control subjects without epilepsy (Berg et al. 2011). This suggests that factors unrelated to cognition also contribute to the learning difficulties of children with epilepsy and/or to those who receive special education services. Among these factors, parent anxiety (Dunn et al. 2010) and family environment (Mitchell et al. 1991; Fastenau et al. 2004) are significantly related to academic achievement and neuropsychological functioning, respectively.

Similarly, as previously mentioned in the section on psychopathology, the presence of psychiatric diagnoses and the type of diagnosis (depression, anxiety, and ADHD) are related to both intelligence (Buelow et al. 2003; Caplan et al. 2004; Caplan et al. 2005b; Hermann et al. 2006) and academic achievement in children with epilepsy (Austin et al. 2010). Worsening of language processing speed, verbal memory and learning, and attention/executive function/construction over a three-year period was found in children with epilepsy with poor self-esteem and self-report symptoms of depression (Austin et al. 2010). Similarly, in children with recent onset epilepsy, there is an association between cognitive dysfunction and comorbidities (ADHD, learning problems) at baseline (Oostrom et al. 2003; Hermann et al. 2006), as well as at the two- (Hermann et al. 2008), three- (Dunn et al. 2010), and four-year follow-up (Oostrom et al. 2005).

SUMMARY
- Frequent subtle-to-mild cognitive deficits in children with epilepsy underscore the need to apply the developmental guidelines when interviewing young children with epilepsy.
- Cognitive deficits play an important role in young children's academic performance.
- Behavior (inattentiveness) and emotional problems (anxiety, depression) might be early signs of cognitive difficulties.

LANGUAGE

What We Know

- From 27% to 68% of children with epilepsy with average intelligence have linguistic deficits.
- These deficits include basic linguistic skills (syntax, semantics) and higher-level impaired language (poor use of language to formulate and communicate thoughts in an organized way).
- Unless associated with intellectual disability or autism, linguistic deficits often go undiagnosed and treated.
- Impaired language skill in children with epilepsy is related to illness severity.
- The long-term negative implications of linguistic deficits on literacy, social function, vocation, and behavior emphasize the importance of early detection and treatment.

Relevance for the Interview of Young Children with Epilepsy

The studies reviewed below provide evidence for the impact of seizures and having epilepsy on language development in children with average intelligence. When interviewing a young child with epilepsy, the interviewer should be sensitive to signs suggesting that the child might have linguistic difficulties. As described in the developmental guideline, *work to understand*, and illustrated in Table 1–4 in chapter 1, these signs include the child responding to questions with repeated "Yes," "No," or "I don't know" answers; one-word sentences, as well as sentences with grammatical errors, incorrect word choice, and/or unclear reference to people, objects, or events. The need for early identification and treatment of language difficulties in young children with epilepsy cannot be overstated for the following reasons.

First, language plays a central role in literacy and academic achievement (Catts et al. 2002; Schuele 2004), as well as in the social competence of children without epilepsy. Children in the general population with language impairment also have problem behaviors (van Daal et al. 2007), anxiety (Corapci et al. 2006; Voci et al. 2006) and a wide range of psychiatric disorders (Im-Bolter and Cohen 2007). Furthermore, the adult communication, cognitive/academic, educational attainment, and occupational outcome (Johnson et al. 2010) as well as the behavior outcome (Brownlie et al. 2004) of these children with language disorders is poor.

Second, pediatric epilepsy is also associated with impaired basic and higher-level language, as well as cognitive and academic performance deficits, a wide range of psychiatric diagnoses, behavior/emotional problems, and social problems (see section to follow). Untreated, these comorbidities can contribute to the poor adult educational, vocational, behavioral, and social outcome of childhood epilepsy (see reviews in Caplan 2010 and Hamiwka et al. 2011a).

Third, from the practical perspective, young children are unaware of their linguistic difficulties. Since parents are also not aware that their children have problems with language if they speak, they do not seek out the necessary treatment. Fourth, pediatric professionals do not refer children with epilepsy for language testing because they receive no training on how to identify language problems in young children. To address this health-care gap, the developmental guidelines, interview techniques, and practical tools the reader can acquire through the clinical examples that follow will help identify children who need language assessment.

Clinical Examples

Rule out Language-related Learning Problems: Isabella, aged 6 years, had experienced one nocturnal seizure involving the right side of her mouth and face with EEG evidence for centrotemporal interictal spikes (Rolandic area) (Table 11–1). Her pediatric neurologist diagnosed benign Rolandic epilepsy and did not prescribe an antiepileptic drug because Isabella had had only one seizure (Shields and Snead 2009). The parents were glad that Isabella needed no medication because she loved her ballet classes, and they were concerned that an antiepileptic drug might negatively impact her coordination and gracefulness.

Isabella was selected to be one of the young children in the Nutcracker Ballet of her dance school, and she needed to attend ballet rehearsals almost every day after school. She had missed a few days of school because of the rehearsals, and on days that she was at school she was tired. The parents reported that Isabella's teacher said she was only in kindergarten and there was no need to worry.

Nevertheless, the father was concerned because he had read that sleep deprivation can induce seizures and that nocturnal epileptic activity in children with benign Rolandic epilepsy was related to language, math, and attention problems (Piccinelli et al. 2008; Ebus et al. 2011). Although the mother felt reassured by the teacher's comment, the father wanted the pediatric neurologist to tell them if Isabella should continue with the rehearsals into the evening for the upcoming ballet performance. To better understand how the child was functioning from the child's perspective, the physician had the following conversation with her:

Rule Out Language-Related Learning Problems
INTERVIEWER: *Isabella, your T-shirt says, "I love to dance." What do you dance?*
ISABELLA: *Ballet.*
INTERVIEWER: *And you love to dance.*
Isabella nods yes.
INTERVIEWER: *What's fun about dancing?*
ISABELLA: *The Nutcracker.*
INTERVIEWER: *Did you see the Nutcracker?*
Isabella nods yes.
INTERVIEWER: *What's your favorite part?*
ISABELLA: *I dance.*
INTERVIEWER: *Do you dance in the ballet?*
Isabella nods yes.
INTERVIEWER: *You must be a good dancer.*
Isabella smiles.
INTERVIEWER: *What do you do in the ballet?*
Isabella dances around the room.

INTERVIEWER: *Oh, thank you for showing me. Remind me, what is the name of the step when you turn?*

Isabella demonstrates a pirouette.

INTERVIEWER: *I forgot what it's called.*

Isabella turns to her mother.

MOTHER: *You know that is a pirouette.*

INTERVIEWER: *That's a hard word.*

Isabella nods yes.

INTERVIEWER: *And what do you like about kindergarten?*

ISABELLA: *My teacher.*

INTERVIEWER: *What's nice about her?*

ISABELLA: *I dance for the kids.*

INTERVIEWER: *Oh, so she lets you dance in class. Is she nice when she teaches reading?*

ISABELLA: *Boring.*

INTERVIEWER: *And when she teaches spelling?*

ISABELLA: *Boring.*

INTERVIEWER: *And math?*

ISABELLA: *Nice.*

INTERVIEWER: *Does boring mean that reading and spelling are easy or hard?*

ISABELLA: *Hard.*

INTERVIEWER: *So, it is hard to read the words?*

ISABELLA NODS YES.

INTERVIEWER: *I bet she also gives homework.*

ISABELLA: *A lot.*

INTERVIEWER: *Reading or spelling?*

ISABELLA: *Every day.*

INTERVIEWER: *And math?*

ISABELLA: *That's easy.*

INTERVIEWER: *So ballet is easy, math is easy, but reading and spelling are hard.*

Isabella nods yes and looks at her mother.

INTERVIEWER: *How about writing?*

ISABELLA: *I write pretty.*

INTERVIEWER: *Isabella, you are doing a very good job talking to me. So before we are done, can you tell me the Nutcracker story? I saw it a long time ago.*

ISABELLA: *It's long.*

INTERVIEWER: *Tell me just a little not the whole story.*

ISABELLA: *The girl and nutcracker.*

INTERVIEWER: *What did they do?*

ISABELLA: *Dance.*

INTERVIEWER: *And then what happens?*

ISABELLA: *The big mouse.*

INTERVIEWER: *What does he do?*

ISABELLA: *Fight.*

INTERVIEWER: *And then what happens?*

ISABELLA: *She woke up?*

INTERVIEWER: *Who woke up?*

ISABELLA: *The girl.*

INTERVIEWER: *And how did the story end?*

ISABELLA: *Merry Christmas.*

INTERVIEWER: *Oh, I see she woke up, and it was Christmas day. Thank you for reminding me about the story.*

The pediatric neurologist established rapport with the child by remarking about her ballet T-shirt, talking to her first about her strengths (dancing), and then gradually moving to talk about school using "What" questions. Complimenting Isabella on her dancing and telling her that the word she could not think of, *pirouette*, is a difficult word helped consolidate the interviewer's rapport with the child. The interviewer's use of short action-based questions and her request to hear the story of the ballet helped identify the child's language difficulties.

This example is instructive since most people might not recognize that this child has language difficulties because she is speaking. However, she does not speak in full sentences—a skill children usually acquire by age 2–3 years. She has difficulty retrieving the word "pirouette" even though she is frequently exposed to this word. She finds both reading and spelling hard to do already at the kindergarten level. Her storytelling skills are poor compared to other 6-year-old children who have relatively good narrative skills in terms of both content (details of the story) and form (sentence structure). The pediatric neurologist recommended to the parents that the child have speech and language testing. She also emphasized that Isabella should continue her ballet rehearsals and that the parents need to encourage this skill as it is an experience of mastery and enjoyment for her.

Behavior Disorder vs. Undiagnosed Language-related Learning Disorder: Grace is a 7-year-old girl whose mother brought her to the pediatric epileptologist, Dr. Doyle, because of intractable seizures. Grace had her first seizure 6 months after a mild head trauma that she experienced while on a jungle gym at a park at age 4 years. She had lost consciousness briefly and was observed for 24 hours in the hospital due to vomiting. After an additional seizure, she was treated with an antiepileptic drug, and she had no subsequent seizures until six months ago. Her recent EEG showed a left temporal focus and an MRI identified a left temporal lobe lesion. She then underwent surgical removal of a low-grade astrocytoma.

Subsequent to the surgery she began to have frequent uncontrolled seizures despite multiple attempts at different antiepileptic drug combinations. The mother was very concerned about her daughter's resistance to going to school and the child's claim that the teacher and the children were mean to her. She worked intensely on a daily basis with the child on reading, spelling, and arithmetic, but Grace began having daily temper tantrums.

Behavior Disorder vs. Undiagnosed Language-Related Learning Disorder

DR. DOYLE: *Grace, let's see ... I think I saw you last in the summer before school started.*

GRACE: *My school is new.*

DR. DOYLE: *Did they just build it?*

GRACE: *No, it's new.*

DR. DOYLE: *Oh, you mean you changed schools.*

Grace nods yes.

DR. DOYLE: *What wasn't good in the old school?*

GRACE: *The teacher.*

DR. DOYLE: *What did she do?*

GRACE: *Mean.*

DR. DOYLE: *What mean things did she do?*

GRACE: *Yell.*

DR. DOYLE: *About what?*

GRACE: *I don't know.*

DR. DOYLE: *That's hard to talk about.*

Grace nods yes.

DR. DOYLE: *What do you like about the new school?*

GRACE: *Recess.*

DR. DOYLE: *What do you like to do in recess?*

GRACE: *Play.*

DR. DOYLE: *Who are your friends?*

GRACE: *Kids.*

DR. DOYLE: *What are their names?*

GRACE: *I don't remember.*

DR. DOYLE: *What don't you like about your new school?*

GRACE: *It's boring.*

DR. DOYLE: *So does that mean the work is hard?*

Grace nods yes.

DR. DOYLE: *What else is boring at school?*

GRACE: *Homework.*

DR. DOYLE: *So what do you do when you come home from school?*

GRACE: *She makes me read.*

DR. DOYLE: *Who does?*

GRACE: *My mom.*

DR. DOYLE: *Sounds like you don't like reading.*

GRACE: *Boring.*

DR. DOYLE: *What's good about being at home?*

GRACE: *Dolls.*

DR. DOYLE: *What do you do with your dolls?*

GRACE: *Clothes.*

DR. DOYLE: *You like to dress them. What clothes do your dolls have?*

GRACE: *Cool clothes.*

DR. DOYLE: *Just like your clothes.*

Grace smiles.

DR. DOYLE: *So you get to play with your dolls when you are at home?*

GRACE: *No.*

DR. DOYLE: *Oh, I thought that's what you like to do.*

GRACE: *Only work, work, work!*

DR. DOYLE: *You mean homework?*

GRACE: *Homework, homework, homework.*

DR. DOYLE: *Sounds like that makes you angry.*

GRACE: *She's mean.*

DR. DOYLE: *Who is?*

GRACE: *Mom.*

DR. DOYLE: *She makes you do the work at home.*

Grace nods yes.

DR. DOYLE: *So what do you do when your mom makes you work and you don't want to?*

GRACE: *Get mad.*

DR. DOYLE: *And then what?*

GRACE: *Hit.*

DR. DOYLE: *Your mom?*

Grace nods yes and looks down.

DR. DOYLE: *That probably doesn't make you feel too good.*

GRACE: *She doesn't listen.*

DR. DOYLE: *Did you tell her the work is hard for you?*

GRACE: *She doesn't listen.*

DR. DOYLE: *Is it all the work?*

GRACE: *Reading and vocabulary list.*

DR. DOYLE: *When you read is it hard to figure out the words?*

Grace nods yes.

DR. DOYLE: *How about the spelling?*

Grace nods yes.

DR. DOYLE: *And math?*

GRACE: *Not so hard.*

DR. DOYLE: *At your new school, is it hard like at your old school?*

Grace nods yes.

DR. DOYLE: *Thanks, Grace, for helping me understand what is making you mad. Let me speak now with your mom and see how I can help.*

Despite the child's linguistic and cognitive limitations, Dr. Doyle obtained important information from Grace about the problems she has with learning, peers, and her mother. Dr. Doyle achieves this by rapport-building techniques (empathy, compliments to the child). Dr. Doyle also checked if he correctly understood Grace's frustration and anger at school and at home from the child's action-based concrete statements such as "Work, work, work," and "Boring."

This clinical example illustrates how language problems might present as behavior problems that reflect the child's language-related learning difficulties with reading and spelling. It also underscores the difficulties parents have "hearing" when their children let them know that they are having problems with learning. Although Grace's mother meant well in her efforts to fix the problem, this increased the child's frustration to the point of being aggressive toward her mother and resisting going to school.

Grace clearly was at risk for language-related learning problems due to the involvement of language-related brain regions in the left temporal lobe by her astrocytoma and because of her uncontrolled seizures. Detailed speech and language testing, as well as cognitive tests shortly after diagnosis of children with epilepsy and other disorders involving the brain, can help determine the appropriate intervention and school/class placement. It can also prevent the related behavior problems. The next chapter presents the psychosocial impact on the child, her parents, and the functioning of the family in the clinical example entitled *Unrealistic Expectations* in the section on Parents.

Impaired Language and High Functioning Autism: Jose was 3-years-old when he started having staring spells, sometimes followed by a generalized tonic-clonic seizure (see Table 10–1 in chapter 10). His EEG confirmed a diagnosis of atypical childhood absence epilepsy (staring spells that are not induced by rapid breathing and with abnormal EEG findings in between seizures). On lamotrigine his parents noticed no staring spells and he had his last generalized tonic-clonic seizures over a year ago.

Now at age 8 years, his parents reported that he had developed tics and seemed to also have difficulty getting his words out. They also noted that they had recently divorced, and he was now in a new school that was equidistant between both parents' homes. The transition to this school and to a regular third grade class had been difficult for him, and he became quite resistant to going to school in the morning and to doing his homework. He also complained that the children in his class were mean.

The parents felt that his tics were stress-induced because they got worse when he was upset. However, they wanted to be sure that they were not seizures. When Jose walked into the pediatrician's office, he went straight to the corner of the room, grabbed a pencil that was on the pediatrician's desk, and started to twirl it. He did not make eye contact with the pediatrician, spoke very slowly with unusual prosody (musical quality of the speech), pronunciation, and inflexion of some words.

Impaired Language and High Functioning Autism

INTERVIEWER: *Hi, Jose. How is your new school?*
JOSE: *Bad.*
INTERVIEWER: *What is the worst part about it?*
JOSE: *The kids.*
INTERVIEWER: *What do they do?*
JOSE: *Call names.*
INTERVIEWER: *What names?*
JOSE: *Retard.*
INTERVIEWER: *Oh sorry to hear that. Do they say that also about other kids?*
Jose shrugs his shoulders.
INTERVIEWER: *That must make you feel bad.*
JOSE: *Yeah.*
INTERVIEWER: *So, they are mean only to you.*
JOSE (with tears in his eyes): *Yesssss.*
INTERVIEWER: *What do you do when they do that?*
JOSE: *Tell them they should be suspended.*
INTERVIEWER: *Does that make them stop?*
JOSE: *No.*
INTERVIEWER: *Are you also living in a new house now?*
JOSE: *It's old.*
INTERVIEWER: *I thought you moved.*
JOSE: *We did.*
INTERVIEWER: *Oh, so the new house you are staying in now is old?*
JOSE: *What?*
INTERVIEWER: *Sorry I am not talking clearly.*
Jose's eyes start to rapidly blink.
INTERVIEWER: *Are your eyes feeling okay?*
JOSE: *Yessss.*

INTERVIEWER: *So what just happened?*
JOSE: *Nothing.*
INTERVIEWER: *I am a little confused. Can you remind me what were we talking about?*
JOSE: *The house.*
INTERVIEWER: *That's right and I was not talking clearly.*
JOSE: *I hate them.*
INTERVIEWER: *Sounds like the kids really upset you. How about your teacher?*
JOSE: *No good.*
INTERVIEWER: *Because?*
JOSE: *She doesn't punish them.*
INTERVIEWER: *How are you finding the work at school?*
JOSE: *Can't do it. They should go home.*
INTERVIEWER: *What else do they do?*
JOSE: *Say I read slowly.*
INTERVIEWER: *That must really bother you.*
JOSE: *They laugh when I tell the teacher I don't understand.*
INTERVIEWER: *What do you do when they do all these mean things?*
JOSE: *Tell them to get suspended.*
INTERVIEWER: *What do your mom and dad say?*
JOSE: *I can't be mad.*
INTERVIEWER: *What was good about second grade in your old school?*
JOSE: *No names and laughing, and the work.*
INTERVIEWER: *So now the work is harder for you?*
JOSE: *Too much reading, writing, spelling.*
INTERVIEWER: *Okay, you have really helped me understand how to help you.*
JOSE: *So, will you suspend the kids?*
INTERVIEWER: *No, I don't work at your school.*

The pediatrician's interview of Jose illustrates how action-based "What" questions, short simple sentences, empathy for the child's problems, and repeat clarification of what the child means to say help the child speak and provide important diagnostic information. Although this child's main complaint was name-calling by peers, his placement in a regular class together with his slow speech, expressive difficulties, slow processing of language, unusual prosody, twirling of objects, poor eye contact, and repeated criticism of the children, made him a target for their ridicule. In addition, he seemed to get by with the work in second grade, but the increased language-related demands of third grade might be tapping into his language difficulties. His use of short concrete sentences, his difficulties with the motor aspects of speech, as well as with reading, writing, and spelling, might reflect an undiagnosed speech and language disorder.

The blinks he experienced seemed to be tics as they were unrelated to a change in consciousness and awareness. His lack of awareness for the blinks is not unusual in young children and in children with autism who do not pay much attention to their bodies. Alternatively, he may have been attempting to change the topic when the pediatrician asked about the blinking. The pediatrician recommended that the child undergo speech and language testing as well as educational testing to determine the optimal classroom placement for him.

Brief Literature Review

Children with epilepsy have basic linguistic skills in the normal, mild deficit, and marked deficit range (Henkin et al. 2003; Fastenau et al. 2004; Byars et al. 2007; Hermann et al. 2008; Caplan et al. 2009b). In a large sample of 182 children with epilepsy with average intelligence aged 6–8, 8–12, and 12–15 years, 22% of the young, 37% of the intermediate, and 68% of the adolescent subgroups had linguistic deficits (Caplan et al. 2009b). These deficits included a wide range of language skills, such as syntax, semantics, phonology, expressive and receptive language, as well as reading.

Although risk factors for low overall language scores varied across age groups, significant epilepsy variables included the type of epilepsy (childhood absence epilepsy) and a longer duration of illness in the young group, a history of prolonged seizures in the intermediate group, and both poor seizure control and a longer duration of illness in the adolescent subgroup. Additional risk factors included demographic variables (minority and low socioeconomic status), low Performance IQ, and anxiety disorder diagnoses.

In addition to basic linguistic deficits, children with epilepsy with average intelligence have impaired higher-level discourse skills (Caplan et al. 2002; Caplan et al. 2006) also known as thought disorder and described in chapter 7. More specifically, during conversation they demonstrate poor organization of their thoughts (at the level of the paragraph), under-use of linguistic devices that help the listener follow who and what the child is talking about across sentences, as well as poor monitoring and repair of communication breakdowns that occur at the level of the paragraph and/or within and across sentences. As a result, the listener has difficulty making sense of what the child is talking about. Risk factors for these discourse deficits include seizure variables (frequency, duration of illness, number and type of antiepileptic drugs), low verbal IQ, ADHD, social problems, and school problems (Caplan et al. 2006).

From the developmental perspective, these findings might reflect the effects of seizures on the normal ongoing development of language-related brain regions from childhood through adolescence (Lenroot and Giedd 2006). The previously described evidence for the most severe linguistic deficits in the adolescent subgroup, the association of both basic linguistic and discourse deficits with seizure variables (Caplan et al. 2009b), and the relationship of these impairments with structural (Caplan et al. 2008a; Caplan et al. 2009a) and functional abnormalities (O'Neill et al. 2011; You et al. 2011) in language-related brain regions imply a cumulative effect of having seizures on language skill. Thus, language skill and linguistic deficits in children with epilepsy with average intelligence reflect both the underlying neuropathology as well as the effects of ongoing seizures.

The apparent predilection of epilepsy for language brain regions is highlighted by prevalent delayed language development, severe linguistic impairment, and marked pragmatic deficits in children with early onset difficult-to-control epilepsy and intellectual disability. More recently, terms such as autism and autistic regression have been used to describe these children (Tuchman et al. 2010). As noted in the Psychopathology section above, some children with epilepsy also have high functioning autism (see review in Tuchman et al. 2010). From a linguistic perspective, children with epilepsy, intellectual disability, and autism have delayed language development, impaired basic linguistic and discourse skills, as well as poor pragmatic skills. In contrast, high-functioning children with an autism diagnosis have mainly discourse and pragmatic deficits.

Impaired language and delayed language development also play a central role in two epilepsy syndromes associated with intellectual disability, relatively easy-to-control seizures, and behavior described as autistic. Children with Landau-Kleffner syndrome (see review in Hughes 2011) have word deafness (despite normal hearing, they do not comprehend the meaning of speech and non-speech sounds, such as a doorbell ring). They typically have focal epileptic activity in the temporal lobe with or without overt seizures. Children with continuous spike and wave during sleep, also known as electrical status epilepticus, have basic and higher level linguistic impairment, as well as relatively easy-to-control seizures (Debiais et al. 2007; Nickels and Wirrell 2008; Loddenkemper et al. 2011).

Delayed language development, language impairment, intellectual disability, and autism are also found in several epilepsy syndromes with early onset intractable seizures, including infantile spasms (Riikonen 2010), Lennox-Gastaut (Camfield 2011), and Doose syndrome (Kelley and Kossoff 2011). The interested reader is also referred to a recent review that examines speech and language disorders, as well as related genetic findings in children with epilepsy (Pal 2011).

SUMMARY

- Language deficits are frequently undiagnosed and untreated in children with epilepsy with average intelligence.
- Interviewers should, therefore, apply the developmental guidelines when talking about emotions, behavior, and illness with children with epilepsy.
- Language plays a central role in children's literacy and academic performance that, in turn, affect children's self esteem and behavior.
- Behavior and emotional problems might be early signs of undiagnosed language problems.

SOCIAL COMPETENCE

What We Know

- About 40% of children with epilepsy with average intelligence have poor social competence.
- Poor social competence in pediatric epilepsy is multifactorial involving:
  - IQ, neuropsychological deficits, and learning difficulties
  - Psychiatric diagnoses
  - Stigma associated with learning difficulties
  - Lack of independence related to poor seizure control
  - Family functioning
- Children with epilepsy experience bullying and are not chosen by peers to be best friends.
- Parents are concerned about the social skills of their children with epilepsy.
- The interview of every child with epilepsy should include questions on social skills.

Relevance for the Interview of Young Children with Epilepsy

Although research on social skills in children with epilepsy is a relatively new field, the poor long-term social outcome of childhood onset epilepsy (Sillanpää et al. 2004; Camfield and Camfield 2009) emphasizes the importance of this comorbidity of pediatric epilepsy. These follow-up studies reveal lower rates of marriage and living independently, as well as social isolation in these individuals. This is particularly important because one of the main concerns of parents of children with epilepsy is that their children have poor social skills. To address this important need, this section provides the reader with guidelines for asking young children with epilepsy about their social skills.

The best way to assess a child's social skills is to observe the child interacting with peers and to obtain information from multiple informants including parents, teachers, and peers (Hamiwka et al. 2011a). Although parents have the opportunity to observe their children in social situations, particularly in younger children, they do not see their children's social behavior at school both in the class and at recess. Teachers are also limited in the information they can provide because children usually work by themselves in class (except for certain group projects), and teachers usually do not spend time on the playground. If they do, they monitor the behavior of many children rather than that of an individual child.

The one-on-one setting of a clinical interview provides limited information on a child's social skills other than observation of how the child interacts with the interviewer and the opportunity to ask the child about his/her social skills. Since social skill impairment is a core symptom of externalizing disruptive psychiatric disorders (hyperactive-impulsive ADHD, oppositional defiant disorder, conduct disorder), internalizing disorders (social phobia and mood disorders), autism, and psychosis, the presence of these diagnoses might imply that a child has social difficulties.

Furthermore, the thought processes of children with these diagnoses might influence how they perceive their social skills. More specifically, depressed children might feel that everyone dislikes them and does not want them as a friend. Children with ADHD hyperactive-impulsive type, oppositional defiant disorder, conduct disorder, and bipolar disorder usually blame others for any social difficulties they might have. Those with psychosis might have auditory hallucinations and delusions that other children are speaking about them, out to get them, or doing bad things to them.

With these limitations in mind, Table 11–2 presents examples of questions that clinicians can use to ask young children about their social skills. A central premise underlying the formulation of these questions is that young children are embarrassed to say they have social difficulties and to acknowledge that they do not have friends. To help young children talk about these difficulties, one needs to ask a series of questions with two main aims. The first aim is to make the child feel comfortable enough to share this information with the interviewer. Clinicians can achieve this aim by first asking the child neutral informative questions about friends (Table 11–2) before posing questions related to rejection by peers. The second aim is to validate the information the child provides and find out if, in fact, the child does or does not have friends and what might sound like social difficulties.

Table 11–2. Questions for Young Children on Social Skills

Topics	Questions	Comments
FRIENDS		
Presence	Are you the type of kid with a lot of friends or a few friends?	Young children might say they have a lot of friends and mean everyone in their class. Even if they say they have a few friends, that does not mean they have friends. The subsequent questions help clarify this.
Names	Who are your friends? What are your friends' names?	If young children have trouble mentioning the names of their friends, this suggests they might not have friends. Again, if they rattle off a whole lot of names, they might be naming the children in their class and that does not mean that these children are their friends.
LOCATION		
School, home, place of worship, at clubs, teams, etc.	Are these your friends at school? How about near your house (in your neighborhood)? Who are your friends? Which kids at ... are your friends?	Follow up the child's answers to these questions by asking for the children's names. Children with difficulty coming up with the names might not have friends.
ACTIVITIES WITH FRIENDS		
What?	What do you like to do with your friends? What kinds of things do you all play?	Young children will often say, "Play." Clarify what they play to ensure that the child is, in fact, playing with other children.
Where?	So where are you playing ... with these friends? Do some kids come over to your house to play? Do you go over to other kids to play?	These questions help confirm the child's prior answers regarding location and that the child has friends at school, in the neighborhood, or other places.
Who decides?	When you all play, who chooses what to play? Is that good or not so good?	These questions provide information on how active the child is in the decision-making process, and whether this causes friction between the child and peers.

Table 11–2. (CONTINUED)

Topics	Questions	Comments
SOCIAL ISOLATION		
Rejection	When all the kids are playing, sometimes are you by yourself?	This question should not precede the above questions because children find it difficult to acknowledge that they are having social difficulties.
Feelings	How does that make you feel?	For children who are often alone, this question helps them open up and talk about their social difficulties, particularly if the interviewer empathizes with "That's not a good feeling."
Reasons	What makes them not want to play with you (let you play)? Are the kids like that to other kids or only to you? What makes them play with the others and not with you?	Most children will say they do not know or that the children are mean. Empathizing again with the child might help him/her provide a reason. If the child answers that the children will play with other children but not with her/him, the next question might help clarify the reason.
Actions	So when they don't want to play with you, what do you do? How does that make you feel?	If children say they play by themselves, ask the next question. Children often answer, "I don't know."

Brief Review of Literature

The reader can find reviews on social skills in children with epilepsy in Drewel and Caplan 2007 and in Hamiwka et al. 2011a. Impaired social competence is found in about 40% of a large sample of 177 children with epilepsy who have average intelligence based on parent reports (Caplan et al. 2011). As a group, however, the mean social competence score of these children was within the normal range when controlling for IQ (Caplan et al. 2005a; Caplan et al. 2011).

The presence of mild cognitive deficits plays a role in the poor social skills of children with epilepsy. Additional risk factors for impaired social competence include deficits in overall language skill, discourse deficits, and ADHD, but not seizure variables (Caplan et al. 2011). Drewel et al. (2009) found that neuropsychological functioning deficits, as well as symptoms of anxiety and inattention are associated with peer difficulties in a large sample of children with epilepsy. Other studies have also shown that learning disabilities and poor family functioning, not seizure variables, were related to impaired social skills (Tse et al. 2007). Thus, as the case with children in the general population (Parker et al. 2006) and in those with traumatic brain injury (Yeates et al. 2004), cognition and academic skills, as well as the use of language for social communication, also play a role in the social skills of children with epilepsy.

Suffering from a chronic illness has been considered to be an additional factor that might impact children's social skills. A recent study reported that children with epilepsy and those with chronic kidney disease had impaired social skills compared to healthy controls, but there were no significant differences between the patient groups on their social skill scores (Hamiwka et al. 2011b). In contrast to children with chronic medical illnesses that do not involve the brain, those with central nervous system disorders, such as head trauma (Muscara et al. 2009), brain tumor (Barrera et al. 2008), neurofibromatosis (Noll et al. 2007), multiple sclerosis (Goretti et al. 2010), as well as those undergoing treatment for primary cancer involving the brain (cranial radiotherapy, intrathecal treatment) (Vannatta et al. 2007) have poor social competence. Of note, with the exception of head trauma (Muscara et al. 2009), similar to pediatric epilepsy, severity of illness is not associated with the social skill impairment of children with these central nervous system disorders.

From the methodological perspective, using state of the art social skill measures that include peer ratings in the classroom environment, Hamiwka (2011) has shown that children with epilepsy are not regarded as different from their peers, but peers would not choose children with epilepsy to be their best friends. Children with epilepsy also undergo more bullying than those without epilepsy and this finding is not associated with seizure variables (Hamiwka et al. 2009).

Semi-structured and open-ended interviews with surgically and medically treated children with intractable epilepsy that focused on the impact of epilepsy on the children's social functioning reveal that the children often feel they cannot engage in social activities because of constant parent monitoring (Elliott et al. 2005). However, once they obtain freedom from seizures after surgery, they acquire more independence from their parents, and engage in more social activities than those with intractable seizures who do not undergo surgery. Children with epilepsy who undergo surgery and those who have medically treated difficult-to-control seizures also report that they are bullied and teased because of their learning difficulties more than because of their seizures (Elliott et al. 2005).

In terms of informants, parent reports on a large study of 226 children with epilepsy and 128 siblings revealed significantly worse social competence scores in the patients than in the siblings (Berg et al. 2007). However, a recent study on the same sample demonstrated a worse quality of life for children with epilepsy than their siblings, based on parent reports, despite similar quality-of-life ratings by the epilepsy patients and their siblings (Baca et al. 2011). These findings underscore the importance of obtaining information from the child as well as from the parent about social skills, an important component of children's quality of life.

Summary

- Frequent poor social competence in children with epilepsy emphasizes the importance of including questions on social skills in the interviews of these children.
- Young children have difficulty acknowledging social problems.
- Corroborative information from parents and other informants is important.
- The poor long-term social outcome of adults with childhood-onset epilepsy highlights the need for early identification and treatment of poor social competence.

ADVERSE DRUG EFFECTS ON COGNITION, LANGUAGE, AND BEHAVIOR

What We Know

- Antiepileptic drugs can have adverse effects on children's behavior and cognition.
- Risk factors for drug-induced behavior problems include:
  - High doses of multiple antiepileptic drugs
  - Psychiatric diagnosis
  - Past negative behavioral response to an antiepileptic drug
  - Family history of psychopathology
- Increased risk for adverse cognitive effects are found in:
  - Children with epilepsy on high doses of multiple antiepileptic drugs
  - Children with epilepsy and learning and/or intellectual disability

Brief Literature Review

A large number of older and newer antiepileptic drugs are used to control seizures in children, and are reviewed in Chu-Shore and Thiele 2010; Hussain and Sankar 2011; and Verrotti et al. 2011. Some of these drugs have adverse effects on cognition, language, and behavior, and children also differ in their sensitivity to these side effects (see review in Loring and Meador 2004). Risk factors for side effects with these antiepileptic drugs in children with epilepsy include high doses of antiepileptic drug polytherapy and prior adverse cognitive or behavioral responses to antiepileptic drugs, as well as poor seizure control (Fastenau et al. 2009) and learning disability (Depositario-Cabacar and Zelleke 2010). Findings in adults suggest that a psychiatric diagnosis (Mula and Monaco 2009), family history of psychopathology (Mula and Monaco F 2009), and rapid titration also increase the likelihood of behavioral adverse effects (Mula et al. 2009).

Effects on cognition include slowing and increased reaction time (see review in Loring and Meador 2004). Impaired word retrieval is described in children treated with topiramate (Gross-Tsur and Shalev 2004). Attentional dysfunction, above and beyond the effects of the illness, is reported in children with absence epilepsy (Table 11–1) treated with valproate compared to those on ethosuximide (Glauser et al. 2010). Behavioral effects such as depression, irritability, hyperactivity, increased anxiety, psychosis, and insomnia have been reported in children treated with phenobarbital, primidone, levetiracetam, gabapentin, felbamate, zonisamide, topiramate, and vigabatrin.

Although typically viewed as a metabolic rather than as a neuropsychiatric adverse effect of the antiepileptic drugs, the weight gain found in children treated with antiepileptic drugs can have a negative impact on children's body image and self-esteem, as well as on the parent–child relationship. Parents who are concerned about their children's weight gain might monitor their eating habits and limit certain foods. The resulting tension further increases the difficulty for both the child and the parents to deal with the illness.

Relevance for the Interview of Young Children with Epilepsy

It is important for the interviewer to determine if a young child with epilepsy who presents for behavior and/or cognitive difficulties is experiencing adverse medication effects. This is a challenge because young children are typically unable to monitor possible adverse effects of medications. At the same time, parents are often concerned that sedation, moodiness, irritability, and any other changes in the behavior and functioning of children with epilepsy are due to their antiepileptic drugs. To deal with this challenge, the interviewer should ask the parents when the reported changes began (in relationship to when the child started the medication or had a dose increase), if they have improved or worsened over time, and what seems to make them worse or mitigate them. The interviewer should also find out whether the child has any of the risk factors for either the cognitive or behavioral side effects of antiepileptic drugs.

Interviewers should be cognizant of the fact that young children who experience cognitive slowing or other difficulties might become frustrated when faced with what they perceive as cognitive challenges. They might act out their frustration with a wide range of symptoms including anger, irritability, crying, sadness, and aggression. Unaware of the cognitive slowing, parents might report that their children have behavior problems.

The following clinical examples demonstrate how to differentiate behavior, cognitive, and linguistic side effects of antiepileptic drugs from other possible causes, such as seizures, the comorbidities associated with epilepsy, and the child's psychosocial response to the illness. The examples highlight the importance of obtaining a careful history of the chronology of the development of the symptoms from the parent, together with a developmentally based interview of the child.

Clinical Examples: Behavior

Psychosis: Olivia, aged 8 years, had a single generalized tonic-clonic seizure (Table 11–1) at age 5 years with no recurrence until four months ago. Despite treatment by her pediatric neurologist with carbamazepine, she continued to have weekly seizures. Olivia's pediatrician has been treating her with methylphenidate for the past six months because the teachers reported problems with attention. The pediatric neurologist crossed over her treatment to levetiracetam over the past six weeks and Olivia has had no subsequent seizures. Her mother brought her to see the pediatric neurologist due to an emergency. Olivia's teacher sent her home from school after calling the mother and reporting that Olivia began talking to herself in class toward the end of the day and that this recurred as soon as school began again. While the mother was talking, Olivia looked like she was talking to herself, with her gaze fixed on the far corner of the room.

Antiepileptic Drugs and Psychosis
INTERVIEWER: *Hi, Olivia. Who are you talking to?*
Olivia looked at her pediatric neurologist and quickly directed her gaze to the corner of the room.

INTERVIEWER: *Please talk a little louder so I can also hear.*

OLIVIA: *Stop saying bad stuff about me.*

INTERVIEWER: *Who is saying these bad things?*

OLIVIA: *The ugly witch.*

INTERVIEWER: *How mean! How do you know she is a witch?*

OLIVIA: *Her pointed black hat,*

INTERVIEWER: *What bad things is she saying?*

OLIVIA: *She's telling the other witch that I am stupid and very bad.*

INTERVIEWER: *Oh that is not nice. She says you are stupid?*

OLIVIA: *And a seizure girl.*

INTERVIEWER: *What bad things does she say you do?*

OLIVIA: *Lie.*

INTERVIEWER: *About what?*

Olivia gets a scared look in her face and runs to her mother (who has been crying while the child has been speaking).

INTERVIEWER: *What are the witches trying to do to you?*

OLIVIA (looking very scared and crying): *Kill me.*

INTERVIEWER: *I am going to help you get rid of those mean witches and make them stop bothering you.*

Olivia's answers to her pediatric neurologist's "Who," "What," and "How" concrete questions indicate that she is experiencing auditory and visual hallucinations. The levetiracetam (Verrotti et al. 2010) and stimulant medications (Mosholder et al. 2009) that she is receiving can both cause psychosis. In Olivia's case, increasing doses of levetiracetam together with the stimulant seem to have triggered an acute psychosis with auditory and visual hallucinations in this child. So her pediatric neurologist decided to decrease the levetiracetam, start valproate, and stop the methylphenidate until resolution of the psychotic symptoms. Although Olivia had been on methylphenidate for several months without overt psychotic symptoms, the pediatric neurologist also planned to do a comprehensive assessment to determine if Olivia meets criteria for ADHD. In addition, the physician intended to find out more from the child about the negative perception she appears to have of herself and her epilepsy based on the content of her auditory hallucinations.

Depression: Otis is a 10-year-old boy with childhood absence seizures and generalized tonic-clonic convulsions (Table 11-1) who has been treated with valproate since age 8 years. About two months ago, the mother reported recurrent staring spells. Despite higher doses of valproate, these events continued. His pediatrician started him on ethosuximide and gradually stopped his valproate. The mother reported no additional seizures but noted marked changes in his behavior. He had outbursts of anger and crying in which he complained that she was criticizing him, and his appetite had decreased.

Antiepileptic Drugs, Depression, and Parent Anxiety

INTERVIEWER: *When I saw you last time, things were not too good with your seizures. How about now?*

OTIS: *Ask my mom, she knows.*

INTERVIEWER: *Do you think you have had any?*

OTIS: *She says I can't go to my friends because I might have a seizure.*

INTERVIEWER: *And then what happens?*

OTIS: *I tell her I am fine.*

INTERVIEWER: *What does your father say about that?*

OTIS: *Nothing.*

INTERVIEWER: *How does that make you feel?*

OTIS: *I also didn't get to go on the class trip.*

INTERVIEWER: *How did that make you feel?*

OTIS: *I don't get to do anything fun.*

INTERVIEWER: *Because?*

OTIS: *She won't let me. She says I might have a seizure.*

INTERVIEWER: *Sounds like you are angry and that your mom is worried about the seizures.*

Otis begins to cry.

INTERVIEWER: *All this really makes you upset.*

OTIS: *She won't listen to me.*

INTERVIEWER: *What else has been bothering you?*

OTIS CRYING: *I might have a seizure and then she won't let me do anything with my friends.*

INTERVIEWER: *Does that mean you think things won't get better?*

OTIS: *I hate my life.*

INTERVIEWER: *You sound really sad. Do you sometimes feel sad or start to cry, and you don't know what is making this happen?*

OTIS NODS YES.

INTERVIEWER: *So when you are so sad and crying, have you ever felt so bad that you wanted to die?*

OTIS: *If she continues to do this, I will.*

INTERVIEWER: *Will what?*

OTIS: *Kill myself.*

INTERVIEWER: *How?*

OTIS: *I don't know.*

INTERVIEWER: *Is this sadness, crying, and wanting to die new feelings or going on for a while?*

OTIS: *Before she wasn't so strict. Now we fight everyday.*

INTERVIEWER: *Is it okay if I talk to your mom and dad about how upset you are about not doing things with your friends?*

OTIS: *She'll get mad at me.*

INTERVIEWER: *How do you know?*

OTIS: *Okay. You can try.*

This child's responses to his pediatrician's developmentally sensitive questions highlight an important diagnostic problem. Although he has symptoms of depression (anger/irritability, crying and sadness, hopelessness, and suicidal ideation), these behaviors also appear to be in response to the restrictions his mother has imposed on his social life because of her concern that he might have a seizure. But, the change in Otis's behavior is recent and parallels increasing ethosuximide doses. Furthermore, frequent seizures that go unnoticed might also make him irritable and moody.

To tease out the role of these different factors, the pediatric neurologist asked the mother how the child's breakthrough seizures have affected the mother's anxiety level. The physician also collected details from both parents on the chronology of changes in Otis's behavior and medication. The mother reported that she has been treated for both anxiety and depression since late adolescence. When Otis was first diagnosed with epilepsy, she became quite anxious and monitored him constantly, but she was relieved when his seizures were controlled, and she thought that he was cured. The occurrence of breakthough seizures "shattered her complacency," and she again began to worry that he might get hurt if he has a seizure when he is not with her. Although Otis's father disagreed with her approach, he did not prevail because the arguments with his wife increased her anxiety. He also thought that Otis's behavior changes were in response to hearing the arguments between his parents.

The mother's detailed diaries on the child's seizures, medications, and behavior helped the pediatric neurologist determine if there was also a possible antiepileptic drug effect. Based on the diaries, Otis first began to be angry and irritable when the ethosuximide was started and the valproate was decreased. During the subsequent crossover, there was a parallel increase in the boy's anger, irritability, crying, and sadness and no subsequent change once he reached the therapeutic ethosuximide dose and stopped the valproate. Given the mother's high anxiety level and the current seizure control, the doctor was reluctant to make any further changes in his antiepileptic drug regimen lest he have a seizure.

Since a family history of psychopathology is a risk factor for an adverse effect of antiepileptic drugs on behavior (and this child has both a family history and current depression), the physician recommended that Otis be treated for depression with a selective serotonin reuptake inhibitor (SSRI) and that he continue on the ethosuximide. In addition, the physician suggested that the mother and child relationship would benefit if the mother received treatment for her anxiety. She also spoke with both parents about the difficulties involved in parenting a child with epilepsy and the developmental advantages and disadvantages of normalizing the child's life despite parental anxiety.

Since the parents were open to all the recommendations, the pediatric neurologist then met with the parents and Otis to summarize for the child what she thought were underlying the problems for him and his parents, the treatment plan for him and for his mother, and how his parents would work together with him to figure out a way that he would be safe, do things with his friends, and they would not be worried.

Anxiety: Madison is a 9-year-old girl, with recent onset complex partial seizures (Table 11-1) that have been treated for the past two months with carbamazepine. Her mother brought her to the pediatric epilepsy clinical nurse specialist for her routine follow-up visit. Madison and her siblings have been staying at an aunt and uncle's house for the past ten days while the parents were out of town on a trip. During this period, Madison had no seizures. But she cried a lot, wanted to call the parents, and frequently asked the aunt and uncle what day the parents were coming back and at what time.

Two hours before their planned arrival, Madison began to worry that something had happened to them. Although this is the first time the parents left her and her siblings for ten days, they had gone on shorter trips before. The mother felt that this was a marked change in the child's behavior. Prior to this trip, Madison had no problems separating from her parents. The mother asked the clinical nurse specialist if these changes in the child's behavior could be due to the carbamazepine.

Antiepileptic Drugs and Anxiety

INTERVIEWER: *Madison, last time I saw you, I gave medicine for your seizures. Is this a good or not so good medicine for you?*

MADISON: *I swallow it quickly so it's okay.*

INTERVIEWER: *And what about seizures?*

MADISON: *I didn't have any at school.*

INTERVIEWER: *That must make you feel good.*

MADISON: *Yes, no more ambulances.*

INTERVIEWER: *How is school going?*

MADISON: *Okay, but I had to get up very early to go to school from my aunt's house.*

INTERVIEWER: *What were you doing at your aunt's house?*

MADISON: *My parents went away.*

INTERVIEWER: *How was that for you?*

MADISON: *I'm glad they're back.*

INTERVIEWER: *Did you not feel comfortable in your aunt and uncle's house?*

MADISON: *I love their house. They have a pool and a big backyard to play in.*

INTERVIEWER: *And how about your cousins?*

MADISON: *They're cool.*

INTERVIEWER: *Did you miss your parents or your house?*

MADISON: *I got to do things my parents don't let me do.*

INTERVIEWER: *Sounds like fun. Some kids think when they are not with their parents that something might happen to them or to their parents. How about you?*

MADISON: *Yeah, a little.*

INTERVIEWER: *Do you think something bad might happen to them or to you?*

MADISON: *Them.*

INTERVIEWER: *Like what?*

MADISON: *Plane accident, car accident.*

INTERVIEWER: *And have you been scared about these accidents since you were little?*

MADISON: *No.*

INTERVIEWER: *So this is a new thing for you.*

Madison nods yes.

INTERVIEWER: *Do you think about this everyday?*

MADISON: *If my mom is there when school is over, that's okay.*

INTERVIEWER: *Oh, so your mom picks you up every day.*

Madison nods yes.

INTERVIEWER: *And if she is late?*

MADISON: *I think she got in an accident.*

INTERVIEWER: *It's not fun to be thinking scary thoughts like that.*

Madison shakes her head no.

The information the nurse practitioner obtained by applying the developmental guidelines to the child's interview ("What" questions, working on making sense of what the child is communicating and her related feelings, expressing empathy for the child's feelings) suggests that Madison had recent onset of separation anxiety symptoms. She does not appear to have experienced a trauma while at her relatives' house. Although separation anxiety symptoms have not been reported in children with epilepsy treated with carbamazepine, the nurse practitioner crossed Madison over to levetiracetam. The child's separation anxiety symptoms subsequently subsided.

Hyperactivity and Irritability: Many antiepileptic drugs can cause ADHD-like symptoms and irritability, particularly when given in high doses and together with other antiepileptic drugs. Although reports on these symptoms are found more typically for phenobarbital and benzodiazepines, both the older antiepileptic drugs (carbamazepine, valproate) and more recently developed anticonvulsants (gabapentin, levetiracetam, felbamate, topiramate) have been associated with these symptoms.

As described earlier, young children do not typically have the insight to monitor changes in their behavior and figure out the causes, or to verbalize them. Parents, teachers, and other adults interacting with the child observe ADHD symptoms and irritability and they, rather than the child, are typically the best informants. The parents can usually confirm if the reported symptoms began in parallel to starting the medication and whether they started or became more pronounced as the dose increased.

When children present with hyperactivity and irritability, it is important to determine if these behaviors reflect tiredness due to the onset of antiepileptic drug treatment, a rapid rather than gradual dose increase, and/or the combined sedative effects of multiple antiepileptic drugs. If parents report that their child has become hyperactive and irritable following any of these medication adjustments, the clinician should ask the parents to describe the child's typical "tired behavior" and how that compares to the current complaint of hyperactivity and irritability. Due to the relatively few drug choices available for the treatment of difficult-to-control seizures, it is important to first rule out sedation as a possible cause of hyperactive and irritable behavior as it can be prevented by slower titration of the drug.

Clinical Examples: Cognition

Antiepileptic Drugs, ADHD, and Cognition: See Box 11–1.

Box 11–1.

ANTIEPILEPTIC DRUGS, ADHD, AND COGNITION

Alyssa, aged 10 years, was diagnosed with childhood absence epilepsy (Table 11–1) at age 5 years. Prior to this diagnosis, she underwent testing because her preschool teacher felt she was hyperactive and inattentive. Her parents did not accept the test results of an ADHD diagnosis. Even though Alyssa's seizures were well controlled on valproate, her parents had great difficulty coming to terms with her diagnosis of epilepsy and the need for medication. From kindergarten through third grade, Alyssa's teachers complained of hyperactivity, inattention, and poor academic achievement. They also noted that

(Continued)

> *(Continued)*
>
> other children did not want to play with her because of her disruptive behavior.
>
> Although the school administration suggested to the parents that she be treated for ADHD, the parents refused. However, they were open to her physician increasing her valproate for what they described as recurrent staring spells.
>
> The child's behavior and learning problems continued, and the parents agreed for her to be put on a stimulant after the school threatened to make her repeat third grade. Treatment with low dose methylphenidate in the morning and at noon targeted her hyperactivity and inattention. However, the child appeared slowed down even after the physician reduced the stimulant to the lowest possible dose. Alyssa continued to have difficulties with all her school subjects and had no friends. The physician gradually discontinued Alyssa's valproate because of seizure control and a normal EEG for the past two years when Alyssa was 10. At Alyssa's follow-up visit three months later, she presented as a happy, calm, and alert child who was proud of her school accomplishments and friends at school. Her beaming parents informed the physician that the child was doing very well at school and that they had also stopped the methylphenidate about one month after discontinuing the valproate because they felt that she did not need it.

Glauser and colleagues (2010) recent prospective drug study demonstrates that valproate can cause inattention in children with absence epilepsy, and Alyssa's preschool "ADHD" diagnosis might have made her more vulnerable to this possible adverse effect. This case highlights the importance of taking into consideration a child's behavior problems prior to the onset of seizures when choosing an antiepileptic drug to minimize possible adverse effects on behavior. Careful monitoring of subsequent changes in the child's behavior and emotions based on parents' report and a developmentally based child interview are needed to help prevent the negative impact of behavioral side effects of antiepileptic drug treatment on a child's academic performance and self-esteem, and how this might impact the child-parent relationship and functioning of the family.

Clinical Examples: Language

Antiepileptic Drugs and Language: Natalie, a 9-year-old girl with complex partial seizures (Table 11–1) from age 7, experienced breakthrough seizures after a seizure-free period of about one year while on levetiracetam. Her mother reported to the pediatric neurologist that, despite the recent addition of topiramate to the levetiracetam, Natalie continues to have a seizure every two weeks.

In addition, Natalie's teacher has complained about the child's schoolwork, particularly in language-related subjects (writing, reading, comprehension). The teacher also noted that Natalie has not been handing in her homework, she participates much less in the class, and she did poorly on a recent vocabulary test. The teacher asked the mother if Natalie was having more seizures at home or was on more medication, because she seemed to be much slower in everything she was doing in class.

The mother had noticed that Natalie seemed to spend more time watching TV in the afternoon and evening, but Natalie would say that she had already finished her homework. Since Natalie had always been a conscientious student, the mother believed her. After the teacher called, the mother spoke with Natalie, who began to cry and say that she hated school. Both parents felt they had been too lenient by relying on Natalie to be in charge of her homework. They decided that one of them would sit with her every day to make sure she did her work, and take it to school every morning.

Antiepileptic Drugs and Language

INTERVIEWER: *Hi, Natalie. You are not looking happy today.*

Natalie gave the interviewer a faint smile.

INTERVIEWER: *What's been making you feel sad?*

NATALIE (slowly): *School.*

INTERVIEWER: *What about school is not good?*

Natalie shrugs her shoulders.

INTERVIEWER: *Is it the work, the kids, or the teacher?*

NATALIE NODS YES.

INTERVIEWER: *Does that mean all of them?*

NATALIE: *A little.*

INTERVIEWER: *So let's talk about the work first. What subject is hard for you?*

NATALIE: *Writing.*

INTERVIEWER: *You used to like writing. Last year you got a prize at school for writing about what it's like to have epilepsy.*

NATALIE (slowly): *No more.*

INTERVIEWER: *What else is hard for you in the class?*

NATALIE (taking a while to respond): *When she asks me.*

INTERVIEWER: *Asks you what?*

NATALIE (thinking a long time and then slowly): *You know.*

INTERVIEWER: *Do you mean the teacher asks you questions?*

Natalie nods yes.

INTERVIEWER: *When she asks questions, what happens?*

NATALIE: *It's hard.*

INTERVIEWER: *Natalie, is it also hard for you to answer my questions?*

Natalie nods yes with tears in her eyes.

INTERVIEWER: *Natalie you usually talk to me with lots of words. Is it hard for the words to come out?*

Natalie nods yes, and starts to sob.

INTERVIEWER: *Do your parents know how hard it is for you?*

Natalie shrugs her shoulders.

INTERVIEWER: *Let me try and explain that to them now, okay?*

Natalie nods yes.

After conducting this developmentally sensitive interview using mainly "What" questions and clarification of the emotions the child expressed during the interview, the pediatric neurologist met with the parents and asked them if they had noticed that Natalie is talking less. They said that now that the doctor mentioned it, she has not been her usual talkative self and they thought that she was having a hard time dealing with the fact that she was still having seizures. The physician reminded them that when he added topiramate to the levetiracetam, he had told the parents that some children have difficulties with language when they are given topiramate. At the time, he had explained that this mainly involves the child's ability to retrieve words or come up with the words he/she needs. He then added that Natalie seemed to be having difficulty finding the words she needs, she was speaking and thinking slower, and she also was sad. He thought that the sadness might be due to the topiramate and/or the difficulties Natalie has experienced with her schoolwork.

The parents felt bad that they had forgotten about the possible language side effect of topiramate, and attributed it to their being focused on Natalie's seizures. Together with the parents, the pediatric neurologist then explained to Natalie that the medicine had caused her difficulties, and that she would regain her language skills and be able to do schoolwork like before once they stop the topiramate, and started another drug to control her seizures.

SUMMARY
- A developmentally oriented interview of the young child with epilepsy helps differentiate adverse antiepileptic drug effects from other causes for problems with behavior, cognition, and language.
- Parents are important informants on the chronology of the development of adverse effects involving behavior and cognition if the child has risk factors for these side effects.
- It is important to rule out drug-induced sedation as a possible cause for hyperactivity and irritability.

DIFFERENTIATING BETWEEN SEIZURES AND BEHAVIOR/EMOTIONAL SYMPTOMS

The Challenge

Before (preictal), during (ictal), and after a seizure (postictal), the child's cognitive, linguistic, and behavioral/emotional functioning, as well as level of consciousness, might be wholly or partially impaired. In addition, the clinical manifestations of some seizures might mimic psychiatric symptoms. Although ongoing epileptic discharges on the EEG might not be associated with an observable seizure, they might impact cognition, language, and behavior. Understanding how seizures affect a child's functioning is essential for the comprehensive assessment of the child with epilepsy. To do this, the clinician needs to take a careful seizure history from the parents, as most seizures do not occur in the clinician's office. Young children are not a valid source of information on their seizures due to the change in state of consciousness during a seizure.

In terms of preictal phenomena, parents often sense that their child will have a seizure from a change in the child's behavior involving increased irritability. Tiredness and/or confusion are the main postictal manifestations. As described below, several ictal phenomena may mimic psychiatric symptoms, depending on the type of seizure. When sensory (hallucination, illusion, déjà phenomena) and psychic phenomena (fear, dread) precede a generalized tonic-clinic seizure, as in an aura (Table 11–1), it is easy to differentiate them from psychiatric symptoms. However, if these phenomena occur alone without being followed by a full-blown seizure (whether a generalized tonic-clonic or a complex partial seizure), this differentiation might be more challenging.

Three main features distinguish seizure manifestations from psychiatric symptoms. First, seizure-related behaviors are typically stereotyped and look the same in each seizure. Second, they are brief and last 1–2 minutes. Third, the child is unaware of the seizure and does not remember it unless it is an isolated aura.

Regarding types of seizures, primary generalized epilepsy with generalized tonic-clonic seizures, also known as grand mal (Table 11–1), are clearly differentiated from psychiatric symptoms. In some cases, however, what appear to be grand mal seizures might, in fact, be non-epileptic seizures (NES) (seizure-like phenomena that are not epileptic seizures). In addition to a lack of evidence for epileptic activity during one of these events on video-EEG, the presence of a specific psychiatric profile helps differentiate NES from primary generalized and other types of seizures as described in chapter 8 on somatization and summarized in Loddenkemper and Wyllie 2009 and Caplan and Plioplys 2009.

The momentary stare or cessation of ongoing activity of children with absence epilepsy (Table 11–1) without falling or subsequent tiredness or confusion might be perceived as the distractibility or inattention of a child with ADHD. Observation of a child very briefly zoning in and out or appearing to lose attention during the clinical assessment should suggest a need for EEG with hyperventilation to rule out childhood absence epilepsy.

The seizures of children with focal epilepsy (Table 11–1) originating in the temporal lobe can include sensory phenomena such as a rising unpleasant epigastric (upper middle region of the abdomen) sensation (often associated with fear), hallucinations, visual illusions, forced thinking, and illusion of familiarity involving vision (déjà vu) and hearing (déjà entendu). Complex partial seizures of temporal origin present with a blank stare, lip smacking or chewing (oroalimentary automatisms), clumsy hand movements (fumbling, touching, or pulling clothes), followed by postictal confusion, tiredness, and amnesia (no memory for what was experienced during a seizure). As previously mentioned, the brevity of these phenomena, their stereotypic presentation, and the presence of postictal changes help differentiate these behavioral symptoms from those of psychiatric disorders.

Children with focal epilepsy, whose seizures start in the frontal lobe, present with inattention, hyperactivity, impulsivity, aggression, and mood instability (laughing, crying) and more rarely with psychotic symptoms (see review in Braakman et al. 2011). They are sometimes given a psychiatric rather than a neurological diagnosis, because their behavioral symptoms might appear to be continuous as they can occur during, after, or between seizures, and the EEG might not show epileptic activity (focal frontal lobe spikes or sharp waves).

Although relatively rare, the autonomic symptoms of children with occipital epilepsy should be considered in young children who present with nausea and vomiting, as well as other autonomic symptoms (see Table 10–1 in chapter 10). Similarly, the visual symptoms of later onset occipital epilepsy (Gastaut syndrome) (Kivity et al.

2000), hallucinations and illusions, need to be differentiated from psychosis (see chapter 7). These visual symptoms are brief and followed by eye and head deviation, vomiting, loss of consciousness, and seizures involving one side of the body with or without a headache. The visual hallucinations of Gastaut syndrome are typically stereotyped and elemental (colors, lines, shapes) but can also be complex (visual scenes). Visual illusions, in which things are seen as small (micropsia), and blindness also occur during these seizures. In contrast, children with psychosis have complex visual hallucinations that change in their form and content and are not stereotyped. Psychotic children also have auditory hallucinations, which are not found in Gastaut syndrome.

Clinical Examples

Anxiety vs. Seizures: Vince, a 5-year-old boy, was seen by a child psychiatrist because of separation anxiety disorder and school phobia, and he has been treated with a selective serotonin reuptake inhibitor (SSRI). Despite this treatment, he began shadowing his mother and following her everywhere in the house including into the shower. If she protested, he had a temper tantrum and cried inconsolably. The frequency of crying episodes increased and they now occur even when he is with his mother. Clinging to his mother, Vince is being seen by a pediatric neurologist.

Anxiety vs. Seizure

INTERVIEWER: *Hi, Vince. I am going to ask your mother a few questions about you and I need you to help me. Sometimes moms don't know everything about their kids. So can you listen real carefully to what she tells me? If she says something that is not quite right, please tell me.*

Vince makes eye contact and nods yes.

INTERVIEWER: *Please tell me what happened from the beginning, when Vince first started to get scared.*

MOTHER: *About two months ago, he cried out and came running to me one day looking very fearful. I asked him what was wrong and he said, "It's scary." About two weeks later, this happened again, and he answered, "It can get me" when I asked him what was wrong. He lay down on the couch and watched television. This started to happen every evening, and when I tried to find out what he was scared of, he would cry and scream and then lie down in a fetal position and go to sleep. So I took him to a child psychiatrist who said he was anxious and gave him Zoloft. But he became more and more scared every day, refused to go to school, and wouldn't let me go to work. So the psychiatrist increased his medication dose. Vince then would not separate from me for a second, and I am now with him 24/7. I don't see any improvement in his condition.*

The mother's eyes welled up with tears, and Vince hugged her.

VINCE: *Don't cry mommy.*

INTERVIEWER: *Vince it sounds like something has been scaring you. We need to figure out what it is, and make it go far away. Should we try doing that?*

Vince looks at the doctor and nods yes.

INTERVIEWER: *Can you try giving me a hint about this very scary thing?*

Vince nods yes.

INTERVIEWER: *Is it something that makes a noise or a sound?*

VINCE: *No.*

INTERVIEWER: *Does it look scary?*

VINCE: *Yes.*

INTERVIEWER: *Is it a person?*

Vince shakes his head no.

INTERVIEWER: *Does it look like an animal?*

Vince shakes his head no.

INTERVIEWER: *What about a monster or something like a monster?*

Vince shakes his head no.

INTERVIEWER: *Well I am not doing a very good job guessing. Maybe you can help me by drawing what it looks like.*

Vince nods yes.

Interviewer gives him paper and pencil and he draws a detailed geometric structure.

INTERVIEWER: *Oh, that does look scary. Is that how it looks every time or just sometimes?*

VINCE: *Every time.*

INTERVIEWER: *And when you can see it, is there anything you can do to make it go away?*

Vince shakes his head no, and suddenly grabs his mother really hard with a fixed look in his eyes that immediately passes.

INTERVIEWER: *Vince, what just happened?*

Vince falls asleep on his mother's lap.

On the assumption that Vince was experiencing a seizure presenting with a visual hallucination of a fixed geometric figure, followed by postictal tiredness, he underwent an EEG. The EEG demonstrated a right occipital epileptic focus. The child was started on an antiepileptic drug with resolution of his separation anxiety symptoms and school phobia as he achieved seizure control.

Finally, it is important to note that Vince was the essential source for the information that lead to the definitive diagnosis, treatment, and resolution of his symptoms. The physician's empathy for the child's fear, concrete action-based questions that helped the child describe how he was experiencing the symptoms, and use of drawing revealed that Vince was experiencing visual hallucination.

Dizziness, Car Accident, Anxiety, or Seizures: Nina, aged 10 years, had her fist seizure at age 3 years while taking a bath, and was saved by her mother from drowning in the bath because she knew CPR. Her complex partial seizures (Table 11–1) were well controlled until age 8 years when she had breakthrough seizures. Subsequent dose changes and the addition of a second antiepileptic drug resulted in seizure control. She comes today to the pediatric epilepsy nurse practitioner with what the mother describes as episodes of dizziness or not feeling well during the past month.

About three weeks ago, Nina was in a car accident during which her head hit the back seat of her grandmother's car without loss of consciousness. Nina's mother has always made sure that Nina led a "normal" life, and was planning to send her to her first summer sleepaway hip-hop camp. The nurse practitioner has the following conversation with Nina to find out if she is aware of the dizziness reported by the mother, if she has any neurological or emotional symptoms following the car accident, and if she is anxious about the upcoming sleepaway camp.

Dizziness, Trauma, Anxiety, or Seizures

INTERVIEWER: *Nina, how have you been feeling since I last saw you?*

NINA: *Fine.*

INTERVIEWER: *Have any parts of you, your body or your head, not been feeling good?*

NINA: *I got hit on the head in my grandmother's car.*

INTERVIEWER: *Oh wow, did she have an accident?*

NINA: *Yes, but I only got hit on the head.*

INTERVIEWER: *I bet that hurt and was scary.*

NINA: *No, it wasn't a big deal.*

INTERVIEWER: *Did the car get messed up?*

NINA: *No, just a big scratch.*

INTERVIEWER: *And is your grandmother okay?*

NINA: *Yes, but she feels bad that I was in the accident and hurt my head.*

INTERVIEWER: *I can understand that. I know you both are very close.*

NINA: *Yes, she's the best.*

INTERVIEWER: *So when you stand or sit or do hip-hop, which I know you love, do your head and other parts of you feel okay?*

NINA: *Yeah.*

INTERVIEWER: *What will you be doing in the summer?*

NINA: *Sleepaway camp.*

INTERVIEWER: *This your first time, right?*

NINA: *Yes, and for three whole weeks.*

INTERVIEWER: *Is that a long or a short time to be away from home?*

NINA: *Not short.*

INTERVIEWER: *You know a lot of kids get scared and worry about going to sleepaway camp. How about you?*

NINA: *I will miss my dog.*

INTERVIEWER: *Who takes care of him?*

NINA: *Me, but my sister when I am gone.*

INTERVIEWER: *Do you worry that she might not do a good job?*

NINA: *No, but my dog will really miss me.*

INTERVIEWER: *Sounds like you will also miss your dog and home.*

NINA: *Yes, but I will be glad to get a break from my sister.*

INTERVIEWER: *How about your parents?*

NINA: *I guess I might miss them a little.*

INTERVIEWER: *You said you would worry about your dog. What else is scary about going to camp?*

NINA: *We go swimming every day. My mom will speak to the lifeguards about my epilepsy and make sure they watch me all the time.*

INTERVIEWER: *Are you also scared of swimming when you are not at camp?*

NINA: *No, because my mom is always there to make sure I don't have a seizure while I'm in the water.*

INTERVIEWER: *And she will make sure that the lifeguards do the same thing.*

NINA: *I guess so.*

INTERVIEWER: *It's tough worrying about these seizures.*

NINA: *Yeah, I had one when I was 3 in the bath.*

INTERVIEWER: *Oh, wow, scary, and what happened then?*

NINA: *I would have drowned, but my mom did CPR.*

INTERVIEWER: *You know lifeguards also know how to do CPR.*

NINA: *That's what my parents say.*

INTERVIEWER: *So even though you are a little scared, it helps to know that the life-guards will watch you carefully and that they know CPR.*

NINA: *I guess camp will be a lot of fun.*

To clarify the mother's report about Nina's dizziness, the nurse practitioner asked Nina "What" questions to rule out seizures by finding out if Nina was aware of these episodes. Using this technique and empathy, she also determined if the head trauma was related to the dizziness and if Nina had posttraumatic stress symptoms following the car accident. The nurse practitioner's subsequent "What" questions were aimed at finding out if the dizziness was an expression of Nina's concerns about having a seizure while swimming when at summer camp. The child did not appear to have any emotional after effects of the car accident and had coping tools to deal with the fear that she might have a seizure at camp. Since she did not report dizziness, this suggests that she was unaware of the "dizziness episodes."

While walking Nina out to the waiting room to her mother, Nina suddenly stopped, had a fixed gaze, and became pale. This lasted a second. The mother who had observed the episode asked Nina if she had just felt dizzy. Nina slowly answered, "Yes," but it took about ten minutes until she seemed to be back on her baseline behavior. The incident in the waiting room suggested that she was experiencing a seizure. Subsequent adjustment of her antiepileptic drug regimen lead to seizure control. This case highlights the importance of obtaining information both from the child and the parent to tease out the nature of the presenting problem. More specifically, the mother's incorrect interpretation of the child's episode as dizziness underscores the value of the clinical interview of the child.

SUMMARY

- Some manifestations of seizures mimic behavior and emotional symptoms and vice versa.
- Since most seizures do not occur in the doctor's office, collecting detailed information from both the parents and the child is essential to differentiate seizures from behavior/emotional symptoms.
- The following features of seizures help make this differentiation:
  - Sudden onset and offset
  - Short duration
  - Stereotyped
  - Tiredness, sleep, confusion, or amnesia (but not in childhood absence epilepsy) following the seizure

CONCLUSIONS ON THE BIOLOGICAL ASPECTS OF PEDIATRIC EPILEPSY

This chapter has exposed the reader to the complex impact of the biological variables of epilepsy (seizure variables including antiepileptic drugs, underlying brain structure/function, family history of seizures and psychopathology) on the behavior, cognition, language, and social skills of children with epilepsy. The clinical examples underscore the important role the child has in providing the interviewer with the information needed to tease out which of the multiple factors underlie the presenting problem for which the child is brought to a pediatric professional. These examples also expose the reader to techniques that apply the developmental guidelines to the comprehensive assessment of the impact of the illness on the child's functioning. In the next chapter the reader will become familiar with the psychosocial aspects of the illness and how they contribute to the child's functioning.

REFERENCES

Akman CI (2011). Nonconvulsive status epilepticus and continuous spike and slow wave of sleep in children. *Semin Pediatr Neurol* 17: 155–162.

Aldenkamp A, Alpherts WCJ, De Bruine-Seeder D, and Dekker MJA (1990). Test–retest variability in children with epilepsy—a comparison of WISC-R profiles. *Epilepsy Res* 7: 165–172.

Aldenkamp A, Weber B, Overweg-Plandsoen WC, Reijs R, and van Mil S (2005). Educational underachievement in children with epilepsy: A model to predict the effects of epilepsy on educational achievement. *J Child Neurol* 20: 175–180.

Austin JK, Dunn DW, Caffrey HM, Perkins SM, Harezlak J, and Rose DF (2002). Recurrent seizures and behavior problems in children with first recognized seizures: A prospective study. *Epilepsia* 43: 1564–1573.

Austin JK, Perkins SM, Johnson CS, Fastenau PS, Byars AW, DeGrauw TJ, and Dunn DW (2010). Self-esteem and symptoms of depression in children with seizures: Relationships with neuropsychological functioning and family variables over time. *Epilepsia* 51: 2074–2083.

Austin JK, Perkins SM, Johnson CS, Fastenau PS, Byars AW, deGrauw TJ, and Dunn DW (2011). Behavior problems in children at time of first recognized seizure and changes over the following 3 years. *Epilepsy Behav* 21: 373–381.

Baca C, Vickrey BG, Caplan R, Vassar D, and Berg AT (2011). Psychiatric and medical comorbidity and quality of life outcomes in childhood-onset epilepsy. *Pediatrics* 128: 1532–1543.

Baker BL, Neece CL, Fenning RM, Crnic KA, and Blacher J (2010). Mental disorders in five-year-old children with or without developmental delay: Focus on ADHD. *J Clin Child Adolesc Psychol* 39: 492–505.

Barnes AJ, Eisenberg ME, and Resnick MD (2010). Suicide and self-injury among children and youth with chronic health conditions. *Pediatrics* 125: 889–895.

Barrera M, Schulte F, and Spiegler B (2008). Factors influencing depressive symptoms of children treated for a brain tumor. *J Psychosoc Oncol* 26: 1–16.

Berg A, Langfitt JT, Testa FM, Levy SR, Dimario F, Westerveld M, and Kulas J (2008). Global cognitive function in children with epilepsy: A community-based study. *Epilepsia* 49: 608–614.

Berg A, Vickrey BG, Testa FM, Levy SR, Shinnar S, and DiMario F (2007). Behavior and social competency in idiopathic and cryptogenic childhood epilepsy. *Dev Med Child Neurol* 49: 487–492.

Berg AT, Hesdorffer DC, and Zelko FAJ (2011). Special education participation in children with epilepsy: What does it reflect? *Epilepsy Behav* 22: 336–341.

Berry-Kravis E, Raspa M, Loggin-Hester L, Bishop E, Holiday D, and Bailey DB (2010). Seizures in fragile X syndrome: Characteristics and comorbid diagnoses. *Am J Intellect Dev Disabil* 115: 461–472.

Braakman HMH, Vaessen MJ, Hofman PAM, Debeij-van Hall MHJA, Backes WH, Vles JSH, and Aldenkamp AP (2011). Cognitive and behavioral complications of frontal lobe epilepsy in children: A review of the literature. *Epilepsia* 52: 849–856.

Brownlie EB, Beitchman J, Escobar M, Young A, Atkinson L, Johnson C, Wilson B, and Douglas L (2004). Early language impairment and young adult delinquent and aggressive behavior. *J Abnorm Child Psychol* 32: 453–467.

Buelow J, Austin J, Perkins S, Shen J, Dunn D, and Fastenau P (2003). Behavior and mental health problems in children with epilepsy and low IQ. *Dev Med Child Neurol* 45: 683–692.

Byars A, deGrauw TJ, Johnson CS, Fastenau PS, Perkins SM, Egelhoff JC, Kalnin A, Dunn DW, and Austin JK (2007). The association of MRI findings and neuropsychological functioning after the first recognized seizure. *Epilepsia* 48: 1067–1074.

Camfield C and Camfield PR (2009). Juvenile myoclonic epilepsy 25 years after seizure onset: A population-based study *Neurology* 73: 1041–1045.

Camfield PR (2011). Definition and natural history of Lennox-Gastaut syndrome. *Epilepsia* 52: 3–9.

Caplan R (2010). Pediatric epilepsy: A developmental neuropsychiatric disorder. In: *Epilepsy: Mechanisms, Models, and Translational Perspectives*, J Rho, R Sankar, and J Cavazos (eds.). Boca Raton, FL.: RC Press—Taylor & Francis Group, 535–549.

Caplan R (in press). Depressive disorders in children and adolescents with neurological disorders. In: *Depression in Neurologic Disorders*, A Kanner (ed.). Oxford, UK: John Wiley & Sons.

Caplan R, Guthrie D, Komo S, Siddarth P, Chayasirisobhon S, Kornblum H, and Sankar R (2002). Social communication in pediatric epilepsy. *J Child Psychol Psychiatry* 43: 245–253.

Caplan R, Levitt J, Siddarth P, Taylor J, Daley M, Wu KN, Gurbani S, Shields WD, and Sankar R (2008a). Thought disorder and fronto-temporal volumes in pediatric epilepsy. *Epilepsy Behav* 13: 593–599.

Caplan R, Levitt JG, Siddarth P, Wu KW, Gurbani S, Donald WD, and Sankar R (2009a). Language and fronto-temporal volumes in pediatric epilepsy. *Epilepsy Behav* 50: 2466–2472.

Caplan R and Plioplys S (2009). Psychiatric features of children with psychogenic nonepileptic seizures. In: *Gates & Rowan's Non-epileptic Seizure*, 3rd Ed, S Schachter and W LaFrance (eds.). Cambridge, UK: Cambridge University Press.

Caplan R, Sagun J, Siddarth P, Gurbani S, Koh S, Gowrinathan R, and Sankar R (2005a). Social competence in pediatric epilepsy: Insights into underlying mechanisms. *Epilepsy Behav* 6: 218–228.

Caplan R, Siddarth P, Gurbani S, Hanson R, Sankar R, and Shields WD (2005b). Depression and anxiety disorders in pediatric epilepsy. *Epilepsia* 46: 720–730.

Caplan R, Siddarth P, Gurbani S, Lanphier E, Koh S, and Sankar R (2006). Thought disorder: A developmental disability in pediatric epilepsy. *Epilepsy Behav* 8: 726–735.

Caplan R, Siddarth P, Gurbani S, Ott D, Sankar R, and Shields WD (2004). Psychopathology in pediatric complex partial seizures: Seizure-related, cognitive, and linguistic variables. *Epilepsia* 45: 1273–1286.

Caplan R, Siddarth P, and Gurbani SR (2011). Social competence in pediatric epilepsy. Annual Meeting of American Academy of Child and Adolescent Psychiatry, Toronto, Canada.

Caplan R, Siddarth P, Stahl L, Lanphier E, Vona P, Gurbani S, Koh S, Sankar R, and Shields WD (2008b). Childhood absence epilepsy: Behavioral, cognitive, and linguistic comorbidities. *Epilepsia* 49: 1838–1846.

Caplan R, Siddarth P, Vona P, Stahl L, Bailey CE, Gurbani S, Sankar R, and Donald WD (2009b). Language in pediatric epilepsy *Epilepsia* 50 2397–2407.

Catts H, Fey ME, Tomblin JB, and Zhang X (2002). Longitudinal investigation of reading outcomes in children with language impairments. *J Speech Lang Hear Res* 45: 1142–1157.

Chu-Shore CJ, and Thiele EA (2010). New drugs for pediatric epilepsy. *Semin Pediatr Neurol* 17: 214–223.

Corapci F, Smith J, and Lozoff B (2006). The role of verbal competence and multiple risk on the internalizing behavior problems of Costa Rican youth. *Ann NY Acad Sci* 1094: 278–281.

Daley M, Levitt J, Siddarth P, Mormino E, Hojatkashani C, Gurbani S, Shields WD, Sankar R, Toga A, and Caplan R (2007). Frontal and temporal volumes in children with complex partial seizures. *Epilepsy Behav* 10: 470–476.

De Bildt A, Sytema S, Kraijer D and Minderaa R (2005). Prevalence of pervasive developmental disorders in children and adolescents with mental retardation. *J Child Psychol Psychiatry* 46: 275–286.

Debiais S, Tuller L, Barthez M-A, Monjauze C, Khomsi A, Praline J, De Toffol B, Autret A, Barthelemy C, and Hommet C (2007). Epilepsy and language development: The Continuous Spike-Waves during Slow Sleep Syndrome. *Epilepsia* 48: 1104–1110.

Depositario-Cabacar DF, and Zelleke TG (2010). Treatment of epilepsy in children with developmental disabilities. *Dev Disabil Res Rev* 16: 239–247.

Drewel E and Caplan R (2007). Social difficulties in children with epilepsy: Review and treatment recommendations. *Expert Rev Neurother* 7: 865–873.

Drewel EH, Bell DJ, and Austin JK (2009). Peer difficulties in children with epilepsy: Association with seizure, neuropsychological, academic, and behavioral Variables. *Child Neuropsychol* 15: 305–320.

Dunn DW, Johnson CS, Perkins SM, Fastenau PS, Byars AW, deGrauw TJ, and Austin JK (2010). Academic problems in children with seizures: Relationships with neuropsychological functioning and family variables during the 3 years after onset. *Epilepsy Behav* 19: 455–461.

Ebus S, Overvliet GM, Arends JBAM, and Aldenkamp AP (2011). Reading performance in children with rolandic epilepsy correlates with nocturnal epileptiform activity, but not with epileptiform activity while awake. *Epilepsy Behav* 22: 518–522.

Elliott IM, Lach L, and Smith ML (2005). I just want to be normal: A qualitative study exploring how children and adolescents view the impact of intractable epilepsy on their quality of life. *Epilepsy Behav* 7: 664–678.

Fastenau PS, Johnson CS, Perkins SM, Byars AW, deGrauw TJ, Austin JK, and Dunn DW (2009). Neuropsychological status at seizure onset in children: Risk factors for early cognitive deficits. *Neurology* 73: 526–534.

Fastenau PS, Shen J, Dunn DW, Perkins SM, Hermann BP, and Austin JK (2004). Neuropsychological predictors of academic underachievement in pediatric epilepsy: Moderating roles of demographic, seizure, and psychosocial variables. *Epilepsia* 45: 1261–1272.

Ferro M and Speechley KN (2009). Depressive symptoms among mothers of children with epilepsy: A review of prevalence, associated factors, and impact on children. *Epilepsia* 50: 2344–2354.

Ferro MA, Avison WR, Karen Campbell M, and Speechley KN (2011). The impact of maternal depressive symptoms on health-related quality of life in children with epilepsy: A prospective study of family environment as mediators and moderators. *Epilepsia* 52: 316–325.

Glauser TA, Cnaan A, Shinnar S, Hirtz DG, Dlugos D, Masur D, Clark PO, Capparelli EV, and Adamson PC (2010). Ethosuximide, valproic acid, and lamotrigine in childhood absence epilepsy. *N Engl J Med* 362: 790–799.

Gonzalez-Heydrich J, Whitney J, Waber D, Forbes P, Hsin O, Faraone SV, Dodds A, Rao S, Mrakotsky C, MacMillan C, DeMaso DR, de Moor C, Torres A, Bourgeois B, and Biederman J (2010). Adaptive phase I study of OROS methylphenidate treatment of attention deficit hyperactivity disorder with epilepsy. *Epilepsy Behav* 18: 229–237.

Goretti B, Ghezzi A, Portaccio E, Lori S, Zipoli V, Razzolini L, Moiola L, Falautano M, De Caro MF, Viterbo R, Patti F, Vecchio R, Pozzilli C, Bianchi V, Roscio M, Comi G, Trojano M, and Amato MP (2010). Psychosocial issue in children and adolescents with multiple sclerosis. *Neurol Sci* 31: 467–470.

Gross-Tsur V, and Shalev RS (2004). Reversible language regression as an adverse effect of topiramate treatment in children. *Neurology* 62: 299–300.

Hamiwka L Jones JE, Salpekar J and Caplan R (2011a). Child psychiatry: Special edition on the future of clinical epilepsy research. *Epilepsy Behav* 22: 38–46.

Hamiwka LD (2011). Social functioning among children with epilepsy. Annual Meeting of the American Academy of Child and Adolescent Psychiatry, Toronto, Montreal.

Hamiwka LD, Hamiwka LA, Sherman EMS, and Wirrell E (2011b). Social skills in children with epilepsy: How do they compare to healthy and chronic disease controls? *Epilepsy Behav* 21: 238–241.

Hamiwka LD, Yu CG, Hamiwka LA, Sherman EMS, Anderson B, and Wirrell E (2009). Are children with epilepsy at greater risk for bullying than their peers? Epilepsy Behav 15: 500–505.

Hanssen-Bauer K, Heyerdahl S, and Eriksson AS (2010). Mental health problems in children and adolescents referred to a national epilepsy center. *Epilepsy Behav* 20: 255–262.

Henkin Y, Kishon-Rabin L, Pratt H, Kivity S, Sadeh M, and Gadoth N (2003). Linguistic processing in idiopathic generalized epilepsy: An auditory event-related potential study. *Epilepsia* 44: 1207–1217.

Hermann B, Jones J, Sheth R, Dow C, Koehn M, and Seidenberg M (2006). Children with new-onset epilepsy: Neuropsychological status and brain structure. *Brain* 129: 2609–2619.

Hermann B, Jones JE, Sheth R, Koehn M, Becker T, Fine J, Allen CA, and Seidenberg M (2008). Growing up with epilepsy: A two-year investigation of cognitive development in children with new onset epilepsy. *Epilepsia* 49: 1847–1858.

Hesdorffer D, Caplan R, and Berg A (2012). Familial clustering of epilepsy and behavioral disorders: Evidence for a shared genetic basis. *Epilepsia* 53: 301–307.

Hoie B, Mykletun A, Sommerfelt K, Bjornaes H, Skeidsvol H, and Waaler PE (2005). Seizure-related factors and non-verbal intelligence in children with epilepsy. A population-based study from Western Norway. *Seizure* 14: 223–231.

Hughes JR (2011). A review of the relationships between Landau–Kleffner syndrome, electrical status epilepticus during sleep, and continuous spike–waves during sleep. *Epilepsy Behav* 20: 247–253.

Hussain S and Sankar R (2011). Pharmacologic treatment of intractable epilepsy in children: A syndrome-based approach. *Semin Pediat Neurol* 18: 171–178.

Im-Bolter N and Cohen N (2007). Language impairment and psychiatric comorbidity. *Pediatr Clin North Am* 54: 525–542.

Johnson CJ, Beitchman JH, and Brownlie EB (2010). Twenty-year follow-up of children with and without speech-language impairments: Family, educational, occupational, and quality of life outcomes. *Am J Speech Lang Pathol* 19: 51–65.

Jones J, Watson R, Sheth R, Caplan R, Koehn M, Seidenberg M, and Hermann B (2007). Psychiatric comorbidity in children with new onset epilepsy. *Dev Med Child Neurol* 49: 493–497.

Jones JE, Jackson D, Kessler A, Caplan R, and Hermann B (2011). A 2-year prospective study of DSM-IV axis I disorders in children with recent onset epilepsy Annual Meeting of American Academy of Child and Adolescent Psychiatry, Toronto, Canada.

Jones JE, Siddarth P, Gurbani S, Shields WD, and Caplan R (2010). Cognition, academic achievement, language, and psychopathology in pediatric chronic epilepsy: Short-term outcomes. *Epilepsy Behav* 18: 211–217.

Kavros P, Clarke T, Strug LJ, Halperin JM, Dorta NJ, and Pal DK (2008). Attention impairment in rolandic epilepsy: Systematic review. *Epilepsia* 49: 1570–1580.

Kelley SA and Kossoff EH (2011). Doose syndrome (myoclonic–astatic epilepsy): 40 years of progress. *Dev Med Child Neurol* 52: 988–993.

Kernan CL, Asarnow R, Siddarth P, Gurbani S, Lanphier EK, Sankar R, and Caplan R. Neurocognitive profiles in children with epilepsy (revise and resubmit).

Killory BD, Bai X, Negishi M, Vega C, Spann MN, Vestal M, Guo J, Berman R, Danielson N, Trejo J, Shisler D, Novotny Jr EJ, Constable RT, and Blumenfeld H (2011). Impaired attention and network connectivity in childhood absence epilepsy. *Neuroimage* 56: 2209–2217.

Kivity S, Ephraim T, Weitz R, and Tamir A (2000). Childhood epilepsy with occipital paroxysms: Clinical variants in134 patients. *Epilepsia* 41: 1522–1533.

Lenroot RK and Giedd J (2006). Brain development in children and adolescents: Insights from anatomical magnetic resonance imaging. *Neurosci Biobehav Rev* 30: 718.

Loddenkemper T, Fernández IS, and Peters JM (2011). Continuous spike and waves during sleep and electrical status epilepticus in sleep. *J Clin Neurophysiol* 28: 154–164.

Loddenkemper T and Wyllie E (2009). Diagnostic issues in children. In: *Gates and Rowan Nonepileptic Seizures*, 3rd Ed, SC Schachter and JW Curt LaFrance (eds.). Cambridge, UK: Cambridge University Press, 110–120.

Loring DW and Meador KJ (2004). Cognitive side effects of antiepileptic drugs in children. *Neurology* 62: 872–877.

Lundy S, Silva, GE, Kaemingk KL, Goodwin JL, and Quan SF (2010). Cognitive functioning and academic performance in elementary school children with anxious/depressed and withdrawn symptoms. *Open Pediatr Med Journal* 4: 1–9.

Mitchell W, Chavez JM, Lee H, and Guzman BL (1991). Academic underachievement in children with epilepsy. *J Child Neurol* 6: 65–72.

Mosholder AD, Gelperin K, Hammad TA, Phelan K, and Johann-Liang R (2009). Hallucinations and other psychotic symptoms associated with the use of attention-deficit/hyperactivity disorder drugs in children. *Pediatrics* 123: 611–616.

Mula M, Hesdorffer DC, Trimble M, and Sander JW (2009). The role of titration schedule of topiramate for the development of depression in patients with epilepsy. *Epilepsia* 50: 1072–1076.

Mula M and Monaco F (2009). Antiepileptic drugs and psychopathology of epilepsy: An update. *Epileptic Disord* 11: 1–9.

Muscara F, Catroppa C, Eren S, and Anderson V (2009). The impact of injury severity on long-term social outcome following paediatric traumatic brain injury. *Neuropsychol Rehabil* 19: 541–561.

Nickels K and Wirrell E (2008). Electrical status epilepticus in sleep. *Semin Pediatr Neurol* 15: 50–60.

Noll R, Reiter-Purtill J, Moore BD, Schorry EK, Lovell AM, Vannatta K, and Gerhardt CA (2007). Social, emotional, and behavioral functioning of children with NF1. *Amer J Medical Genet A* 143: 2261–2273.

O'Neill J, Seese R, Hudkins M, Siddarth P, Levitt J, Tseng PB, Wu KN, Gurbani S, Shields WD, and Caplan R (2011). 1H MRSI and social communication deficits in pediatric complex partial seizures. *Epilepsia* 52: 1705–1714.

Oostrom K, Schouten A, Kruitwagen CL, Peters AC, Jennekens-Schinkel A, and the Dutch Study Group of Epilepsy in Childhood (DuSECH) (2001). Epilepsy-related ambiguity in rating the child behavior checklist and the teacher's report form. *Epileptic Disord* 3: 39–45.

Oostrom K, Smeets-Schouten A, Kruitwagen CL, Peters AC, Jennekens-Schinkel A, and the Dutch Study Group of Epilepsy in Childhood (2003). Not only a matter of epilepsy: Early problems of cognition and behavior in children with "epilepsy only"—a prospective, longitudinal, controlled study starting at diagnosis. *Pediatrics* 112: 1338–1344.

Oostrom K, van Teeseling H, Smeets-Schouten A, Peters A, Jennekens-Schinkel A, and the Dutch Study of Epilepsy in Childhood (2005). Three to four years after diagnosis: Cognition and behaviour in children with "epilepsy only." A prospective, controlled study. *Brain* 128: 1546–1555.

Ott D, Siddarth P, Gurbani S, Koh S, Tournay A, Shields WD, and Caplan R (2003). Behavioral disorders in pediatric epilepsy: Unmet psychiatric need. *Epilepsia* 44: 591–597.

Pal DK (2011). Epilepsy and neurodevelopmental disorders of language. *Curr Opin Neurol* 24: 126–131.

Parker J, Rubin KH, Erath S, Wojslawowicz JC, and Buskirk AA (2006). Peer relationships and developmental psychopathology. In: *Developmental Psychopathology: Risk, Disorder, and Adaptation*, D Cicchetti and D Cohen (eds.). New York: Wiley, 2: 419–493.

Piccinelli P, Borgatti R, Aldini A, Bindelli D, Ferri M, Perna S, Pitillo G, Termine C, Zambonin F, and Balottin U (2008). Academic performance in children with rolandic epilepsy. *Dev Med Child Neurol* 50: 353–356.

Pulsipher D, Seidenberg M, Guidotti L, Tuchscherer VN, Morton J, Sheth RD, and Hermann B (2009). Thalamofrontal circuitry and executive dysfunction in recent-onset juvenile myoclonic epilepsy. *Epilepsia* 50 1210–1219.

Riikonen RS (2010). Favourable prognostic factors with infantile spasms. *Eur J Paediatr Neurol* 14: 13–18.

Rodenburg R, Meijer AM, Dekovic M, and Aldenkamp AP (2005). Family factors and psychopathology in children with epilepsy: A literature review. *Epilepsy Behav* 6: 488–503.

Schoenfeld J, Seidenberg M, Woodard A, Hecox K, Inglese C, Mack K, and Hermann B (1999). Neuropsychological and behavioral status of children with complex partial seizures. *Dev Med Child Neurol* 41: 724–31.

Schuele C (2004). The impact of developmental speech and language impairments on the acquisition of literacy skills. *Ment Retard Dev Disabil Res Rev* 10: 176–183.

Scott KM, Hwang I, Chiu W-T, Kessler RC, Sampson NA, Angermeyer M, Beautrais A, Borges G, Bruffaerts R, de Graaf R, Florescu S, Fukao A, Maria Haro J, Hu C, Kovess V, Levinson D, Posada-Villa J, Scocco P, and Nock MK (2010). Chronic physical conditions and their association with first onset of suicidal behavior in the world mental health surveys. *Psychosom Med* 72: 712–719.

Sherman E, Slick DJ, Connolly MB, and Eyrl K (2007). ADHD, Neurological correlates and health-related quality of life in severe pediatric epilepsy. *Epilepsia* 48: 1083–1091.

Shields WD and Snead C (2009). Benign epilepsy with centrotemporal spikes. *Epilepsia* 50: 10–15.

Shore CP, Austin JK, Huster GA, and Dunn DW (2002). Identifying risk factors for maternal depression in families of adolescents with epilepsy. *J Spec Pediatr Nurs* 7: 71–80.

Sillanpää M, Haataja L, and Shinnar S (2004). Perceived impact of childhood-onset epilepsy on quality of life as an adult. *Epilepsia* 45: 971–977.

Steffenburg S, Gillberg C, and Steffenburg U (1996). Psychiatric disorders in children and adolescents with mental retardation and active epilepsy. *Arch Neurol* 53: 904–912.

Tosun D, Siddarth P, Seidenberg M, Toga A, Caplan R, and Hermann B (2011). Intelligence and cortical thickness in children with complex partial seizures. *Neuroimage* 15: 337–346.

Tosun D, Siddarth P, Seidenberg M, Toga A, Hermann B, and Caplan R (2010). Effects of childhood absence epilepsy on associations between regional cortical morphometry and aging and cognitive abilities. *Hum Brain Mapp* 32: 580–591.

Tse E, Hamiwka L, Sherman EMS, and Wirrell E (2007). Social skills problems in children with epilepsy: Prevalence, nature and predictors. *Epilepsy Behav* 11: 499–505.

Tuchman R, Cuccaro M, and Alessandri M (2010). Autism and epilepsy: Historical perspective. *Brain Dev* 32: 709–718.

van Daal J, Verhoeven L, and van Balkom H (2007). Behaviour problems in children with language impairment. *J Child Psychol Psychiatry* 48: 1139–1147.

Vannatta K, Gerhardt CA, Wells RJ, and Noll RB (2007). Intensity of CNS treatment for pediatric cancer: Prediction of social outcomes in survivors. *Pediatr Blood Cancer* 49: 716–722.

Verrotti A, D'Adamo E, Parisi P, Chiarelli F, and Curatolo P (2010). Levetiracetam in childhood epilepsy. *Pediatric Drugs* 12: 177–186

Verrotti A, Loiacono G, Coppola G, Spalice A, Mohn A, and Chiarelli F (2011). Pharmacotherapy for children and adolescents with epilepsy. *Expert Opin Pharmacother* 12: 175–194.

Voci SC, Beitchman JH, Brownlie EB, and Wilson B (2006). Social anxiety in late adolescence: The importance of early childhood language impairment. *J Anxiet Disord* 20: 915–930.

Wu KN, Lieber E, Siddarth P, Smith K, Sankar R, and Caplan R (2008). Dealing with epilepsy: Parents speak up. *Epilepsy Behav* 13: 131–138.

Yeates KO, Swift E, Taylor HG, Wade SL, Drotar D, Stancin T, and Minich N (2004). Short- and long-term social outcomes following pediatric traumatic brain injury. *J Int Neuropsychol Soc* 10: 412–426.

You X, Adjouadi M, Guillen MR, Ayala M, Barreto A, Rishe N, Sullivan J, Dlugos D, VanMeter J, Morris D, Donner E, Bjornson B, Smith ML, Bernal B, Berl M, and Gaillard WD (2011). Sub-patterns of language network reorganization in pediatric localization related epilepsy: A multisite study. *Hum Brain Mapp* 32: 784–799.

Psychosocial Impact
of Pediatric Epilepsy

In this chapter, we describe the potential psychosocial impact of epilepsy on the child, the parents, the siblings, and on family functioning. Understanding how seizures, the illness, the comorbidities, and the stigma of epilepsy impact the emotional functioning of children with epilepsy and their family is essential for the comprehensive assessment of these children for several reasons. First, behavior that might appear to reflect a psychiatric diagnosis could simply be a "normal" response to dealing with the unpredictability of seizures together with the impact of ongoing seizures and the illness on the child's cognitive, linguistic, and academic functioning. Second, the child's behavior might be a reaction to how the parents and/or siblings cope with the seizures, the comorbidities (described in the previous chapter), and the potential long-term impacts of the illness.

To provide the interviewer with the background needed to talk to young children with epilepsy about the psychosocial impact of their illness, we first describe the stressors children with epilepsy face. We then discuss how these same stress factors impact the parents of children with epilepsy, along with the additional epilepsy-related stressors with which parents have to cope. The third section of the chapter focuses on risk factors for how parents deal with the illness and with the child's responses to the illness. In the last section, we put this all together with clinical examples of dialogues between interviewers and children that illustrate how to apply the developmental guidelines and the suggested techniques to identify the psychosocial impact of epilepsy on the child and parents; how to differentiate between psychosocial and biological effects of the disorder; and how to determine the interaction between the biological and psychosocial factors on the child's behavior.

THE CHILD

What We Know

- Dealing with the psychosocial impact of having seizures is emotionally taxing for young children.

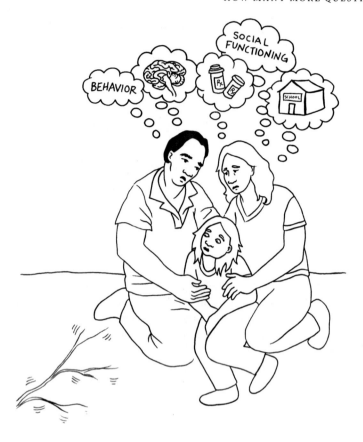

- Stressors include:
  - Unpredictable seizures
  - Loss of control during a seizure
  - Negative or intrusive peer responses to seizures
  - Absences from school
  - Adverse medication effects
  - Illness-related fears
  - Stigma of epilepsy
  - Impact of the illness on siblings
- The unpredictability of seizures and the need to be a "normal" child might increase a child's baseline anxiety.
- Young children might act out how they are feeling rather than talk about these stressors.

Relevance for the Interview of Young Children with Epilepsy

Epilepsy is both an acute and chronic illness. As an acute illness, children experience *unpredictable* sudden onset seizures that can occur anywhere and, during which, they might be taken to an emergency room by an ambulance. As a chronic illness, children have to contend with variable seizure control, daily medication, repeat blood tests, visits to the doctor, and the comorbidities described in chapter 11.

Table 12-1. EMOTIONAL DEVELOPMENT IN YOUNG HEALTHY CHILDREN AND IN
CHILDREN WITH SEIZURES

Seizures	No Seizures
Control	Lack of control
Competence	Fearful, anxious
Self-esteem	Unsure
Independence	Dependence

The unpredictability of seizures, a hallmark of epilepsy, is a significant stressor for which a young child cannot prepare. During a seizure, a child also loses control of consciousness, thoughts, actions, and bodily functions including sphincter control (bladder, bowel), and might sustain bodily harm. The loss of control, fear of bodily harm, and exposure to negative comments made by spectators (particularly children at school) about how the child looks during a seizure are also stressful. Being driven off to the emergency room by ambulance and missing schoolwork due to a seizure are additional social and academic stressors for the young child with epilepsy.

As described in the previous chapter, children with epilepsy on antiepileptic drugs might experience adverse effects on their behavior, cognition, and language. While adults and adolescents can monitor possible changes that they experience when they start a new medication or have a dose increase, this is typically not the case in young children. Additional stressors for young children include the need to deal with the impact of cognitive slowing; sedation-related poor emotional control with hyperactivity, irritability, anger, and/or temper tantrums; and the resulting negative response by parents or others to these behaviors. Furthermore, possible cognitive slowing, as well as the occurrence of seizures in clusters, and the need to catch up on missed schoolwork because of trips to the emergency room and visits to doctors significantly increase the child's academic burden.

Thus, the acute stress of unpredicted seizures, the chronic stress of their recurrence, negative peer responses, medication effects, school absences, and the cumulative effects of having to make up missed school work can increase a child's baseline level of anxiety. Furthermore, other than the clearly visible manifestations of generalized tonic-clonic seizures (See Table 11–1 in chapter 11), most people would not know that a child has epilepsy. In the absence of external signs suggesting a child might have an illness such as epilepsy, the environment expects children with epilepsy to be similar to others (Heisler and Friedman 1981). Following a seizure or a cluster of seizures, the child's parents and the school also often expect the child to return to baseline functioning.

As a result, rather than proceeding on the developmental trajectory with a sense of mastery and competence toward achieving independence (Table 12–1), children with epilepsy might feel that they have little control over what happens (external locus of control). The resulting fear and anxiety ("I might get hurt, laughed at" and the like), dependence ("I need help"), and poor self-esteem ("I can't do it") can be viewed as "normal" coping responses to the psychosocial impact of the illness. The need to toe the line and be "just like everyone else" when a child has an illness that is not readily apparent to others—the marginality status (Heisler and Friedman 1981)—can be quite daunting and emotionally demanding for a young child. Coping with the psychosocial impact of the disorder is further complicated by the direct effects of seizures and the underlying neuropathology on brain function and by the comorbidities described in chapter 11.

The child's seizure-related fear and anxiety are sometimes exacerbated as professionals do not adequately explain the illness to the child, or they give an explanation that is not commensurate with the child's developmental level. Inappropriate examples include "an electrical short in your brain makes all the lights go out" or the "electrical wires in your brain work too much at the same time and cause a seizure." Given young children's lack of understanding about the workings of electrical systems and warnings from the toddler period that electricity can be dangerous, these explanations can intensify children's fears and fantasies about what could go wrong in their brains during a seizure.

Young children understand the external aspects of disease, such as they fall and their arms and legs move (generalized tonic-clonic seizure), they do something without knowing about it like when they are sleep (complex partial or absence seizures), they take medicine and have blood tests. Explanations about the illness should, therefore, be concrete and action-based ("When you have a seizure, you suddenly stop talking and stare"), rather than abstract (as in the previously described electric explanations of epilepsy).

Given their lack of control and the possibility of sustaining harm during a seizure, most children are scared that they might hurt themselves or die during a seizure. Hearing physicians and adults around them mention that seizures involve their brain can invoke fears that they might become "stupid" or "weird." Yet, clinicians and most parents might not discuss these fears with children with epilepsy. This might be because young children usually keep these fears to themselves for the following two reasons. First, they might avoid sharing these fears with their parents to protect their parents from additional worry. Second, they might harbor the magical belief that talking about fears might make them happen.

Physicians might not talk to children with epilepsy about their illness-related fears because they are unaware of these fears or they feel untrained to do this. Some clinicians might also actively avoid this topic due to the erroneous belief that bringing up these fears to children will make them have the fears or make them worse in children who are already fearful. Parents, overburdened by their own fears regarding the child's illness, might not think their child has any fears. They, too, might be concerned that they could introduce these fears to their child. Struggling with the same fears as the child, parents might feel unable to discuss this difficult topic with their child. Furthermore, discussions about fears are not normative in all families, so it simply might not occur to anyone in the family to have these conversations.

Harboring these fears without an outlet increases the young child's sense of lack of control and baseline anxiety. To understand the impact of these fears on the child's emotional functioning, a comprehensive evaluation should determine if the child has fears related to having seizures, the nature of these fears, who the child has told about these fears, and what the response was. If the child has not spoken to anyone about his fears, clarifying the reasons for this is important. It can provide the clinician with information on how the child deals with overwhelming feelings and whether internal child-based or external family-based reasons prevent him from sharing the information with his parents.

An additional, often unspoken, stressor with which some children with epilepsy have to deal is the stigma of epilepsy (Austin et al. 2002). A negative attitude toward epilepsy, greater worry, poorer self-concept, and more depression symptoms were associated with higher scores on a stigma scale in a large group of children with new onset seizures (Austin et al. 2004). Stigma-related bullying of children with epilepsy, another significant stressor, is not uncommon (Hamiwka et al. 2009). In some cases, however, children with epilepsy who have poor social and/or communication skills might misdirect blame for their social functioning difficulties on the stigma of epilepsy (Caplan et al. 2005).

The stigma of epilepsy varies across cultures and subcultures, making it not apparent in some cultures but a significant social obstacle in others. Assessing the child's perception of stigma and attitude toward epilepsy, as well as his/her social and communication skills, together with the cultural perception of epilepsy within the family (both nuclear and extended), and at school (if the child has seizures at school), is an important part of the comprehensive assessment of young children with epilepsy.

Within the family, the child with epilepsy is faced with the response of the parents (described in the next section) and siblings to the illness. Siblings might experience posttraumatic symptoms if they see and/or hear their brother or sister have a seizure. They might be envious and angry because the parents pay more attention to the child with epilepsy and are more lenient when it comes to discipline than with their children without epilepsy. In an environment in which epilepsy is regarded as a stigma, siblings might feel embarrassed that they have a sibling with this illness. They might not want to be seen with their sibling or might withdraw from the child when their friends come over. When older siblings have to take care of their sibling with epilepsy to help their parents, they might become resentful and direct their anger toward the child with epilepsy. Siblings might also have to deal with the stress of living with a child with epilepsy who has behavioral, cognitive, linguistic, or social comorbidities.

Due to their developmental limitations, young children are not cognizant of how these multiple stressors affect them—or they cannot verbalize it. They might respond to their increasing stress through externalizing behaviors (hyperactive, angry, irritable, aggressive, explosive) or internalizing behaviors (sad, anxious, withdrawn), which might be misinterpreted and misdiagnosed. As demonstrated in the following clinical examples, the interviewer can help the child describe the stressors that underlie these behaviors through age-appropriate questions.

Clinical Examples

Fears about Seizures: Jamal, aged 7 years, was first diagnosed with complex partial seizures with secondary generalized tonic-clonic seizure (Table 11-1) three months ago. At his follow-up visit today, his mother reports that he has had no seizures for the past month since the last dose increase in his antiepileptic drug, and that he is doing well at school. He has been clinging to her quite a lot. She thinks he simply has liked all the attention he has received due to his epilepsy and tries to get more by being clingy. When the mother started to speak about the clinging behavior, Jamal smiled bashfully at the pediatrician, Dr. Abassian, and then looked at the floor. The mother denied any family problems and felt that she, her husband, and Jamal were all coping well with the epilepsy, particularly during the past four weeks in which he had no seizures. The pediatrician interviewed Jamal separately to find out his perspective on the clinging behavior.

Fears about Seizures

DR. ABASSIAN: *Jamal, thank you for being so quiet and patient while I talked with your mother. Was that easy or hard for you?*

JAMAL: *Hard.*

DR. ABASSIAN: *I thought so, so thanks very much.*

Jamal smiles.

DR. ABASSIAN: *I see lots of kids with seizures and they tell me that the seizures make things hard for them. What have they made hard for you?*

JAMAL: *I hate the shots.*

DR. ABASSIAN: *That's what other kids also tell me. What else do you hate about seizures?*

JAMAL: *The medicine.*

DR. ABASSIAN: *The taste or something else about it?*

JAMAL: *I can only take it with applesauce otherwise I want to throw up.*

DR. ABASSIAN: *Throwing up doesn't sound like a lot of fun. How about applesauce?*

JAMAL: *I love it.*

DR. ABASSIAN: *Okay so if you take the medicine with applesauce, it sounds like you don't mind.*

JAMAL NODS.

DR. ABASSIAN: *What else don't you like about the seizures?*

Jamal shrugs his shoulders

DR. ABASSIAN: *Let me tell you some things other kids tell me about seizures. Some kids become scared.*

JAMAL: *Of what?*

DR. ABASSIAN: *Different things.*

JAMAL: *What kind of things?*

DR. ABASSIAN: *Some think that seizures might make them stupid.*

JAMAL: *They get stupid.*

DR. ABASSIAN: *I'm not sure what you mean by stupid.*

JAMAL: *My dad says that when I have a seizure, they talk to me and I just stare and don't answer. That's stupid.*

DR. ABASSIAN: *Did your dad say that is stupid?*

JAMAL: *No, I know it's just dumb.*

DR. ABASSIAN: *It's not a good feeling to feel like that.*

Jamal nods.

DR. ABASSIAN: *Should I tell you about other things kids with seizures are scared of?*

JAMAL: *Okay.*

DR. ABASSIAN: *Some kids worry that something really bad can happen to them while they are having a seizure.*

JAMAL: *Like what?*

DR. ABASSIAN: *Falling and hurting themselves.*

JAMAL: *I fell once but nothing happened to me. What else?*

DR. ABASSIAN: *Some even are scared that they might die in a seizure.*

JAMAL: *Not if you are with your mom.*

DR. ABASSIAN: *So does that mean that when you are not with mom you are scared you might die if you have a seizure?*

JAMAL (tearful): *Where's my mom?*

DR. ABASSIAN: *Should we go get her and you can tell her what you are scared of?*

JAMAL: *Okay, but you tell her.*

DR. ABASSIAN: *Because?*

JAMAL: *She will cry.*

The mother joined them and Jamal sat on her lap.

DR. ABASSIAN: *Jamal has helped me understand what bad things he thinks the sei-zures are doing to him.*

MOTHER: *I had no idea about this.*

DR. ABASSIAN: *Well, it's difficult for kids to talk about it and sometimes even to think about it.*

Jamal nods yes.

DR. ABASSIAN: *First of all, he feels stupid and dumb, because when he has a seizure, he just stares.*

MOTHER: *How can he know that he stares if he is having a seizure?*

JAMAL: *Dad said that to grandma when she babysat me.*

MOTHER: *Honey, it's not being stupid. It's like not paying attention when someone talks to you; is that stupid?*

JAMAL: *You do that.*

MOTHER: *So am I stupid and dumb?*

JAMAL: *No.*

DR. ABASSIAN: *The other scary thing for Jamal, like for other children with seizures, is that he is scared that he might die during a seizure.*

Mother starts to tear.

DR. ABASSIAN: *By being very close to you, Jamal feels protected. So can he let you know when he has these fears so you can help him feel protected?*

MOTHER: *Jamal will you please tell dad or I when you feel like that?*

JAMAL: *But then you'll cry?*

MOTHER: *No, now that I understand, I won't.*

As suggested by Jamal's smile, Dr. Abassian established good rapport with the child by telling him that it must have been difficult to be in the room during the mother's interviewer. Subsequent "What" questions and examples of fears other children with epilepsy experience helped Jamal talk about feeling stupid and that he might die during in a seizure.

This example demonstrates how knowledge about the impact of the disorder on children's emotions, together with developmentally crafted questions, can help identify the fears that young children with epilepsy harbor. Knowledge about these fears, in turn, can help parents make sense of the young child's behavior (clinging behavior in this case) and know how to help the child cope with these fears.

School-related Stress: Noah, aged 9 years, has clusters of complex partial seizures (Table 11-1) for a few days that occur every three to four months. His seizures are fol-lowed by post-ictal tiredness that can last up to twenty-four hours. He did not attend school the whole of last week because of a cluster of seizures. The mother told the pedi-atric epilepsy nurse practitioner that since the beginning of this week Noah started complaining about stomachaches in the morning before school. She brought him in to see the nurse practitioner, Ms. Sharifi, because his stomach pain was so bad this morn-ing that he could not go to school. The mother thought this might be due to the new anti-epileptic drug the nurse practitioner started last week when the cluster began.

Ms. Sharifi found out from the mother and Noah that he is a hard-working, good fourth grade student when seizure-free. Last year, his teacher had a good understanding for epilepsy and worked with him after each cluster to help him catch up on the material he had missed. This is the first cluster of seizures he has experienced this school year. His new teacher seems to know little about epilepsy and has not been willing to read any of the articles about epilepsy that the mother had given to her and Noah's teacher last year. During Noah's physical exam, Ms. Sharifi had the following conversation with him.

School-Related Stress

MS. SHARIFI: *A lot has been going on for you with the seizures and stomachaches.*

NOAH (looking sad): *The seizures stopped.*

MS. SHARIFI: *Good, and we need to fix these stomachaches, too. Are they happening every morning?*

Noah nods yes.

MS. SHARIFI: *Weekends as well?*

Noah shakes his head no.

MS. SHARIFI: *What's happens on weekends that doesn't happen during the week?*

NOAH: *School.*

MS. SHARIFI: *How is school going for you?*

NOAH: *Horrible.*

MS. SHARIFI: *Sorry to hear that. When I saw you last year, I remember you liked school and did really well.*

NOAH: *No more.*

MS. SHARIFI: *Is it the work, the kids, or the teacher that makes it horrible?*

NOAH: *Not the kids.*

MS. SHARIFI: *So then it is the teacher and the work?*

NOAH: *She's so mean.*

MS. SHARIFI: *What mean things is she doing to you?*

NOAH: *Too much work.*

MS. SHARIFI: *For you, or for all the kids?*

NOAH: *They don't have epilepsy.*

MS. SHARIFI: *This might sound like a stupid question, but it is important for me to understand. How does epilepsy make it bad for you at school?*

NOAH: *I miss too much school.*

MS. SHARIFI: *So then it is difficult to keep up and understand what the teacher is teaching?*

Noah nods yes, and tears well up in his eyes.

MS. SHARIFI: *I see that makes you really sad.*

NOAH: *She says I am lazy.*

MS. SHARIFI: *That must make you feel really bad. What makes her say that?*

NOAH: *I haven't done all my work sheets.*

MS. SHARIFI: *Is that in all subjects?*

NOAH: *Math.*

MS. SHARIFI: *Do your mom and dad know how upset you are about this?*

NOAH: *Yes, they say I am smart in math and I can do it.*

MS. SHARIFI: *And what do you think?*

NOAH: *It's too hard.*

This case demonstrates that the parents' focus on the child's seizures and medications, together with their perception that their son is a good student, prevented them from understanding his call for help. The nurse practitioner's concrete "What" questions, verbalization of what the child might be feeling, and her empathy identified the child's difficulty relatively easily. With the mother's permission, Ms. Sharifi wrote a letter to the teacher explaining the need to help him understand the math work he missed given the cumulative demands of math. She also emphasized to the mother the importance of encouraging Noah to communicate with her and her husband about his difficulties and how to problem-solve. Stress-related somatic symptoms, such as abdominal pains, are more frequent among those with ineffective coping skills and can become a lifelong pattern (see chapter 8 on Somatization and chapter 14 on Pediatric pain).

Sibling-related Stress: Felipe, aged 10 years, has primary generalized epilepsy with tonic-clonic seizures (Table 11-1) that occur about once a month. He had a seizure about three weeks ago. Dr. Curtner, a clinical psychologist, is seeing him today because he has been both verbally and physically aggressive toward his younger 8-year-old brother. The mother reported that he has never had a problem with aggression at home or at school and that he always played well with his brother. She has given Felipe no consequences for his behavior toward his brother because she is concerned that this would stress him out and cause a seizure. However, her husband disagrees with her and says that Felipe should be punished. The mother thinks that Felipe's medicine is making him lose his temper easily and get out of control, although Felipe has shown no aggression with her and her husband or at school. She is concerned about her younger son, because Felipe is much stronger than him and can hurt him.

Sibling-Related Stress

DR. CURTNER: *Felipe, how are things going with your seizures?*

FELIPE: *Okay I guess.*

DR. CURTNER: *Is that a not so okay or a fine?*

FELIPE: *Not so okay.*

DR. CURTNER: *In what way?*

FELIPE: *Because I had one; my mom says my brother has to watch me when I take a shower.*

DR. CURTNER: *And how does that make you feel?*

FELIPE: *Like a baby. He told his friends that I am a baby and can't even take a shower by myself.*

DR. CURTNER: *That can make someone angry.*

FELIPE: *He is a smarty-pants.*

DR. CURTNER: *What does he do that makes you say that?*

FELIPE: *He says he can read better than me even though he is in second grade and I am in fourth.*

DR. CURTNER: *Oh, that must make you really mad.*

FELIPE: *He also hangs out with my friends when they come over and no one does stuff with me.*

DR. CURTNER: *Have you told your parents about all these things he does to you?*

FELIPE: *They say someone has to watch me in the shower.*

DR. CURTNER: *What about how he brags and takes your friends away?*

FELIPE: *They hear and see it but do nothing.*

DR. CURTNER: *So when your brother does all these mean things to you, what do you do?*
FELIPE: *I hit him and then he goes and cries to my mom.*
DR. CURTNER: *How about we invite your mom to come in so you can tell her about all of this?*
FELIPE: *Only if she won't be mad at me.*
DR. CURTNER: *Let's try.*

This developmentally based dialogue between Dr. Curtner and Felipe with its initial focus on seizures (not the presenting behavior problem), concrete action-based and nondirectional "What" questions, as well as empathy for the child's problems, identifies the source of Felipe's anger. It also emphasizes that parents of children with epilepsy have their hands full, especially if they have several children but need to observe the child with epilepsy in situations, such as taking a shower. Siblings might not understand epilepsy and its possible impact on the learning skills of the child with epilepsy. They might be scared and have posttraumatic anxiety symptoms because of seizures they have observed or heard. They also might resent the attention the parents and they themselves (as parent surrogates) need to give to the child with epilepsy. Ideally, Dr. Curtner should have also spoken with Felipe's brother (who did not come with his mother and brother) to clarify the difficulties he is experiencing due to Felipe's epilepsy.

SUMMARY
- A developmentally oriented sensitive assessment of epilepsy-related stressors and the impact of the child's emotions and behavior should include the following topics:
- Seizures
  - What happens to the child during a seizure
  - When and where seizures occur
  - How others respond
  - The child's fears related to having seizures
- Relationships at home with:
  - Parents
  - Siblings
- School
  - Easy and difficult work/subjects
  - Friends and social activities
  - Teacher understanding and accommodations

THE PARENTS

What We Know

- Parents of children with epilepsy face multiple psychosocial stressors related to:
  - Features of the illness
  - The medical system and the school system
  - Parenting the child with epilepsy and siblings and their illness-related stressors

- Different coping styles of the parents
- Cultural biases about epilepsy among family members and friends
- Risk factors for difficulty coping with these stressors include:
  - Demographic variables (female gender, low socioeconomic status)
  - Past history of a psychiatric diagnosis, particularly, depression and anxiety disorder
  - Family dysfunction

Relevance for the Interview of Young Children with Epilepsy

Similar to their children, the parents of children with epilepsy have to deal with a large number of stressors related to having a child with epilepsy (see review in Austin and Caplan 2007). These include the unpredictability of seizures, uncertainty related to the illness, the medical and school systems, economic burden of the illness, stigma and cultural approaches to the illness, parenting of the healthy siblings, and illness-related stress on the parental relationship and functioning of the family. In addition, parents have to deal with the responses of the child with epilepsy and their healthy children to the stressors. Factors that play a role in how parents deal with these stressors include the severity of the child's illness, the presence or absence and severity of comorbidities, the mental health of the parent, demographic variables (female gender, socioeconomic status, parent education, marital status, parent age), and available social support. (Detailed reviews can be found in Austin and Caplan 2007, Rodenburg et al. 2011, and Ferro and Speechley 2009.)

Stressors

Coping with the hallmark of the illness, unpredictable seizures, is probably the most challenging aspect of the illness. Parents need to tread a fine line between what they (and others) might perceive as being either negligent or overprotective of their child. Parents who want to normalize their children's lives make sure that their children engage in the same activities as other children, including swimming, riding a bicycle, climbing trees, having sleepovers, going to sleepaway camp, and the like. But if a child experiences a seizure while biking, climbing, or swimming, it is potentially dangerous. And should a child have a seizure during a sleepover or at a sleepaway camp, this might upset the other children and their parents. The parents of the child with epilepsy might also be perceived as "negligent."

In contrast, some parents of children with epilepsy might be considered "overprotective" if they do not allow their child to engage in "normal" childhood activities because of harm the child might sustain if he or she has a seizure. The decision parents make on how they will tread this fine line between normalizing the child's life and restricting activities affects the child's developmental trajectory toward independence. With normalization and participation in the same activities as peers, children feel more in control of their lives and less anxious. In contrast, dependence and fear of separating from parents, anger and resentment toward parents, and feeling different from peers are all common responses that might characterize the behavior of children whose parents are "overprotective." Thus, parental response to the challenge of unpredictable seizures can play an important role in how children cope with their illness in terms of their sense of competence (mastery), self-esteem, social skills, and development toward independence.

In addition to influencing the normal emotional development of the child, differences in how parents handle this problem might lead to disagreement and arguments. Overhearing their parents argue about how to deal with their epilepsy, children might feel guilty about all the problems they cause between their parents. They might also learn to take advantage of these differences in their parents' approaches by asking the "normalizing" parent for permission to engage in activities with peers or by asking the "overprotective" parent for permission to avoid an activity. This behavior is called "splitting" (between the "normalizing" and "overprotective" parent). It can increase the tension between the parents and might make them with the child.

Uncertainty about illness-related complications and the long-term outcome of the illness is an additional stressor parents need to deal with. Like children with epilepsy, parents worry that their child might die during a seizure (Shore et al. 1998), or has died (Besag et al. 2005), and refrain from talking about this fear even with their spouse. Parents also feel that professionals do not provide them with information about the long-term outcome and comorbidities of epilepsy (Wu et al. 2008). Most parents want to know about sudden unexpected death related to epilepsy (SUDEP), according to a recent survey (Gayatri et al. 2011). Knowledge about SUDEP and its risk factors might help all parents of children with epilepsy. Yet, some clinicians suggest that this information be provided only to parents whose children might be at risk for SUDEP (young age, frequent tonic-clonic convulsions, medical intractability) (Brodie et al. 2008). The stress of all this uncertainty can have a negative impact on how parents cope with the illness (see review in Duffy 2011).

The medical system and the school system are also major sources of stress for parents (Wu et al. 2008; Wagner et al. 2009). Medical system stressors include the acute and chronic economic hardships of having a child with epilepsy: the burden of medical bills for doctors' appointments, ambulance trips, emergency room visits, medications, blood tests, MRIs, hospitalizations for video-EEGs, and other medical procedures—all of this is often coupled with a decrease in salary because of the need to take time off from work.

Noneconomic stressors invoked by the medical system can be equally overwhelming for parents, particularly the difficulty in getting an appointment or the wait to hear back from the child's physician after an acute event, such as breakthrough seizures or adverse medication effects. Dealing with cumbersome and unpredicted medical bills, as well as the need to obtain insurance authorization for the child's medical services, can be time consuming and emotionally depleting. The need for time off from work to take the child to doctor's visits is an additional emotional stressor, particularly if only one parent bears this burden, and the work environment has little understanding for what it means to have a child with epilepsy. In terms of career development, parents might not be able to accept better positions in other companies after the child develops epilepsy because they fear not being able to get a new health care plan due to their child's illness.

The school system poses additional problems. The school administration might call an ambulance and send the child to an emergency room when he has a seizure. In addition to this being unnecessary, creating a frightening "drama" for the child, and wasting time at the emergency room, parents must leave work and are then faced with expensive bills for both the emergency room visit and the ambulance.

At the level of the teacher(s) and school principal, misconceptions about epilepsy, as well as fear that the child might have a seizure in class, can underlie overt or covert resistance to having the child in the classroom or at school. Some teachers think children with epilepsy have intellectual disability and expect them to be poor students, while others attribute the same learning skills to children with epilepsy as their other students. Teachers' expectations and their behavior toward children in their class is related to how well the child does in the class (see review in Hornstra et al. 2010). Therefore, lower teacher expectation for children with epilepsy is a relevant parental concern (Wu et al. 2008).

Alternatively, teachers might be unrealistically demanding with little understanding for the stress the child with epilepsy experiences due to the need to catch up on missed work because of absences during a cluster of seizures or when experiencing medication-related sedation. The resulting stress might negatively affect the relationship between the parents and child if, when trying to help their child, parents become surrogate teachers, and pressure the child to get the work done. Similar to dealing with the unpredictability of seizures, differences in how parents handle school-related demands might increase the tension between the parents. This, in turn, adds to the child's guilt about the burden his illness puts on the parents.

Parenting the siblings of children with epilepsy is a stressor for parents. Given the attention and time parents need to spend on their ill child, they often feel guilt-ridden because they do not have the time or the emotional resources for care of their other children. Findings on a large sample of siblings of children with chronic illness demonstrate good adjustment in the majority of siblings despite increased emotional symptoms compared to the general population (Taylor et al. 2001). However, better sibling adjustment is associated with higher maternal awareness of sibling attitudes and perceptions about the sick child's illness. Taylor et al. concluded that their findings emphasized the role of relationship (communication between mothers and siblings) and attitude variables in sibling adjustment to chronic physical disorder. Clinicians often overlook this topic, and there have been no studies to date on how mothers perceive their parenting of the healthy siblings of children with epilepsy.

However, a study of coping, adjustment, and mental health in a large sample of siblings of children with epilepsy as compared to a healthy control group demonstrated increased reports by teachers of behavior problems in the siblings of the children with epilepsy (Aronu and Iloeje 2011). There was a significant relationship between sibling behavior problems and poor seizure control in the children with epilepsy. The mothers of children with epilepsy reported increased somatic complaints in their children without epilepsy (Freilinger et al. 2006). The siblings of children with new onset seizures, however, experienced both increased school problems and somatic complaints based on fathers' reports. Siblings who had witnessed their siblings' seizures also had increased social problems.

Although Wood et al. (2008) found internalizing problems (depression, anxiety, somatic complaints) in 25% of the siblings of children with intractable epilepsy, based on mother reports, data on sibling self-report of depression, anxiety, and quality of life indicated overall good functioning and quality of life. Inconsistent findings in these sibling studies probably reflect different methods and study designs.

From the social perspective, parents are also faced with the response of their extended family and friends to the child's illness. This response varies across cultures from acceptance and support to shame, guilt, and the need to keep the illness a secret. Given the previously described difficulties parents have dealing with their child's epilepsy, adding cultural stigma and the associated lack of social support by extended family and friends to the mix can deplete the parents' emotional resources for coping with the illness and being emotionally available for the child with epilepsy and the siblings.

Summary: In addition to stressors experienced by parents of children with chronic illness (severity of illness, the medical and school systems, parenting and family functioning, different parent coping styles), the unpredictability and stigma of epilepsy add heavily to the coping burden of these parents. Knowledge about these stressors is relevant for the interview of young children with epilepsy whose emotions and behavior might reflect how their parents deal with these stressors.

Risk Factors

Among the multiple factors that play a role in how parents cope with these stressors, maternal mental health has been well studied. Hoare and Kerley (1991) demonstrated that maternal psychopathology is associated with behavior disturbances in children with epilepsy, as well as with the need to deal with the school system in mothers whose children also have learning difficulties. Other early studies reported that lack of independence in children with epilepsy was related to maternal psychopathology (Carlton-Ford et al. 1997) and to problems in the mother-child interaction (Pianta and Lothman 1994; Sbarra et al. 2002).

In terms of the type of maternal mental health problems, understanding the relationship between parent anxiety and the emotional well-being of children with epilepsy is important in light of evidence from an excellent meta-analysis that has shown that children without epilepsy, who have anxious and controlling parents, are themselves anxious (Van der Bruggen et al. 2008). As previously described in the child section, the unpredictability of seizures can increase the child's baseline anxiety and impact the child's sense of competence and independence. The child's response to this unpredictability is associated with the mental health of each parent. Thus, children with epilepsy whose parents are anxious, overly directive, and who do not allow normalization of their children's lives have poor adaptive functioning (Chapieski et al. 2005) and quality of life (Williams et al. 2003).

There appear to be gender-related differences in the level of concern and illness-related burden parents of children with epilepsy experience (Ramaglia et al. 2007). Mothers are more worried and bear a larger burden than fathers, both at the onset of the disorder and over time (Shore et al. 1998). Access to information about anti-epileptic drugs and their side effects is associated with less anxiety in parents of children with epilepsy irrespective of gender (Hirfanoglu et al. 2009).

From 12% to 49% of the mothers of children with epilepsy have depression, similar to findings in the mothers of children with pediatric chronic illness and developmental disabilities (see review in Ferro and Speechley 2009). Uncertainty related to the outcome of the illness for both mothers (Mu et al. 2001) and fathers (Mu 2005), as well as behavior problems and/or disabilities (Shore et al. 2002; Mu 2005; Adewuya

2006) in their children with epilepsy are associated with parental depression. Above and beyond possible distorted reports about children's behavior by mothers due to their own depression (Gartstein et al. 2009), there appears to be a two-way relationship between maternal depression and child behavior problems that is moderated by maternal rejection of the child with epilepsy (Rodenburg et al. 2006).

Parent intrusiveness, criticism, and rejection of the child are related to behavior problems, poor self-esteem, depression, internalizing problems, antisocial behavior, and dependence in children with epilepsy (Hodes et al. 1999; Rodenburg et al. 2006). Thus, the mental health of parents is associated with the emotional resources they have available to cope with their child's illness and support their children. Their support or lack thereof plays an important role in their children's behavior and emotions.

Furthermore, family adaptive resources (socioeconomic status, parent education), family cohesion, extended family social support, family members' beliefs and perceptions of epilepsy, as well as family organization, reflect parental psychopathology and play an important role in the child's behavior (see review in Austin and Caplan, 2007). As described in the previous chapter, family organization and parental anxiety also predict child performance on neuropsychological and academic achievement tests both cross-sectionally (Fastenau et al. 2004) and over time (Dunn et al. 2010) in children with new onset seizures. Therefore, it is important to obtain information on the psychosocial impact of epilepsy on the parents and the related family organization and functioning, and how parents, in turn, interact with the child's psychosocial difficulties, illness comorbidities, and severity of illness to achieve a comprehensive understanding of the child's behavior.

Summary: Parents at risk for difficulty coping with the stress of having a child with epilepsy have a past psychiatric diagnosis, such as depression and anxiety disorder, that might exacerbate with onset of the child's illness. Mothers are more vulnerable and often bear more of the burden than fathers. Child behavior problems, family dysfunction, economic hardships, and lack of social support are additional risk factors.

PUTTING IT ALL TOGETHER

Based on the variable, albeit inevitable stressors that face children with epilepsy and their parents, the comprehensive evaluation of a child with epilepsy should include a separate interview with the child and with the parents. The reason for a separate interview is twofold. It ensures that both the child and parents will be able to openly speak about the impact of the disorder on their lives. In addition, exposing the child to the toll of the illness on the parents and family might make the child feel guilty or increase the child's guilt about having epilepsy.

The aim of the child interview is to shed light on what underlies the parents' main concern regarding the child. To do this, the clinician needs to conduct a comprehensive evaluation of all aspects of the illness from the child's perspective, including the seizures, treatment effects, psychosocial stressors, and the psychiatric, cognitive, linguistic, and social comorbidities described in this and the prior chapter. Table 12–2 provides examples of questions on each of these topics for the young child.

Table 12–2. CHILD INTERVIEW QUESTIONS: SEIZURES AND PSYCHOSOCIAL ASPECTS
OF EPILEPSY

Topics	Questions
Seizures	What is not fun about having seizures?
	What is the worst part about having seizures?
	When do they bother you the most?
	Is there anything good about having seizures?
	What would your parents say if I asked them what is the worst part about you having seizures?
	Is the medicine you are taking for your seizures helping?
	What don't you like about the medicine?
	Kids with seizures are often scared something bad might happen to them because of their seizures. What things are you scared of?
School	What is your favorite subject at school?
	What do you hate doing at school?
	What do the kids at school say about you having epilepsy?
	How about your teacher—what does he/she say?
	What subjects at school are easy … a little difficult … really difficult?
	What do your teacher or your parents say about that?
Social	Are you the type of kid who has a lot of friends or a few friends?
	At school at recess, whom do you play with?
	And, what do you play with … ?
	Do you always have someone to play with?
	Sometimes are you by yourself at recess and all the other kids are playing?
	Do you get to play with other kids when you are not at school?
	At your house or at their house?
	Do you like to have sleepovers?
	At your house or at their house?

The interview with the parents should focus first on the child and then on the parents, because the parents' main concern is usually the child's illness. In addition, while talking to the parents about the child and his/her illness, the clinician establishes rapport with the parents and this helps parents talk more freely about their own difficulties coping with the illness.

After finding out why the parents have brought the child to see the clinician, the clinician should ask about the child's seizures, treatment and treatment effects, behavior, school performance, as well as functioning with siblings and peers. The clinician should then obtain information on how each parent copes with the disease, the impact of the illness on family functioning, and sources of support. Tables 12–3 and 12–4 present the topics and examples of questions that should be covered with the parents.

Table 12-3. PARENT INTERVIEW: QUESTIONS ON SEIZURES AND TREATMENT

Topics	Questions
SEIZURES	
Type	Please describe your child's seizures for me.
Age of onset	From what age does your child have seizures?
Frequency	How often does your child have seizures?
Complicated/ Uncomplicated	Does the child have other neurological or medical illnesses?
Prolonged seizures (5+ min)	How long do the seizures take?
Total	How many seizures has your child had?
Associated behavior changes	What changes occur in your child's behavior before a seizure?
	When do these occur?
	What changes occur in your child's behavior after a seizure?
	For how long do they continue?
Fear	What is your greatest fear when your child is having a seizure?
TREATMENT	
Antiepileptic drugs	What are your child's current antiepileptic drugs and their dosage?
	When were the last drug changes made? Why?
	What was the effect on seizures, behavior, and cognition?
Ketogenic diet[1]	Has your child been on the diet?
	From when and for how long?
	What was the effect on seizures, behavior, and cognition?
Surgery	Did your child undergo surgery for epilepsy?
	When and what type of surgery?
	What was the effect on seizures, behavior, and cognition?

[1] Beyond the scope of this book, see review in Kossoff et al. 2009.

Table 12-4. PARENT INTERVIEW: QUESTIONS ON PSYCHOSOCIAL ASPECT OF PEDIATRIC EPILEPSY

Topics	Questions
Coping	Please describe the main difficulties you experience because of your child's epilepsy.
	Which is the most difficult aspect for you (your spouse)?
	How do you (your spouse) deal with it?
	How has the illness impacted your child with epilepsy, your other children, and your relationship with your spouse?
	How do you and your spouse share the burden of your child's illness?
Parenting	Has your behavior (or your spouse's) changed toward your child with epilepsy?
	Has your behavior (or your spouse's) changed toward your other children?

Table 12–4. (CONTINUED)

Topics	Questions
	How has your child with epilepsy reacted to these changes? And how have your other children reacted?
	Are you (and your spouse) comfortable letting your child with epilepsy play outside with peers, have play dates, go to sleepovers, be alone in the shower or in other parts of the house?
	What do you not let your child with epilepsy do with friends?
	How about your other children?
Support	How do members of your extended family react to your child's illness?
	How do your friends react to your child's illness?
	Who are the people who support you and who you can call upon and who not?
	Who do you talk to about all of this?
School	Are you satisfied with your child's school, teacher(s), and the children in your child's class?
	How do they respond to your child having epilepsy?
	What do they do when your child has a seizure at school?
	Do you feel your child is making adequate progress at school? If not, why not?
	Is your child having difficulty with any of the school subjects?
	Which subjects?
	Is he/she getting help from the school with these subjects?
Future	What has your child's neurologist told you (or your spouse) about the future for children with epilepsy?
	What are your main concerns (and your spouse's) now and for your child's future?
	Have you shared these with anyone? With whom? How did that help?
Economic	Parents are usually worried about the impact the illness has on the family's finances. Has there been a significant impact for your family? If so, what has it been?
Anxiety Depression	Besides worrying that your child might have a seizure, having to deal with all these aspects of the illness takes its toll on parents.
	Has it made you (or your spouse) more anxious, worried, irritable, angry, or sad?
	What aspect of the disease makes you (or your spouse) feel like that?
	Do you lie awake worrying your child will have a seizure during the night?
	Do you (or your spouse) sleep with your child?
	Have worries or anxiety been a problem for you (or your spouse) before your child had epilepsy?
	How do you think your worrying impacts your behavior toward your child with epilepsy?
	How do you think your worrying impacts your behavior toward your other children?
Child's Behavior	Do you have any concerns about the behavior of your child with epilepsy?

Clinical Examples of Stressors

The examples that follow illustrate the interaction between parent and child responses to the illness and how clinicians can tease out which of the multiple aspects of the illness underlie what the parents report as the child's presenting problem.

Undiagnosed Juvenile Myoclonic Epilepsy and Parent Depression: Addison is a 10-year-old girl who was taken to the emergency room because of a generalized tonic-clonic seizure, and then referred to a pediatric neurologist who started treatment with valproate. About 6–8 months earlier, Addison had saved her 5-year-old brother who fell into the family swimming pool while she was supposed to be watching over him. The mother reported that although Addison was a good student, her grades started to go down after she began treatment with valproate. Addison was also having trouble sleeping at night, startled easily, and would be so nervous sometimes at home that dishes frequently fell from her hands. Her parents were concerned and punitive about the change in her grades and felt she was not applying herself to her schoolwork. They also scolded her for breaking dishes because they felt this reflected the same carelessness with which she approached her schoolwork.

Addison's mother appeared quite depressed, cried while she provided the information on her daughter, and indicated that she alone bore the burden of her daughter's illness. She felt her daughter had changed since she was on the valproate and that she had become so high strung that things were falling from her hands.

A child psychiatrist, Dr. Kaminsky, conducted a comprehensive evaluation of Addison to determine if her behavior and learning difficulties were associated with uncontrolled seizures; untreated posttraumatic stress disorder symptoms (insomnia, exaggerated startle) following her brother's near drowning incident; adverse cognitive and emotional effects of the valproate; an undiagnosed learning disorder; her mother's depression; or a combination of all these factors. Part of the interview is presented below.

Undiagnosed Juvenile Myoclonic Epilepsy, Child Anxiety, and Parent Depression

DR. KAMINSKY: *Hi, Addison. I bet you must be tired of seeing so many doctors and being asked many questions.*

ADDISON (smiling): *If it will help, I guess it's okay.*

DR. KAMINSKY: *What would you like help with?*

ADDISON: *School.*

DR. KAMINSKY: *What's not going well at school?*

ADDISON: *My grades.*

DR. KAMINSKY: *You're not happy with them?*

ADDISON: *Before I always got As, now only Cs.*

DR. KAMINSKY: *How does that make you feel?*

ADDISON's (eyes tearing): *Sad and stupid.*

DR. KAMINSKY: *I am sorry to hear that you feel so bad about yourself. Do you feel like this all the time?*

ADDISON: *At school when we have tests and at home when my parents get mad at me.*

DR. KAMINSKY: *So tests are hard?*

ADDISON: *When I do them, I think I did okay. But then I get bad grades.*

DR. KAMINSKY: *Oh that must be hard for you.*

ADDISON CRIES.

DR. KAMINSKY: *Some kids tell me that when they have tests they get scared and think about it a lot.*

ADDISON: *I think about that a lot.*

DR. KAMINSKY: *What do you do to try get the thoughts out your head?*

ADDISON: *They just come back.*

DR. KAMINSKY: *Do your parents know how much you think about this?*

ADDISON: *They just say I am lazy.*

DR. KAMINSKY: *Are there other thoughts that keep on coming into your head even if you don't want to think them.*

ADDISON SOBS.

DR. KAMINSKY: *These thoughts really bother you.*

ADDISON CRIES: *They're pictures not thoughts.*

DR. KAMINSKY: *Pictures of what?*

ADDISON SOBS: *My brother.*

DR. KAMINSKY: *Your brother?*

ADDISON: *In the pool.*

DR. KAMINSKY: *Oh, wow. That must have been so difficult for you.*

ADDISON: *I thought he died.*

DR. KAMINSKY: *What did you do?*

ADDISON: *I jumped in and saved him.*

DR. KAMINSKY: *You saved him—wow! Not too many kids can do that.*

ADDISON: *But they say it is my fault.*

DR. KAMINSKY: *Who does?*

ADDISON: *My parents, because I was watching him.*

DR. KAMINSKY: *And you still think about that a lot.*

ADDISON NODS YES.

DR. KAMINSKY: *When is it the worst for you with all these pictures and thoughts?*

ADDISON: *When I go to bed.*

DR. KAMINSKY: *Is it easy or difficult for you to fall asleep?*

ADDISON: *Difficult.*

DR. KAMINSKY: *Because of the thoughts and pictures about your brother or about school?*

ADDISON: *Both.*

DR. KAMINSKY: *Are there any other thoughts that bother you when you are trying to go to sleep?*

ADDISON: *My parents fight.*

DR. KAMINSKY: *About what?*

ADDISON: *Me.*

DR. KAMINSKY: *That probably makes you feel bad.*

ADDISON CRIES: *My mom always cries when they fight.*

DR. KAMINSKY: *And they fight about you?*

ADDISON: *My mom says I am too much.*

DR. KAMINSKY: *Please help me understand. What does she mean?*

ADDISON: *I have epilepsy, my grades are bad, and I don't look after my brother.*

DR. KAMINSKY: *So you feel that they fight and she cries because of you.*

Addison nods yes.

DR. KAMINSKY: *That's a lot of things for one person to be thinking about.*
Addison nods yes.
DR. KAMINSKY: *Addison you are such a good talker. I know it is not easy to talk about all of this. You are really helping me understand how hard things are for you at home and at school. Help me understand what will make this all better for you?*
ADDISON CRIES: *Nothing can help.*
DR. KAMINSKY: *And that's because?*
ADDISON: *I don't know.*
DR. KAMINSKY: *I know that's a hard question to answer.*

As evident from this dialogue, Addison responded well to the interview techniques Dr. Kaminsky used. Dr. Kaminsky first helped establish rapport with Addison by acknowledging that she might be weary of physicians and their questions. Dr. Kaminsky subsequent empathy for the child's symptoms and positive feedback on the information Addison provided further consolidated the rapport with the child. Dr. Kaminsky's "What" questions yielded information from the child suggesting that she was anxious and worried about her dropping grades, her brother, her mother's crying, and tension between her parents due to her epilepsy. Addison also confirmed symptoms of depression with crying and hopelessness for her future.

Addison's epileptologist ordered an EEG, which revealed ictal rapid spike followed by irregular slow waves, which were commensurate with a diagnosis of childhood onset of juvenile myoclonic epilepsy (see Table 10–1 in chapter 10). Dropping plates, which Addison's parents attributed to "nervousness" and carelessness, occurred during her myoclonic jerks. In addition, Addison's anxiety appeared to be secondary to her poor grades at school that, in turn, might have been due to the adverse effects of valproate on attention (Glauser et al. 2010). The epileptologist gradually stopped the valproate and increased the lamotrigine. Addison's seizures were well controlled and she underwent therapy for her posttraumatic stress disorder following her brother's near drowning. These interventions led to improvement in the child's attention, anxiety, and school performance.

However, Addison continued to feel that her epilepsy was the cause of her mother's sadness and frequent crying. Despite the improvement in Addison's condition, the mother continued to complain to Dr. Kaminsky that her daughter was not doing well and had difficulty coping with her epilepsy. Whereas the mother had focused on the child's nervousness and poor school grades prior to the child's therapy, the mother was unable to provide specific examples of why she felt the child was not doing well, and continued to be tearful as she spoke about her daughter.

In addition, the mother had little understanding about mental health issues, such as depression. Her cultural background made her resistant to the possibility that her complaints about the child might reflect her own depression. Dr. Kaminsky, therefore, explained how difficult it is for parents to deal with their children's epilepsy and the prevalence of depression among parents of children with epilepsy. The psychiatrist also emphasized the possible impact of the mother's depression on her not being emotionally available to support Addison and parent her other two children. This information made it easier for the mother to understand and accept that she, like other mothers of children with epilepsy, was depressed and that treatment for her depression would ultimately benefit her daughter with epilepsy as well as her other children.

Unrealistic Parental Expectations: This case was presented in the previous chapter as a clinical example of a *"Behavior Disorder vs. Undiagnosed Language-related Learning Disorder* (see pages 205-207)." To recap, Grace is a 7-year-old girl with intractable seizures who had her first seizure 6 months after a mild head trauma that she experienced while on a jungle gym at a park at age 4 years. She had lost consciousness briefly and was observed for 24 hours in the hospital due to vomiting. After an additional seizure, she was treated with an antiepileptic drug, and had no subsequent seizures until six months ago. Her EEG showed a left temporal focus, and her MRI identified a left temporal lobe lesion. She underwent surgical removal of a low-grade astrocytoma. Subsequent to the surgery, she began to have frequent uncontrolled seizures despite multiple attempts at different antiepileptic drug combinations.

The mother was very concerned about her daughter's resistance to going to school and the child's claim that the teacher and the children were mean to her. She worked intensely on a daily basis with the child on reading, spelling, and arithmetic, and Grace began having daily temper tantrums. The mother brought Grace for an evaluation by the pediatric epileptologist, Dr. Doyle, because of these problem behaviors. The pediatric epileptologist's interview with the child (see pages 205-207) revealed that Grace had difficulties processing language probably due to the left temporal lobe location of the tumor, incomplete removal of the tumor, and continued uncontrolled seizures.

Grace was in a regular second grade class and clearly was struggling with all her subjects due to her linguistic and cognitive difficulties. Dr. Doyle's feedback on the need for language and cognitive testing, as well as evaluation by the school to determine what special education services she should receive, were received with great shock and sadness by both parents. The mother became tearful and felt that the physician's evaluation was incorrect and that her daughter was much higher functioning than she appeared during the interview. In subsequent appointments she presented Dr. Doyle with examples of Grace's good intuition and information on all the college graduates in both her family and her husband's.

The mother did not schedule the repeatedly recommended language and cognitive testing. This omission confirmed her difficulty in accepting the child's deficits. In parallel, the child began to have severe temper tantrums with increasing aggressive behavior toward the mother. When forced to attend school, she would tear up her worksheets at school and then hit her peers. The father was unable to attend any of the clinic visits, and focused all his energies on his work.

The mother requested additional appointments so that Dr. Doyle could reexamine Grace because of her severe aggression. The interviews with the child confirmed the anger and frustration she experienced because of her language-related learning disorder and continued placement in a regular education class. The frequency of temper tantrums and aggressive outbursts at home increased and the child became depressed, felt nothing would ever get better, said she was a bad girl, and wanted to die. Although the parents were willing for Grace to be treated with an antidepressant medication, they continued the academic pressure on the child.

It took a year of recurrent "urgent" appointments for Grace with Dr. Doyle due to further escalating behavior problems and threats of expulsion from the school before the mother was able to recognize and accept her own need for counseling to help her come to terms with her daughter's illness and related learning deficits. Because of the stress on the marital relationship, both parents subsequently also had couples therapy. Grace began receiving special education services in third grade, and she did all her work only at school. There was marked improvement in the mother–daughter relationship, and the father became more engaged in the child's upbringing.

This case demonstrates the importance of determining to what degree parents' complaints about behavior problems in a child with epilepsy might reflect their own difficulties coping with the illness and its comorbidities. It also emphasizes that for some parents coming to terms with the illness and related deficits takes a while, and might occur only after severe worsening of the child's behavior and/or demands for intervention by external institutions, such as the school.

Parent Anxiety: Jasmine, aged 6 years, is brought to a child psychologist because, since she started to have complex partial seizures (Table 11-1) about three months ago, she has become demanding and irritable with temper tantrums if she does not get her way. The parents are at a loss and want some guidance on how to deal with these behavior problems. They think that she might be having difficulty dealing with the diagnosis of epilepsy because she was an easygoing, calm, happy child before her first seizure.

In his interview with Jasmine, the psychologist found out that the child knew she was taking medicine to stop her from staring, making chewing movements, and then being tired or falling asleep. The child's main concern about her illness was that she might need to have blood tests. Jasmine felt sad because her parents argued every night after she went to bed. She heard them fight about the mother sleeping with Jasmine rather than in the parents' room, and the mother refusing to leave Jasmine with a babysitter so they could socialize with friends. When asked what makes her angry, Jasmine bashfully admitted feeling mad when her mother does not buy her what she wants. The psychologist asked what Jasmine does when that happens and Jasmine said, "I get mad with my mom and she buys it for me."

In a separate meeting with the parents, the psychologist found out that the mother felt she had to be with Jasmine all the time because of her fears that her daughter might get hurt or die during a seizure. Although the father had suggested use of a "baby monitor" so that they could hear if the child had a seizure at night, this was too anxiety-provoking for the mother. When the psychologist asked how they discipline Jasmine, the mother said she did not want the child to get angry or upset because she might have a seizure. The father was not sure about the best approach. He did not want his daughter to have a seizure, but he also felt that giving her whatever she wants would not help her for her future life.

The psychologist explained that parents cope differently when their children are first diagnosed with epilepsy. Some become anxious but are able to separate their anxiety and the child's developmental needs. Parents with overwhelming anxiety might need to keep the child in sight all the time and meet all the child's demands, even when they are inappropriate or excessive. He added that parents are faced with the difficulty of resolving these differences in their approaches. He also noted that in some families this is easily accomplished and in others parents need counseling.

Jasmine's parents agreed to counseling with the psychologist, and the child's behavior and family functioning improved after a few sessions. Thus, as demonstrated in previous clinical examples, the information obtained from the child was key to finding out about the mother's anxiety and related tension between the parents.

Cultural: Elijah is 10 years old and the youngest of triplets (two boys and a girl). He was diagnosed with complex partial seizures (Table 11-1) at age 7 years and has had well-controlled seizures for the past two years. He was stung by a bee ten days ago and had a severe allergic response, and has been treated with prednisone. A child psychiatrist is seeing him as an emergency case because he punched his brother in the face last night during a fight. The parents report that he has been arguing and harassing his brother during the past week, and that he reacts with extreme anger toward the parents when they scold him and tell him to leave the brother alone.

During the child's interview, the child psychiatrist found out that he is angry with his brother, because the brother boasts about his grades at school, plays in the baseball and basketball team, skates, bikes, and swims with his friends, and is allowed to go to sleepovers. In contrast, Elijah's teachers mark him down for stupid things so his grades are not as good as those of his brother, and he never does the "fun stuff" his brother does with friends.

The physician needed to determine if, in fact, the parents were restricting Elijah's sport and social activities and/or if the addition of prednisone to Elijah's medication regime caused him to be irritable and "paranoid" toward his brother. The parents confirmed that Elijah has always had trouble getting along with his brother but that his anger escalated since he started the prednisone. They also acknowledged that they did not want Elijah to have a seizure at school, on the sport's field, or while socializing with other children from the neighborhood school because all the children were from the same community as Elijah's family. The stigma of epilepsy in this community was such that it might stigmatize and socially isolate the family.

In addition to talking to the child's pediatrician about decreasing the prednisone, the child psychiatrist asked the parents if Elijah could attend school with a more diverse population of children. The parents thought that this was not a feasible option, as it would raise too many questions in their community. The child psychiatrist emphasized that, in addition to allowing Elijah to make friends with children who were not his brother's friends, a transition to another school could mitigate the academic competition between Elijah and his brother. The parents felt that the need to prevent excessive competition between the two brothers would be an acceptable explanation for a change in schools in their community.

SUMMARY

- Each child with epilepsy should have a developmentally oriented interview to determine if the child is faced with psychosocial stressors and, if so, how the child deals with them.
- The child's interview might also provide information on difficulties the parents have in dealing with the psychosocial stressors.
- Focused on the parents' presenting complaint regarding the child, the interviewer should obtain information from the parents on the child's seizures; response to treatment; functioning in terms of behavior, emotions, and learning; social activities; and the child's relationship within the family.
- Once the interviewer has established rapport with the parents, the clinician should find out how each parent copes with the illness-related stressors and all aspects of the impact of the illness on the child, as well as assessing the relationship between the parents, their parenting skills, and functioning of the family.

- Providing parents with information on the impact of epilepsy on parents and families helps these parents talk about the difficulties they experience due to their child's illness.
- This comprehensive approach is essential to help children with epilepsy cope with their illness.

REFERENCES

Adewuya AO (2006). Parental psychopathology and self-rated quality of life in adolescents with epilepsy in Nigeria. *Dev Med Child Neurol* 48: 600–603.

Aronu A and Iloeje SO (2011). Behavioral problems of siblings of epileptic children in Enugu. *Niger J Clin Pract* 14: 132–136.

Austin JK and Caplan R (2007). Behavioral and psychiatric comorbidities in pediatric epilepsy: Toward an integrative model. *Epilepsia* 48: 1639–1651

Austin JK, MacLeod J, Dunn DW, Shen J, and Perkins SM (2004). Measuring stigma in children with epilepsy and their parents: Instrument development and testing. *Epilepsy Behav* 5: 472–482.

Austin JK, Shafer PO, and Deering JB (2002). Epilepsy familiarity, knowledge, and perceptions of stigma: Report from a survey of adolescents in the general population. *Epilepsy Behav* 3: 368–375.

Besag FM, Nomayo A, and Pool F (2005). The reactions of parents who think that a child is dying in a seizure—In their own words. *Epilepsy Behav* 7: 517–523.

Brodie MJ and Holmes GL (2008). Should all patients be told about sudden unexpected death in epilepsy (SUDEP)? Pros and Cons. *Epilepsia* 49: 99–101.

Caplan R, Sagun J, Siddarth P, Gurbani S, Koh S, Gowrinathan R, and Sankar R (2005). Social competence in pediatric epilepsy: Insights into underlying mechanisms. *Epilepsy Behav* 6: 218--228.

Carlton-Ford S, Miller R, Nealeigh N, and Sanchez N (1997). The effects of perceived stigma and psychological over-control on the behavioural problems of children with epilepsy. *Seizure* 6: 383–391.

Chapieski L, Brewer V, Evankovich K, Culhane-Shelburne K, Zelman K, and Alexander A (2005). Adaptive functioning in children with seizures: Impact of maternal anxiety about epilepsy. *Epilepsy & Behavior* 7: 246–252.

Duffy L (2011). Parental coping and childhood epilepsy: The need for future research. *J Neurosci Nurs* 43: 29–35.

Dunn DW, Johnson CS, Perkins SM, Fastenau PS, Byars AW, deGrauw TJ, and Austin JK (2010). Academic problems in children with seizures: Relationships with neuropsychological functioning and family variables during the 3 years after onset. *Epilepsy Behav* 19: 455ˆ461.

Fastenau PS, Shen J, Dunn DW, Perkins SM, Hermann BP, and Austin JK (2004). Neuropsychological predictors of academic underachievement in pediatric epilepsy: Moderating roles of demographic, seizure, and psychosocial variables. *Epilepsia* 45: 1261–1272.

Ferro M and Speechley KN (2009). Depressive symptoms among mothers of children with epilepsy: A review of prevalence, associated factors, and impact on children. *Epilepsia* 50: 2344–2354.

Freilinger M, Neussl D, Hansbauer T, Reiter E, Seidl R, and Schubert MT (2006). Psychosocial adjustment, relationship and self-concept in siblings of children with idiopathic epilepsy syndromes. *Klin Padiatr* 218: 1–6.

Gartstein MA, Bridgett DJ, Dishion TJ, and Kaufman NK (2009). Depressed mood and maternal report of child behavior problems: Another look at the depression–distortion hypothesis. *J Appl Dev Psychol* 30: 149–160.

Gayatri NA, Morrall MCHJ, Jain V, Kashyape P, Pysden K, and Ferrie C (2011). Parental and physician beliefs regarding the provision and content of written sudden unexpected death in epilepsy (SUDEP) information. *Epilepsia* 51: 777–782.

Glauser TA, Cnaan A, Shinnar S, Hirtz DG, Dlugos D, Masur D, Clark PO, Capparelli EV, and Adamson PC (2010). Ethosuximide, valproic acid, and lamotrigine in childhood absence epilepsy. *N Engl J Med* 362: 790–799.

Hamiwka LD, Yu CG, Hamiwka LA, Sherman EMS, Anderson B, and Wirrell E (2009). Are children with epilepsy at greater risk for bullying than their peers? *Epilepsy Behav* 15: 500–505.

Heisler AB and Friedman SB (1981). Social and psychological considerations in chronic disease: With particular reference to the management of seizure disorders. *J Pediatr Psychol* 6: 239–250.

Hirfanoglu T, Serdaroglu A, Cansu A, Soysal AS, Derle E, and Gucuyener K (2009). Do knowledge of, perception of, and attitudes toward epilepsy affect the quality of life of Turkish children with epilepsy and their parents? *Epilepsy & Behavior* 14: 71–77.

Hoare P and Kerley S (1991). Psychosocial adjustment of children with chronic epilepsy and their families. *Dev Med Child Neurol* 33: 201–215.

Hodes M, Garralda ME, Rose G, and Schwartz R (1999). Maternal expressed emotion and adjustment in children with epilepsy. *J Child Psychol Psychiatry* 40: 1083–1093.

Hornstra L, Denessen E, Bakker J, van den Bergh L, and Voeten M (2010). Teacher attitudes toward dyslexia: Effects on teacher expectations and the academic achievement of students with dyslexia. *J Learning Disabil* 43: 515–529.

Kossoff EH, Zupec-Kania BA, and Rho JM (2009). Ketogenic diets: An update for child neurologists. *J Child Neurol* 24: 979–988.

Mu PF, Wong TT, Chang KP, and Kwan SY (2001). Predictors of maternal depression for families having a child with epilepsy. *J Nurs Res* 9: 116–126.

Mu PF (2005). Paternal reactions to a child with epilepsy: Uncertainty, coping strategies, and depression. *J Adv Nurs* 49: 367–376.

Pianta RC and Lothman DJ (1994). Predicting behavior problems in children with epilepsy: Child factors, disease factors, family stress, and child-mother interaction. *Child Dev* 65: 1415–1428.

Ramaglia G, Romeo A, Viri M, Lodi M, Sacchi S, and Cioffi G (2007). Impact of idiopathic epilepsy on mothers and fathers: Strain, burden of care, worries and perception of vulnerability. *Epilepsia* 48: 1810–1814.

Rodenburg R, Marie Meijer A, Dekovic M, and Aldenkamp AP (2006). Family predictors of psychopathology in children with epilepsy. *Epilepsia* 47: 601–614.

Rodenburg R, Wagner JL, Austin JK, Kerr M, and Dunn DW (2011). Psychosocial issues for children with epilepsy. *Epilepsy Behav* 22: 47–54.

Sbarra DA, Rimm-Kaufman SE, and Pianta RC (2002). The behavioral and emotional correlates of epilepsy in adolescence: A 7-year follow-up study. *Epilepsy Behav* 3: 358–67.

Shore C, Austin J, Musick B, Dunn D, McBride A, and Creasy K (1998). Psychosocial care needs of parents of children with new onset seizures. *J Neurosci Nurs* 30: 169–174.

Shore C, Austin JK, Huster GA, and Dunn DW (2002). Identifying risk factors for maternal depression in families of adolescents with epilepsy. *J Spec Pediatr Nurs* 7: 71–80.

Taylor V, Fuggle P, and Charman T (2001). Well sibling psychological adjustment to chronic physical disorder in a sibling: How important is maternal awareness of their illness attitudes and perceptions? *J Child Psychol Psychiatry* 42: 953–962.

Van der Bruggen CO, Stams GJJM, and Bögels SM (2008). Research review: The relation between child and parent anxiety and parental control: A meta-analytic review. *J Child Psychol Psychiatry* 49: 1257–1269.

Wagner JL, Sample PL, Ferguson PL, Pickelsimer EE, Smith GM, and Selassie AW (2009). Impact of pediatric epilepsy: Voices from a focus group and implications for public policy change. *Epilepsy Behav* 16: 161–165.

Williams J, Steel C, Sharp GB, DelosReyes E, Phillips T, Bates S, Lange B, and Griebel ML (2003). Parental anxiety and quality of life in children with epilepsy. *Epilepsy Behav* 4: 483–486.

Wood LJ, Sherman E, Hamiwka LD, Blackman M, and Wirrell E (2008). Depression, anxiety, and quality of life in siblings of children with intractable epilepsy. *Epilepsy Behav* 13: 144–148.

Wu KN, Lieber E, Siddarth P, Smith K, Sankar R, and Caplan R (2008). Dealing with epilepsy: Parents speak up. *Epilepsy Behav* 13: 131–138.

Application of the Developmental Guidelines

Specific Communication Challenges in Young Ill Children

Overview to Part IV

WHERE TO NOW?

In the next three chapters the reader will learn how to use the developmental guidelines and interview techniques to conduct developmentally sensitive interviews of young children with pain, iatrogenic trauma symptoms, and terminal illness. Seriously medically ill children struggle with these problems and they pose specific challenges to the interviewer.

In the chapter on pain, we review those biological, psychological, and social factors that comprise the biopsychosocial model of pain, and we present techniques for assessment of these factors in the young child. While pain has been extensively researched, many clinicians and most families have a simplistic understanding of pain processes, tending to dichotomize pain as either physical or psychological. It is important to utilize a biopsychosocial approach to ensure that the evaluation is comprehensive, the pain is thoroughly understood, and that the child and family begin to learn about the many factors that impact pain and disability. It takes effort and practice to become adept at maintaining a more integrated biopsychosocial stance and to use language that reflects the biopsychosocial model. Likewise, children and their parents might be concerned that the interviewer does not believe the pain is "real" if the interviewer prematurely asks questions related to emotional and behavioral functioning. Although the chapter on pain is not a comprehensive review of specific pain disorders, it provides the building blocks for competent interviewing of children with pain. (For a comprehensive review, see Schechter et al. 2003.)

In the chapter on iatrogenic trauma, we review symptoms of medical trauma in the young child and present information on techniques for interviewing this vulnerable group of children. Seriously ill children have typically been exposed to many frightening and painful medical experiences. A subset of these children develop trauma symptoms as a result of these experiences, called iatrogenic trauma symptoms. It is challenging to interview young children with iatrogenic trauma because just thinking or talking about the traumatic experiences can be very distressing to the child (and/or parent). Additionally, the interviewer may be perceived by the traumatized child as an individual who will subject the child to more traumatic experiences. Some children will become nonverbal or simply refuse to speak to professionals. This chapter emphasizes techniques that can be used with a nonverbal child with trauma symptoms.

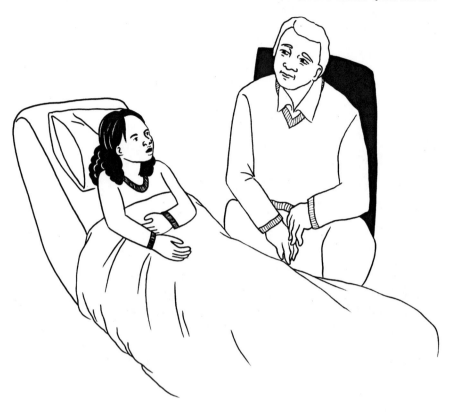

In the chapter on terminal illness, we review common symptoms in the young terminally ill child, present frequent communication challenges, and provide techniques for interviewing these children. Few topics are as distressing as the death of a child. Parents are typically extremely stressed. Clinicians are also deeply affected. The ill child may be quite symptomatic and may be worried about distressing

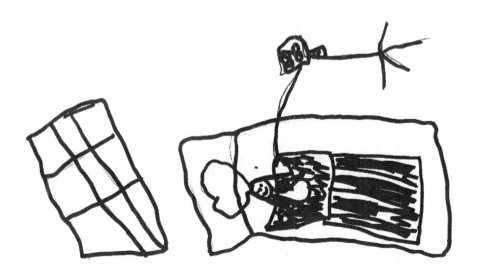

others. Effective communication with the child (about death and associated symp-toms) increases the likelihood that the concerns of the child will be understood and appropriately addressed. Such intervention can significantly improve the quality of life for the child and the family. Additionally, the interviewer who gains expert competency in assessing a terminally ill child may feel an increased sense of satis-faction and ability to make a meaningful contribution to the life of the child and the family.

REFERENCES

Schechter NL, Berde CB, Yaster M, eds. (2003). *Pain in Infants, Children, and Adolescents*, 2nd Ed. Philadelphia: Lippincott, Williams, and Wilkins.

Pediatric Pain Disorders

Pain is defined by the *International Association for the Study of Pain* as "an unpleasant sensory and emotional experience associated with actual or potential tissue damage, or described in terms of such damage."
—(MERSKEY ET AL. 1979)

Pain is a common experience for children, especially among those who are medically ill. Most children experience minor painful injuries and many experience pain when stressed. Developmental differences in reports of chronic pain are seen across the age range, with prepubertal children most likely to report pain in one location, most commonly abdominal pain or headaches (Belmaker et al. 1985; Faull and Nicol 1986; Garber et al. 1991; Garber et al. 1990; Larson 1991; Tamminen et al. 1991).

Community-based studies suggest that recurrent abdominal pain is experienced by 10–15% of school-age children (Apley 1975; Apley and Naish 1958) and that headaches are experienced by 8.3% of children under 10 years of age (Groholt et al. 2003). The gender ratio is equal in early childhood; females are more likely to report pain than males, starting around the time of puberty (Groholt et al. 2003; Stickler and Murphy 1979; Apley and Naish 1958; Spierings et al. 1990; Steinhausen et al. 1989). Chronic pain appears to be more likely in lower socioeconomic groups (Groholt et al. 2003).

Symptoms of pain increase significantly in children who have underlying medical conditions or injuries. Pain may be related to procedures and surgeries, to treatment side effects, and to the underlying medical problem or injury. For example, between 45%–60% of pediatric cancer patients report pain (Forgeron et al. 2006; Jacob et al. 2007; Ljungman et al. 1999), although one study suggested that only 22% received analgesics (Forgeron et al. 2006). Likewise, between 40%–86% of children with arthritis report pain, often well after treatment has been initiated (Lovell and Walco 1989; Petty et al. 2004; Sherry et al. 1990; Schanberg et al. 2003). Children under 15 years old who report pain in an emergency room are significantly less likely to receive pain medication than individuals 15–65 years old (McCaig and Nawar 2006). Thus, pain assessment is an important skill for clinicians working with young medically ill children.

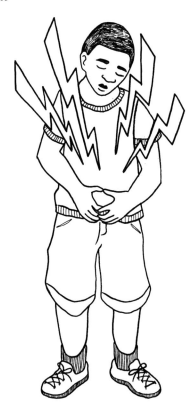

In this chapter, we will present information on the factors related to pain perception and pain-related disability that provide the reader with guidance for assessing a young child with chronic pain.

Factors Related to Pain Perception and Pain Disability

Many biopsychosocial factors related to pain and pain disability have been identified. Biological processes related to pain perception include nervous system reactivity and recovery in response to stress and symptoms. Psychological processes include temperamental tendencies, such as attentional biases toward symptom-related stimuli and coping strategies. Social environmental factors include chronic stressors and parental responses to their children's symptom behavior.

For example, children with recurrent abdominal pain exhibit hyperreactive sympathetic nervous system arousal in response to stress (hypersensitive perception of gastrointestinal stimuli and a lower threshold for pain), disrupted or delayed parasympathetic recovery from stressors (meaning it takes longer than usual for nervous system arousal to abate), and hypervigilance to internal and external pain cues (DiLorenzo et al. 2001; Duarte et al. 1999; Compas and Boyer 2001; Thomsen et al. 2002). Biochemical changes in the sensory neurons of the central nervous system and the enteric nervous system (which controls the gastrointestinal system), influenced by cognitive processes and other sensations, appear to be related to the reduced pain threshold.

The following section briefly reviews some of the factors that have been found to influence pain perception and disability and, therefore, are important to assess in young children with pain.

Past Painful Experiences

Research has provided evidence that newborns are *more* sensitive to pain than older infants, children, and adults (Anand 1998). Repetitive or prolonged pain in the neonatal period can cause long-term changes in pain processing (including pain sensitivity) and may be related to later childhood neurodevelopmental, behavioral, and cognitive deficits (Anand 2000; Bhutta and Anand 2002; Chacko et al. 1999; Grunau 2000; Johnston and Stevens 1996; McLendon et al. 2003; Mitchell and Boss 2002; Rossi et al. 1998; Taddio et al. 2002; Tobiansky et al. 1995; Whitfield and Grunau 2000). Prior medical illness, physical injury, trauma, and hospitalizations have all been found to be related to increased pain sensitivity. The adverse nature of prior pain experiences appears to be a more important variable than the number of past pain episodes. Additionally, as illustrated in the following interview, the pain need not be remembered for it to have had an impact on current pain processing, such as in the case of a premature infant who may experience many medical procedures prior to discharge home.

Past Pain
INTERVIEWER: *Have you had pain when you were younger; before this pain?*
CHILD: *No, I don't remember having bad pain like this before.*
INTERVIEWER: *Do you remember ever being in the hospital before?*
CHILD: *No.*
INTERVIEWER: *What would you say is the worst thing that ever happened to you?*
CHILD: *I don't know. My mom says I was a preemie and she was scared I was going to die.*
INTERVIEWER: *What did she tell you a preemie is?*
CHILD: *She said I was born two months before I was supposed to be born.*
INTERVIEWER: *I see. So, did you stay in the hospital for a while when you were born?*
CHILD: *My mom says I did, but I don't remember it.*

Temperament, Coping, and Psychological Characteristics

Temperament, coping style, and the psychological characteristics of an individual impact that individual's perception of pain, the likelihood of developing a pain disorder, and risk for pain-related disability. Temperament refers to inborn personality traits or the tendency to respond to and cope with stimuli in predictable ways. Temperamental traits include activity level, regularity in habits (eating and sleeping), tendency to approach or withdrawal from a novel situation, adaptability, emotional intensity/reactivity, mood (lability and the tendency to be optimistic or pessimistic), persistence, distractibility, and sensory sensitivity.

Behaviorally inhibited temperament in childhood (restrained, wary, and fearful in response to unfamiliar stimuli) has been associated with variability in stress reactivity (the tendency to activate neural circuits that trigger distress responses to threatening stimuli), anxiety disorders, and somatic complaints (Biederman et al. 1993; Boyce et al. 1992; Campo et al. 2004; Kagan et al. 1988; Manassis et al. 1995). Consequently, for example, an interaction between an inhibited temperamental style and environmental stresses, such as going to a new school, appears to place young children at risk for physical symptoms, such as recurrent abdominal pain (Davison et al. 1986).

Pain sensitivity and disability have been linked with a tendency to fixate on pain and pain-related distress (Bennett-Branson and Craig 1993; Gil et al. 1991). Related catastrophizing (thinking that a situation is far worse than it actually is) has been significantly correlated with increased laboratory pain (usually caused by immersion of an arm into cold water) in healthy child and pediatric pain samples (Gil et al 1993; Keefe et al 2000; Lester et al. 1994; Piira et al. 2002; Sullivan et al. 2001; Thastum et al. 2001; Thastum et al. 1997).

Anxiety sensitivity (defined as the tendency to interpret anxiety-related bodily sensations, such as rapid heartbeat, as dangerous) in adults has been associated with anxiety disorders (Taylor 1999) and chronic pain (Asmundson et al. 1999). Comparable research in pediatric populations has only recently been initiated (Fuss, Pagé and Katz 2011; Pagé et al. 2010). In a community-based study of children, girls with persistent pain reported higher levels of anxiety sensitivity (P<0.001) and pain catastrophizing (P<0.001) than girls without persistent pain and than boys (regardless of pain status) (Fuss et al. 2011). In one pediatric pain laboratory study, measures of anxiety sensitivity, anxiety symptoms, and anticipatory anxiety combined explained 62% of the variance in pain intensity (Tsao et al. 2007).

The following dialogue illustrates how the interviewer can ask a young child about anxiety sensitivity.

Anxiety Sensitivity
INTERVIEWER: *What do you think is causing your pain?*
CHILD: *Maybe cancer.*
INTERVIEWER: *What makes you think it might be cancer?*
CHILD: *My uncle had cancer and he died.*
INTERVIEWER: *I am so sorry to hear that. When did that happen?*
CHILD: *I don't remember. I was a baby.*
INTERVIEWER: *I see. Why do you think you might have cancer?*
CHILD: *Cause they can't figure out why I have pain. My mom thinks it could be cancer.*
INTERVIEWER: *Is that something you are worried about?*
CHILD: *Yeah.*
INTERVIEWER: *Have you told your mom that you are worried about maybe having cancer?*
CHILD: *Yeah. We talk about it all the time. We need to find a doctor who can find it.*

In the dialogue above, it is apparent that the child has learned from the parent to interpret the abdominal pain as potentially life-threatening. The chronic stress and anxiety experienced by this child due to this perception (in both the child and parent) have the potential to increase the child's pain perception.

Perceived coping inefficacy by an individual is associated with increased distress, autonomic nervous system arousal, and plasma catecholamine secretion (stress hormones released into the bloodstream) (Bandura et al. 1982; Bandura et al. 1985). Research on children with recurrent abdominal pain (RAP) reveals that accommodative coping (distraction, acceptance, positive thinking, challenging unhelpful irrational thoughts) is correlated with less pain, while passive coping strategies (denial, cognitive avoidance, behavioral avoidance, wishful thinking) are correlated with increased levels of pain (Thomsen et al. 2002; Walker et al. 1997). Interestingly, active coping strategies (problem solving, emotional expression, emotional modulation, decision making) are inconsistent in their relationship to pain (Thomsen et al. 2002; Walker et al. 1997). Active problem-solving strategies aimed at reducing pain or at a specific stressor are helpful, however, active problem-solving behaviors that are not focused on a changeable problem may be ineffective and frustrating to the child.

The following dialogue illustrates an interviewer asking a young child about coping with pain. As is evident from the dialogue, this child feels unable to reduce pain through self-management skills.

Efficacy of Coping

INTERVIEWER: *So, what kinds of things do you do to try to help yourself when you have pain?*

CHILD: *I tell my mom.*

INTERVIEWER: *Okay, and what else do you do?*

CHILD: *I lie down. Sometimes I cry.*

INTERVIEWER: *Is there anything you do that helps the pain?*

CHILD: *No.*

INTERVIEWER: *Is there anything your mom does that helps the pain?*

CHILD: *No, but she gives me medicine.*

INTERVIEWER: *And anything else?*

CHILD: *She takes me to the ER to be sure I am okay.*

INTERVIEWER: *Have you ever been able to stop the pain?*

CHILD: *No. I just wait.*

Stress

Persistent stressors are thought to result in illness and symptoms, such as pain, due to their impact on the individual's internal response systems (McEwen and Seeman 1999). School, family, social, and illness stressors can all contribute to the development and/or exacerbation of pain. Daily stress appears to be more important than major stressors in triggering episodes of abdominal pain in children (Walker et al. 2001). Potentially stressful common comorbid findings include anxiety disorders, difficulty identifying and expressing emotions, depression, unsuspected learning problems (even in high achieving children), developmental or communication disorders, social problems (such as bullying or social perception deficits), physical or emotional trauma, family illness, and/or prominent family distress (Bursch et al. 2004; Bursch and Zeltzer 2002; Campo et al. 2002; Campo et al. 1999; Egger et al. 1998; Fritz et al. 1997; Garber et al. 1990; Hodges et al. 1985a; Hodges et al. 1985b; Hyman et al. 2002; Lester et al. 2003; Livingston 1993; Livingston et al. 1995; Schanberg et al. 1998; Stuart and Noyes 1999; Zuckerman et al. 1987).

Claar et al. (1999) studied self-perceived academic, social, and athletic competence as moderators between symptoms of irritable bowel syndrome and functional disability in youth with a history of recurrent abdominal pain. The relationship between symptoms and disability was stronger at lower levels of perceived *academic* competence. The same relationship was found for females at lower levels of perceived *social* competence, and for males at lower levels of perceived *athletic* competence. This research shows how chronic stress in the form of lower levels of perceived competence impacts functioning among those with chronic pain.

The following dialogue provides an example of a typical interview with a child with chronic pain. The child initially denies any worries, but detailed and developmentally sensitive questioning by the interviewer elicits a number of worries.

Stress

INTERVIEWER: *What kind of things do you worry about?*

CHILD: *Nothing.*

INTERVIEWER: *I see. Do you ever worry about your family?*

CHILD: *Only if I don't know where they are.*

INTERVIEWER: *And how often does that happen?*

CHILD: *When I get home from school.*

INTERVIEWER: *Every day?*

CHILD: *Pretty much.*

INTERVIEWER: *What kind of things do you worry about?*

CHILD: *A shooting or a car accident.*

INTERVIEWER: *So, almost every day you worry about your family being shot or in a car accident until they get home?*

CHILD: *Yeah.*

INTERVIEWER: *Has that happened to your family before?*

CHILD: *No.*

INTERVIEWER: *Do you know what makes you worry about a shooting or car accident?*

CHILD: *Because it's always on the news.*

INTERVIEWER: *I see. What about school? Do you worry about school?*

CHILD: *Just tests.*

INTERVIEWER: *And what worries you about tests?*

CHILD: *Sometimes I can't breathe when I take a test.*

INTERVIEWER: *Oh my. What else happens when you take a test?*

CHILD: *I feel shaky and sometimes dizzy, too.*

INTERVIEWER: *Do you sometimes worry that something bad could happen to you?*

CHILD: *Only at night or when I can't breathe.*

INTERVIEWER: *What do you worry about at night?*

CHILD: *Noises.*

INTERVIEWER: *I see. Can you tell me more about that?*

CHILD: *Maybe someone could break in and shoot us.*

INTERVIEWER: *Is that something you have also seen in the news?*

CHILD: *It happened to a family that lives by my cousin.*

INTERVIEWER: *Oh my. Was that someone you know?*

CHILD: *No, but my cousin lives near the park and the family in the news lives by the park.*

Family Variables

Parents of pediatric pain patients report higher levels of clinically significant anxiety, depression, and somatization than parents of well children (Campo et al. 2007; Emiroglu et al. 2004; Walker et al. 1991). In children with chronic pain, parental distress predicts poor outcomes measured by functional disability (not going out with friends, not participating in gym class or sports, or not being in school all day) (Logan and Scharff 2005; Wasserman et al. 1988).

Accounting for up to 55% of variance in child distress behavior (Frank et al. 1995), children look to their parents in order to assess the dangerousness of a situation and to learn how to cope with adverse situations. Parents directly impact their children's pain experiences and behavior through modeling responses to painful stimuli (Goodman and McGrath 2003). Parent behaviors that facilitate distraction (using toys, bubble-blowing, party blowers, or cartoons during painful procedures), that encourage the child to employ effective coping strategies, and that utilize humor are all related to decreases in child distress during painful medical procedures (Blount et al. 1989; Blount et al. 1990).

Parent reassurance, empathy, apologies, giving the child excessive control, and criticism of the child, however, are related to increases in children's distress during painful medical procedures. Discouraging children's coping efforts and providing special attention and accommodation to the child, such as breakfast in bed and relief from chores, are related to long-term distress, difficulties coping with pain, and the likelihood of developing chronic pain (e.g., Walker and Zeman 1992; Walker et al. 1993).

In the following dialogue, the interviewer discovers that the child's mother may be modeling and reinforcing pain-related disability. Additionally, the arguments between the parents could be a source of the stress for the child.

Modeling by Parent

INTERVIEWER: *Who helps you the most when you are in pain?*
CHILD: *My mom.*
INTERVIEWER: *And what does your mom do when you are in pain?*
CHILD: *She tells me to stay home from school and she brings me food while I watch TV.*
INTERVIEWER: *And what about your dad?*
CHILD: *He tells me to go to school.*
INTERVIEWER: *So your dad says go to school and your mom says stay home. How do you decide?*
CHILD: *They argue and my mom wins because she knows what it is like to have pain.*
INTERVIEWER: *Does your mom have pain, too?*
CHILD: *Yes. She gets migraines*

Summary

The assessment of children with pain should include developmentally based questions on the following factors related to pain perception and pain disability:

- Prior pain experiences
- Temperament
- Stress

- Coping
- Family variables

Assessment of Pain

GENERAL APPROACH

A biopsychosocial model should be applied to the evaluation and treatment of all types of pain. Clinicians should be alert to their own tendencies toward dualistic thinking and resist pressure from others to revert to dualistic thinking about pain as either a purely mind or body problem. Additionally, it is important for clinicians to be sensitive to concerns by the child or the family that the child is intentionally producing or exaggerating symptoms.

Most children and families will appreciate discussion of the distressing physical symptoms prior to being asked questions of a psychosocial nature. Pain can be classified in many ways, including by location on the body, duration (acute, recurrent, chronic), intensity (mild, moderate, severe), cause (malignant vs. nonmalignant), and presumed physiological mechanism (see Table 14–1).

The following exchange starts off well, but the clinician loses rapport with the child when attempting to use a dualistic approach.

Dualistic Approach

INTERVIEWER: *I understand that pain has been a problem for you. Can you tell me about your pain?*
CHILD: *It is mostly in my tummy.*
INTERVIEWER: *I see. Is it there all the time?*
CHILD: *No. Sometimes my legs hurt.*
INTERVIEWER: *I see. Where else does it hurt sometimes?*
CHILD: *Hmm. Just my tummy and my legs.*
INTERVIEWER: *What helps the pain?*
CHILD: *When my mom rubs my head. And staying home from school.*
INTERVIEWER: *And what makes the pain worse?*
CHILD: *When I have to run too much.*
INTERVIEWER: *When do you have to run too much?*
CHILD: *When I am at school.*
INTERVIEWER: *Seems to me that you say you have pain so you can stay home from school.*
CHILD: *I tell my mom when I have pain and she keeps me home from school.*
INTERVIEWER: *Some kids tell their parents they have pain even when they don't have pain. What about you?*
CHILD: *I don't do that.*
INTERVIEWER: *Well, you know, the doctors haven't found anything wrong with you.*
CHILD: *I am not lying.*
INTERVIEWER: *Let's try to figure out how to get you back to school.*
CHILD: *I don't want to talk to you.*

By contrast, maintaining a more neutral biopsychosocial perspective leads to a better understanding of the leg pain, which sounds neuropathic in nature (see Table 14–1), as in the following example.

Table 14–1. PAIN CLASSIFICATION

Classification System	Types	Description/Common Features
Duration	Acute	• Sudden onset; typically declines over a relatively short time (minutes to days) • A discrete episode that normally follows injury or illness, and resolves as the body heals • Often associated with physical signs of autonomic nervous system activity, such as tachycardia, hypertension, diaphoresis (sweating), pupil dilation, and/or pallor
	Recurrent	• Discrete episodes of pain that are typically brief in duration with complete resolution between episodes
	Chronic	• Persists on a daily basis for weeks to years • May or may not be associated with tissue inflammation or damage • Frequently not associated with physical signs of autonomic nervous system activity
Presumed Physiological Mechanism	Nociceptive pain: *Experienced when an injury or irritation is detected by receptors that respond to heat, cold, vibration, stretch and chemicals released from damaged cells*	• Subtypes: superficial, deep, visceral • Superficial and deep nociceptive pain is usually localized and non-radiating • Visceral pain is more diffuse over the viscera (organs) involved, poorly localized, and often referred (pain that is perceived in a body part that is away from the actual source of the pain)
	Neuropathic pain: *Experienced when peripheral, autonomic or central nervous system structures are injured, irritated, and/or overactive, causing dysfunction in pain signaling*	• Pain may be much greater than expected given the associated injury or illness • Pain may radiate along dermatomal (areas of skin supplied by a spinal nerve) or peripheral nerve distributions • Described as burning and/or deep aching. May include episodes of stabbing, sharp pain • May be associated with other unpleasant abnormal sensations (numbness, tingling, burning), a loss of sensory sensitivity or hypersensitivity (including a painful response to stimuli not normally painful), autonomic changes (sweating, vasomotor abnormalities), motor changes (weakness, dystonia), and/or trophic changes (skin or bone atrophy, hair loss, joint contractures)

Biopsychosocial Approach

INTERVIEWER: *I understand that pain has been a problem for you. Can you tell me about your pain?*

CHILD: *It is mostly in my tummy.*

INTERVIEWER: *I see. Is it there all the time?*

CHILD: *No. Sometimes my legs hurt.*

INTERVIEWER: *I see. Where else does it hurt sometimes?*

CHILD: *Hmm. Just my tummy and my legs.*

INTERVIEWER: *What helps the pain?*

CHILD: *When my mom rubs my head. And staying home from school.*

INTERVIEWER: *And what makes the pain worse?*

CHILD: *When I have to run too much.*

INTERVIEWER: *What started that problem; do you know?*

CHILD: *I tripped one day and now my leg sometimes hurts when I run too much and then my other leg starts to hurt, too.*

INTERVIEWER: *Can you tell me what the pain feels like?*

CHILD: *It hurts real bad and my leg gets hot, hot, hot; I can't even touch it.*

INTERVIEWER: *What about your tummy?*

CHILD: *My tummy doesn't get hot. It just hurts.*

INTERVIEWER: *What do you think about all the time at school you have been missing?*

CHILD: *Well, I am glad I don't have to run, but I miss seeing my teacher and my friends.*

INTERVIEWER: *Let's try to figure out how we can help you so that you can get back to school.*

CHILD: *Sounds good.*

Identification of specific pain symptoms, their typical precipitants and reinforcers, psychosocial stressors, and comorbidities allows for feedback that makes sense to the child and parents, particularly when subsequent treatment recommendations are closely linked to assessment findings. For example, a homebound child with tension headaches, perfectionistic traits, and a bully at school may be anxious about maintaining his straight As and avoiding his aggressor. The effort required for him to maintain his grades might be excessive due to an unrecognized math disorder. His parents, who feared he might have a brain tumor, may have inadvertently exacerbated his anxiety and muscle tension. This type of comprehensive evaluation provides multiple targets for intervention to improve the functioning of the child and potentially decrease his headaches.

Pain is measured by self-report, observational, and/or physiological measures. When possible, pain is best assessed by directly asking the child about his or her pain. However, a number of barriers can limit the assessment. As described in the developmental guidelines for interviewing children, young children might not have the ability to engage in such an assessment. Other children may be reluctant to report pain due to anxiety related to talking to doctors, taking pills, getting an injection of pain medication, being viewed as weak or demanding, distressing others, not being able to stay awake or have clear thinking, or finding out they are sick or in need of going to the hospital. Some children have heard their parents express concern that they will become a "drug addict" if they take pain medication.

Younger children may not understand what this means, but they are aware that it displeases their parents. As a result, they might not be forthcoming regarding their pain.

It can also be difficult for others to report on a child's pain. For example, it can be a challenge to differentiate between distress related to pain and distress related to fear or some other discomfort. Additionally, some children become adept at using distraction or withdrawal/dissociation to cope with pain and therefore might appear comfortable when they are not. This can present a confusing picture for clinicians who might see a child exhibiting extreme pain behaviors alternating with normal play, TV viewing, or sleep.

STRUCTURED PAIN ASSESSMENT TOOLS

Often used in medical settings to evaluate pain severity, structured pain assessment tools have been developed for use with young children (Cohen et al. 2008; Stinson et al. 2008; von Baeyer and Spagrud 2007). It is important for the interviewer to be aware of these scales since children with chronic pain will likely be accustomed to using them to rate the severity of their pain, and because they represent a standardized measurement that can be used over time. Recommended evidence-based measures are summarized in Table 14–2. It is important to use measures that are developmentally appropriate, and it is preferable to rate pain prospectively (in the moment) whenever possible.

Table 14–2. RECOMMENDED EVIDENCE-BASED PAIN ASSESSMENT TOOLS

Type of Measure	Name of Measure	Description of Measure
Child self-report measures	Faces Pain Scale-Revised (Hicks et al. 2001)	• For children 4 to 12 years of age • The Faces Pain Scale—Revised consists of 6 gender-neutral line drawings of faces depicting different intensities of pain
	• Visual analog scale (VAS)	• For children 8 years old or older • A VAS is a line with descriptive or numerical anchors on a continuum of pain intensity, anchored at one end by *no pain* (0) and at the other by their *worst pain imaginable* (10). The child rates their current pain by making a mark across the line.
	Pain diaries	• For children 6 years old or older (ideal age range unknown) • Typically used to assess recurrent or chronic pain, correlates of pain symptoms, and/or response to treatment • Might include rating scales & questions related to pain intensity, disability, perceived triggers, coping strategies used, consequences, medications used, and medication efficacy

Table 14–2. (CONTINUED)

Type of Measure	Name of Measure	Description of Measure
Parent observational (behavioral) measures	Parents' Postoperative Pain Measure (Chambers et al. 1996)	• For children in acute pain who are 1 year old or older, • A 15-item scale; parents observe and report changes from their children's usual behavior
Clinician observational (behavioral) measures	• FLACC Scale • (Merkel et al. 1997)	• For children in the hospital with procedural or postoperative pain who are 1 year old or older • Similar to an APGAR, this is a 5-item scale with scores from 0 to 2 for each item, combined for a total score from 0–10 • Raters score the following five items that have behavioral descriptions anchoring each score: (F) Face; (L) Legs; (A) Activity; (C) Cry; and (C) Consolability
	Children's Hospital of Eastern Ontario Pain Scale (CHEOPS) (McGrath et al. 1985)	• For children in the hospital with procedural or postoperative pain who are 1 year old or older • A 6-item scale; raters choose a score anchored by a behavioral description of the following: crying, facial expression, verbal expression, torso position, touch, and leg position
Clinician observational (behavioral) measures	COMFORT Scale (Ambuel et al. 1992)	• For children in critical care who are 1 year old or older • Uses alertness, calmness/agitation, respiration, physical movement, blood pressure change, heart rate change, muscle tone, and facial tension to assess distress

Because asking the child to focus on pain can exacerbate it, is also important to ask children to rate pain only when necessary. For hospitalized chronic pain patients, it is acceptable for nurses and others to refrain from pain assessment as the fifth vital sign *if this instruction is incorporated into the treatment plan.* Therefore, the interviewer need not feel obligated to ask children to rate their pain if it is clinically contraindicated. Additionally, observational measures are not recommended for assessing chronic or recurrent pain since behavioral signs of chronic pain decrease over time, making them difficult to reliably observe.

CLINICAL INTERVIEW

In addition to soliciting a careful description of the pain described above, the clinical interview of the child should review factors that are related to pain perception and disability. The Piagetian stages of cognitive development in Table 14–3 provide a

Table 14–3. PIAGETIAN STAGES OF COGNITIVE DEVELOPMENT
AND THE EXPERIENCE OF PAIN

Developmental Stage	Typical Implications Related to Pain
Sensorimotor children (birth to about 2 years old)	• They are mostly preverbal, without the capacity to create narratives to explain their experiences • They are most likely to demonstrate pain by social withdrawal or changes in their patterns of sleep, eating, and level of activity • By 18 months of age, most typically developing children will make an effort to localize pain and seek reassurance from adults; 2-year-old children are often able to use specific words to indicate the presence of pain
Preoperational children (about 2–7 years old)	• They use words and understand basic concepts of cause and effect. However, they tend to erroneously see events that are temporally related as causally related. • They may view pain as a punishment for the real or imagined transgression of rules • During this stage, children are not able to use self-generated coping strategies and tend to rely on their environment (i.e., the support of adults) • Children in this developmental stage have difficulty using rating scales of pain. They also have difficulty differentiating pain from anxiety or fear
Concrete operational children (about 7–11 years old)	• They can apply logic to their perceptions in a more integrative manner. However, the logic is literal (concrete) and allows for only one cause for an effect • Interventions that are concrete will make more sense to children at this stage. For example, applying a topical anesthetic to a painful part will make more sense to them than pain relief via oral or IV medication • At this stage, they are likely to be able to use a rating scale for pain assessment, and they will have an increased ability to use self-initiated coping strategies such as distraction or guided imagery
Formal operational children (11+ years old)	• They are able to use abstract reasoning to discuss body systems and can conceptualize multiple causation of pain • They are potentially more aware of the psychological aspects of pain and better able to understand a biopsychosocial model • Their greater ability to focus on future events may lead to greater worries and concerns about the pain • It should not be assumed that all adolescents (or parents) can utilize abstract reasoning. Most adults engage in abstract reasoning only in areas of their own expertise, if at all. And everyone tends to regress under stress

helpful context for understanding a child or adolescent's experience of pain (Gaffney et al. 2003).

There are significant variations in pain sensitivity and the consequent need for analgesics among individuals experiencing pain. Distress and pain severity are not always linearly related among those with either acute or chronic pain. And pain-related disability involves many factors in addition to pain severity and distress.

Regardless of the type of pain, the following domains are helpful to assess: current pain and pain history, other physical symptoms, pain beliefs, coping strategies and consequences, physical functioning, emotional and cognitive functioning, and family functioning. For children with recurrent, uncontrolled, or chronic pain, it is also helpful to carefully assess behaviors outside the hospital setting, such as social functioning and academic functioning. Table 14–4 provides a summary of topics to cover in these domains.

The example that follows illustrates how to ask questions that are related to the location, quality, and intensity of the pain when talking to children in acute or chronic pain. Again, parents might be better able to report duration, variability, predictability, and types of pain under differing circumstances due to young children's developmental limitations.

Questions on Pain for Young Children
INTERVIEWER: *What part of your body hurts?*
CHILD: *Right here (point to legs).*
INTERVIEWER: *Okay. And where else does it hurt?*
CHILD: *Nothing else hurts.*
INTERVIEWER: *Does your whole leg hurt or just part of your leg? Can you show me?*
CHILD: *Right here (points from toe to just above the knee).*
INTERVIEWER: *Okay. Can you tell me what your leg feels like?*
CHILD: *It hurts real bad.*
INTERVIEWER: *What happens when you walk?*
CHILD: *I can't walk. It hurts too much.*
INTERVIEWER: *And what happens when you touch it?*
CHILD: *I can't touch it. It hurts too much. I can't even sleep under the covers or put my pants on!*
INTERVIEWER: *Can you think of any other words to tell me what it feels like?*
CHILD: *Like what?*
INTERVIEWER: *Well, some kids have pain that feels like an elephant is sitting on them and some kids say that their pain is hot or feels like a knife is cutting them. Do any of those things sound like your pain?*
CHILD: *It's like when I got a real bad sunburn at the beach. I can't even touch it. And sometimes it gets red like a sunburn, too.*
INTERVIEWER: *That is very helpful. You did a very good job of telling me about your pain.*

As previously discussed in the chapters on somatization and autism symptoms (chapters 8 and 9), alexithymia (defined as greater than developmentally expected difficulty identifying and/or expressing one's emotional state) is important to assess before asking questions related to children's emotional functioning (De Gucht and Heiser 2003). Most children are capable of assessing their ability to readily identify

Table 14–4. CLINICAL INTERVIEW TOPICS

CURRENT PAIN
- Location, quality, intensity, duration, variability, predictability and types of pain under differing circumstances
- Exacerbating and alleviating factors
- Other associated sensations/symptoms
- Past evaluations, treatment attempts, home remedies, alternative/complementary therapies
- Ability to self-management symptoms, response to pain
- Impact of pain on daily life, including school, social activities, eating, and sleep (onset and maintenance)

BELIEFS ABOUT THE PAIN
- Cause of the pain
- What will and will not help
- Dangerousness
- Prognosis

PHYSICAL FUNCTIONING
- Basic functioning: walking and eating
- Change in participation in P.E., sports, exercise, social outings, school, chores, homework, activities of daily living driving

SOCIAL FUNCTIONING
- Changes in social functioning
- Satisfaction with social life
- Contact with and types of friends
- Types of activities with friends

COGNITIVE DEVELOPMENTAL FUNCTIONING
- Tendency to approach or avoid a problem/challenge
- Few friends or "friends with everyone"
- Impaired social behaviors
- Unusual interests, worries, habits or hobbies
- Early developmental delays
- Sensory hyper- or hyposensitivities

PAIN HISTORY
- Time spent in NICU, procedures, injuries, trauma, other illnesses, sensory overload, opioid use

COMORBID SYMPTOMS
- Other pain or sensory sensitivity
- Sleep disturbance, fatigue
- Nausea, decreased appetite, fear of eating, conditioned aversions, vomiting
- Panic symptoms (with/without panic): heart pounding, sweating, shaking, shortness of breath, choking, lump in throat, chest pain, nausea, dizziness, numbness/tingling, chills/hot flashes

PAIN CONSEQUENCES
- Argue with parents or teachers about school, stay home from school, or switch to home schooling
- Parent stays home from work, quits working, or does not return to work
- Parents get along better or argue more
- Child exempt from chores or homework
- Parent more sympathetic to child or more upset with child

ACADEMIC FUNCTIONING
- Perfectionism and/or near perfect grades
- Heavy workload and/or advanced classes
- Learning disorders or subjects that are more challenging or aversive to the child
- Problems with handwriting, homework, tests
- Changes in school or classroom
- Bullies, relational aggression, isolation
- Problems with teachers
- Problems with athletic ability

Table 14–4. (Continued)

EMOTIONAL FUNCTIONING	PERCEIVED STRESSORS
• Alexithymia • Cognitive vs. somatic symptoms of anxiety • Worry; nervousness; fears; anxiety; obsessiveness; perfectionism; test anxiety; panic; excessive concerns about safety, separation, germs, competence, health, symptoms, routines/rituals, and/or symmetry; tendency to catastrophize • Trauma (including prematurity and medical procedures), grief, changes • Depression, suicidality	• School • Peers • Parents • Other relatives • Siblings • Living arrangements • Health • Extra-curricular activities
FAMILY FACTORS	**MAJOR LIFE EVENTS**
• Parental coping, anxiety, depression • Parental illness, pain or disability • Parental understanding of pain • Marital distress, problems in co-parenting, substance abuse, domestic violence • Discipline styles of parents • Problems with siblings or others at home	• Starting new school • Move to new house • Parent remarried • Birth of sibling • Learning to drive • Menstruation • Important birthday • Death and/or illness of family member • Death of a pet

and express their emotions. Those with alexithymia, however, may describe that when something distressing occurs their emotions get confused with one another, they simply feel overwhelmed, or they do not have an emotional reaction at all. The words young children use to describe these experiences vary, but it is helpful for the interviewer to monitor for attempts at such descriptions. Such children may have an easier time identifying the physical symptoms associated with depression, anxiety, or other feeling states (e.g., "I feel tired," or "I am shaky").

The next clinical example demonstrates how to ask young children about alexithymia.

Alexithymia

INTERVIEWER: *For some kids, it is easy for them to figure if they are feeling mad, sad, scared, or happy. Other kids know they are having feelings, but have a hard time figuring out which one, like their feelings all get jumbled together. What type of kid are you? Is it easy or hard for you to figure out how you are feeling?*

CHILD: *I can tell if I am happy … Sometimes I get confused when I have bad feelings.*

INTERVIEWER: *What happens then?*

CHILD: *I cry and I have to go to my room for a time-out to calm down.*

INTERVIEWER: *Does it help you to have a time-out?*

CHILD: *Yeah, but I don't like it when that happens.*

INTERVIEWER: *Do you remember, do your feelings get confused just when you are upset or do your feelings also get confused when you feel calm?*

CHILD: *I think it is mostly when I am upset or when something bad is happening.*

INTERVIEWER: *I see. When that happens, do you notice what your body is doing?*
CHILD: *What do you mean?*
INTERVIEWER: *Well, do you ever notice your heart starts to go faster ... or your breathing changes ... or your hands get sweaty ... or you feel shaky?*
CHILD: *That happens when I have to get my chemo!*

Among those children who are not attending school due to their pain, psychoeducational testing may be needed to identify learning problems (including specific learning disorders, uneven intellectual development, and/or communication disorders) that might be difficult to characterize through interview alone. Although children may be able to describe which academic subjects are easier or more difficult for them, they might not have a sense of what is considered a reasonable level of difficulty when learning a new subject. For example, one child might spend three hours per night on homework to obtain excellent grades and another might spend just one hour per night. Both children might report excellent grades and no trouble learning. A referral for formal testing should be considered if the child is academically behind, has peer problems including poor social problem-solving skills, or has high overall achievement with a difficulty in a particular area. Children in this latter group may be maintaining high (or perfect) grades despite an undiagnosed learning problem, as in the following example.

Undiagnosed Learning Problem
INTERVIEWER: *Would you say school is easy or hard for you?*
CHILD: *Easy, I guess.*
INTERVIEWER: *I see. What makes it easy?*
CHILD: *I am smart. I get perfect grades.*
INTERVIEWER: *Wow. You must do all your homework.*
CHILD: *Yep.*
INTERVIEWER: *What is your best subject?*
CHILD: *Reading.*
INTERVIEWER: *And what is your hardest subject?*
CHILD: *Math. My mom has to do my math homework for me.*
INTERVIEWER: *What happens when you have to take a test?*
CHILD: *My mom talks to my teacher so I can take the test home.*

CLINICAL EXAMPLE
The following case example illustrates several of the concepts we have described.

Jenny is a 9-year-old girl who reported she has had abdominal pain for her entire life, at least for as long as her mother can remember. She had previously undergone comprehensive medical testing, including an upper gastrointestinal (GI) x-ray series with findings consistent with duodenitis. She also had an endoscopy which showed mild inflammation of her lower esophagus. She was treated for reflux with multiple reflux medications and, finally, a Nissen fundoplication surgery was performed in an effort to prevent her chronic reflux. Jenny reported to her mother that she had some improvement after her surgery, but it was only minimal. She continued to have the sensation of nausea and retching. She also complained of continued periumbilical pain which was exacerbated either by eating too fast, eating too much, or not eating at all. After her anti-reflux surgery, she began taking amitriptyline for pain and insomnia. This seemed to improve her ability to initiate sleep, but she continued to wake multiple times through the night, sleep with her mom, and have nightmares. Her mom believes that her marital problems and ongoing on-and-off divorce proceedings are the result of Jenny's medical difficulties.

Jenny then developed several additional symptoms including intermittent blurry vision, dizziness, fainting, headaches, and weakness, as well as her GI symptoms. Because of fear of her fainting at school, the school would send her home when she did not feel well. She had missed an enormous amount of school.

According to her mother, Jenny's symptoms became worse toward the end of her 2nd grade year resulting in her being sent home constantly by the nurse. She has attempted to go back to school on and off but was eventually unable to attend school at all due to the severity of the symptoms. Jenny likes school and wishes that she could attend regularly.

Jenny's mother reported that Jenny met her developmental milestones on time, but she "always had trouble with her gastrointestinal system." She has always been sensitive to physical pain and her temperament has been irritable. She reportedly cried often as an infant, never ate, would not gain weight, and experienced constipation.

Jenny lives with her mother age 35 and a younger sister who is 6 years old. Her mother and father have been separated on and off over the last two years, and have always had a marriage filled with conflict. They have repeatedly discussed divorce and reconciliation. Her father is a firefighter and her mother works part time as yoga teacher. They have four dogs. Jenny reportedly has many friends whom she sees relatively frequently.

There is a family history of a maternal aunt and a maternal grandmother with panic disorders. Jenny's mother has history of untreated chronic abdominal pain.

During the initial assessment, Jenny appeared extremely sad and guarded. She clung to her mother and cried. She was shy and spoke very little. During part of the interview with her mother, Jenny sat on her mother's lap with her head hidden. She did agree to a separate interview, but had a very difficult time separating from her mother. Her mother also had a hard time with the separation. She cried and hugged Jenny throughout. Her mother did try to comfort Jenny and reassure her that she needed to engage in the assessment and treatment in order to get better.

Interview with Jenny

INTERVIEWER: *Hi Jenny. Thank you for meeting with me separately from your mom. You are being brave.*

Jenny smiles.

INTERVIEWER: *Can you tell me, in your words, about your pain? Where is it?*

Jenny points to location above her belly button.

INTERVIEWER: *And I know you have been asked this before, where on this pain thermometer is your pain right now. This side is no pain and this side is the most pain ever.*

Jenny points to level 7 of 10, a moderately high level of pain.

INTERVIEWER: *You are doing a good job, Jenny. What words would you use to tell me about your pain?*

JENNY: *Bad.*

INTERVIEWER: *Bad. Anything else?*
JENNY: *Boring.*
INTERVIEWER: *Boring. Any other words you can think of?*
JENNY: *Yucky.*
INTERVIEWER: *Good words, Jenny. What makes your pain better?*
JENNY: *Nothing.*
INTERVIEWER: *What makes it worse?*
JENNY: *Eating, or sometimes not eating.*
INTERVIEWER: *What do your parents do when you feel yucky or have pain?*
JENNY: *My dad yells. He tells me to eat. My mom cries.*
INTERVIEWER: *What is that like for you?*
JENNY: *Bad. They are getting divorced.*
INTERVIEWER: *What makes you think they are getting divorced?*
JENNY: *They talk about it all the time, and my dad has a girlfriend.*
INTERVIEWER: *How does it make you feel that your parents are getting a divorce and your dad has a girlfriend?*
JENNY: *He doesn't love us.*
INTERVIEWER: *That sounds sad. Do you feel sad about all this?*
JENNY: *Yeah. I cry every day.*
INTERVIEWER: *Would you say this is the worst thing that ever happened to you?*
JENNY: *No, the worst thing was having a tube in my nose. And surgery on my stomach.*
INTERVIEWER: *Those sound pretty bad, too. What about worries? Are you the type of kid that worries about stuff?*
JENNY: *No, I don't worry.*
INTERVIEWER: *What about your parents, do you worry about them?*
JENNY: *I guess I worry about my mom when she is at work.*
INTERVIEWER: *What do you think could happen to her?*
JENNY: *She could die.*
INTERVIEWER: *How would she die?*
JENNY: *I don't know. Maybe an accident.*
INTERVIEWER: *Do you worry about her in the middle of the night when you are trying to sleep?*
JENNY: *No, we sleep together.*
INTERVIEWER: *What about when you are at a sleepover?*
JENNY: *I would miss my mom too much.*
INTERVIEWER: *I see. No sleepovers?*
JENNY: *No way.*
INTERVIEWER: *Have you ever noticed what your body does when you are worried about your mom?*
JENNY: *Sometimes I feel sick.*
INTERVIEWER: *Jenny, thank you so much for talking with me. You did a great job of helping me understand what it is like for you.*

In the dialogue above, the interviewer learned much from Jenny. By thanking her and giving her praise for talking, Jenny became more verbal over the course of the interview. The interviewer was careful to ask "What" questions, to remain neutral, and to ask specific and concrete questions about worry after Jenny denied general worry. Observations of Jenny and Jenny's descriptions were consistent with each other, suggesting she has a depressed mood and significant separation anxiety. Significant stressors and traumatic events were identified, including her physical symptoms, medical events, worries about her mother, and her parents' marital discord. Jenny and her mother both exhibited and described ineffective coping skills. The detailed information the child gives the interviewer allows the interviewer to develop a comprehensive treatment plan.

Based on the clinical interview with Jenny and the information obtained from her mother, a treatment plan designed to address Jenny's multiple problems was implemented. In addition to initiation of medication (citalopram) for her anxiety, depressive symptoms and abdominal pain, treatment involved psychoeducation with the family, family therapy, and intensive individual cognitive-behavioral therapy with Jenny. Consistent contact was maintained with her elementary school to facilitate school reentry. Psychoeducation consisted of regular meetings with the parents and providing the family with handouts regarding parenting, chronic pain, and anxiety. A behavioral contract was developed for implementation at home to help structure the family environment. In family therapy, sessions focused on improving communication among the family members, constructing appropriate boundaries between the parents and the children (i.e., keeping adult information from the children, such as details of the divorce proceedings and finances), increasing independence among family members (including sleeping in separate bedrooms), decreasing conflict, assisting the parents in progressing with divorce proceedings, and assisting in the development of appropriate behavioral routines and structure for the home environment.

Summary

- All pain is biological, and influenced by complex biological processes, cognitive and psychological factors, and social-cultural context.
- Maintaining an organic versus nonorganic etiology of pain dichotomy is misleading and can be harmful, potentially leading to excessive medical intervention or to a lack of empathy for the child with pain.
- Persistent stressors can result in illness and symptoms due to a disturbance in the internal response systems. Among young children with chronic pain, inadequate coping skills can contribute to life impairing distress and disability.
- Common comorbid findings among children with disabling chronic pain include:
  - anxiety disorders,
  - difficulty identifying and expressing emotions,
  - depression, learning problems (even in high achieving children),
  - developmental or communication disorders,
  - social problems,
  - physical or emotional trauma,
  - family illness, and/or
  - prominent family distress.
- Application of the techniques presented in this chapter, together with the developmental guidelines, help the interviewer query the young child about the multiple factors that may contribute to chronic pain.

REFERENCES

Ambuel B, Hamlett KW, Marx CM, and Blumer JL (1992). Assessing distress in pediatric intensive care environments: The COMFORT scale. J Pediatr Psychol 17: 95–109.

Anand KJS (1998). Clinical importance of pain and stress in preterm neonates. Biol Neonate 73: 1–9.

Anand KJS (2000). Pain, plasticity, and premature birth: A prescription for permanent suffering? Nat Med 6: 971–973.

Apley J and Naish N (1958). Recurrent abdominal pains: A field survey of 1,000 school children. Arch Dis Child Apr 33(168): 165–170.

Apley J (1975). The child with abdominal pain (2nd ed.). Oxford: Blackwell Scientific Publications.

Asmundson GJ, Norton PJ, and Veloso F (1999). Anxiety sensitivity and fear of pain in patients with recurring headaches. Behav Res Ther 37(8): 703–713.

Bandura A, Reese L, and Adams NE (1982). Microanalysis of action and fear arousal as a function of differential levels of perceived self-efficacy. J Pers Soc Psychol 43: 5–21.

Bandura A, Taylor CB, Williams SL, Mefford IN, and Barchas JD (1985). Catecholamine secretion as a function of perceived coping self-efficacy. J Consult Clin Psychol 53: 406–414.

Belmaker E, Espinoza R, and Pogrund R (1985). Use of medical services by adolescents with nonspecific somatic symptoms. Int J Adolescent Med Health 1: 150–156.

Bennett-Branson SM and Craig KD (1993). Postoperative pain in children: Developmental and family influences on spontaneous coping strategies. Can J Behav Sci 25: 355–383.

Bhutta AT and Anand KJS (2002). Vulnerability of the developing brain: Neuronal mechanisms. Clin Perinatol 29: 357–372

Biederman J, Rosenbaum JF, Bolduc-Murphy EA, Faraone SV, Chaloff J, Hirshfeld DR, and Kagan J (1993). Behavioral inhibition as a temperamental risk factor for anxiety disorders. Child Adolesc Psychiatr Clin N Am 2: 667–683

Blount RL, Corbin SM, Sturges JW, Wolfe VV, Prater JM, and James LD (1989). The relationship between adult's behavior and child coping and distress during BMA/LP procedures: A sequential analysis. Behavior Therapy 20: 585–601.

Blount RL, Sturges JW, and Powers SW (1990). Analysis of child and adult behavioral variations by phase of medical procedure. Behavior Therapy 21: 33–48.

Boyce W, Barr R, and Zeltzer L (1992). Temperament and the psychobiology of childhood stress. Pediatrics 90: 483–486

Bursch B, Ingman K, Vitti L, Hyman P, and Zeltzer LK (2004). Chronic pain in individuals with previously undiagnosed autistic spectrum disorders. J Pain 5(5): 290–295

Bursch B and Zeltzer LK (2002). Autism spectrum disorders presenting as chronic pain syndromes: Case presentations and discussion. The Journal of Developmental and Learning Disorders 6: 41–48.

Campo JV, Bridge J, Ehmann M, Altman S, Lucas A, Birmaher B, Di Lorenzo C, Iyengar S, and Brent DA (2004). Recurrent Abdominal Pain, Anxiety, and Depression in Primary Care. Pediatrics 113(4): 817–824.

Campo JV, Bridge J, Lucas A, Savorelli S, Walker L, Di Lorenzo C, Iyengar S, and Brent DA (2007). Physical and emotional health of mothers of youth with functional abdominal pain. Arch Pediatr Adolesc Med 161(2): 131–137.

Campo JV, Comer DM, Jansen-McWilliams L, Gardner W, and Kelleher KJ (2002). Recurrent pain, emotional distress, and health service use in childhood. J Pediatr 141: 76–83.

Campo JV, Jansen-McWilliams L, Comer DM, and Kelleher KJ (1999). Somatization in pediatric primary care: Association with psychopathology, functional impairment and use of services. J Am Acad Child Adolesc Psychiatry 38: 1093–1101.

Chacko J, Ford WD, and Haslam R (1999). Growth and neurodevelopmental outcome in extremely-low-birth-weight infants after laparotomy. Pediatr Surg Int 15: 496–499.

Chambers CT, Reid GJ, McGrath PJ, and Finley GA (1996). Development and preliminary validation of a postoperative pain measure for parents. *Pain* 68: 307–313.

Claar RL, Walker LS, and Smith CA (1999). Functional disability in adolescents and young adults with symptoms of irritable bowel syndrome: The role of academic, social and athletic competence. *J Pediatr Psychol* 24: 271–280.

Cohen LL, Lemanek K, Blount RL, Dahlquist LM, Lim CS, Palermo TM, McKenna KD, and Weiss KE (2008). Evidence-based assessment of pediatric pain. *J Pediatr Psychol* 33(9): 939–955.

Compas BE and Boyer MC (2001). Coping and attention: Implications for children's health and pediatric conditions. *J Dev Behav Pediatr* 22: 1–11.

Davison IS, Faull C, and Nicol AR (1986). Research note: Temperament and behavior in six-year-olds with recurrent abdominal pain: A follow up. *J Child Psychol Psychiatry* 27(4): 539–544.

De Gucht V and Heiser W (2003). Alexithymia and somatisation: A quantitative review of the literature. *J Psychosom Res* 54: 425–434.

Di Lorenzo C, Youssef NN, Sigurdsson L, Scharff L, Griffiths J, and Wald A (2001). Visceral hyperalgesia in children with functional abdominal pain. *J Pediatr* 139(6): 838–843.

Duarte MA, Goulart EM, and Penna FJ (1999). Pain threshold and age in childhood and adolescence. *J Pediatr* (Rio J) 75(4): 244–248.

Egger HL, Angold A, and Costello EJ (1998). Headaches and psychopathology in children and adolescents. *J Am Acad Child Adolesc Psychiatry* 37: 951–958.

Emiroglu F N, Kurul S, Akay A, Miral S, and Dirik E (2004). Assessment of child neurology outpatients with headache, dizziness, and fainting. *J Child Neurol* 19(5): 332–336.

Faull C and Nicol AR (1986). Abdominal pain in six-year-olds: An epidemiological study in a new town. *J Child Psychol Psychiatry* 27(2): 251–260.

Forgeron PA, Finley GA, and Arnaout M (2006). Pediatric pain prevalence and parents' attitudes at a cancer hospital in Jordan. *J Pain Symptom Manage* 31:440–448.

Frank NC, Blount RL, Smith AJ, Manimala MR, and Martin JK (1995). Parent and staff behavior, previous child medical experience, and maternal anxiety as they relate to child distress and coping. *J Pediatr Psychol* 20: 277–289.

Fritz GK, Fritsch S, and Hagino O (1997). Somatoform disorders in children and adolescents: A review of the past 10 years. *J Am Acad Child Adolesc Psychiatry* 36: 1329–1338.

Fuss S, Pagé G, and Katz J (2011). Persistent pain in a community-based sample of children and adolescents. *Pain Res Manag* 16(5): 303–309.

Gaffney A, McGrath PJ, and Dick B (2003). Measuring pain in children: Developmental and instrument issues. In: *Pain in Infants, Children and Adolescents*, 2nd Edition, NL Schechter, CB Berde, and M Yaster (eds.). Philadelphia: Lippincott Williams & Wilkins, 128–141.

Garber J, Walker LS, and Zeman J (1991). Somatization symptoms in a community sample of children and adolescents: Further validation of the children's somatization inventory. *Psychol Assess: J Consul Clin Psychol* 3: 588–595.

Garber J, Zeman J, and Walker L (1990). Recurrent abdominal pain in children: psychiatric diagnoses and parental psychopathology. *J Am Acad Child Adolesc Psychiatry* 29: 648–656.

Gil KM, Thompson RJ, Keith BR, Tota-Faucette M, Noll S, and Kinney TR (1993). Sickle cell disease pain in children and adolescents: Change in pain frequency and coping strategies over time. *J Pediatr Psychol* 18: 621–637.

Gil KM, Williams DA, Thompson RJ Jr, and Kinney TR (1991). Sickle cell disease in children and adolescents: The relation of child and parent pain coping strategies to adjustment. *J Pediatr Psychol* 16(5): 643–663.

Goodman JE and McGrath PJ (2003). Mothers' modeling influences children's pain during a cold pressor task. *Pain* 104(3): 559–565.

Groholt EK, Stigum H, Nordhagen R, and Köhler L (2003). Recurrent pain in children, socioeconomic factors and accumulation in families. *Eur J Epidemiol* 18(10): 965–975.

Grunau RE (2000). Long-term consequences of pain in human neonates. In: *Pain in Neonates* KJS Anand, BJ Stevens, and PJ McGrath (eds.). Amsterdam, Netherlands: Elsevier Science, 55–76.

Hicks CL, von Baeyer CL, Spafford P, van Korlaar I, and Goodenough B (2001). The Faces Pain Scale Revised: Toward a common metric in pediatric pain measurement. *Pain* 93: 173–183.

Hodges K, Kline JJ, Barbero G, and Flanery R (1985a). Depressive symptoms in children with recurrent abdominal pain and in their families. *J Pediatr* 107: 622–626.

Hodges K, Kline JJ, Barbero G, and Woodruff C (1985b). Anxiety in children with recurrent abdominal pain and their parents. *Psychosomatics* 26: 859, 862–866.

Hyman PE, Bursch B, Sood M, Schwankovsky L, Cocjin J, and Zeltzer LK (2002). Visceral pain-associated disability syndrome: A descriptive analysis. *J Pediatr Gastroenterol Nutr* 35(5): 663–668.

Jacob E, Hesselgrave J, Sambuco G, and Hockenberry M (2007). Variations in pain, sleep, and activity during hospitalization in children with cancer. *J Pediatr Oncol Nurs* 24(4): 208–219.

Johnston CC and Stevens BJ (1996). Experience in a neonatal intensive care unit affects pain response. *Pediatrics* 98: 925–930.

Kagan J, Reznick J, and Snidman N (1988). Biological bases of childhood shyness. *Science* 40: 167–171.

Keefe FJ, Lefebvre JC, Egert JR, Affleck G, Sullivan MJ, and Caldwell DS (2000). The relationship of gender to pain, pain behavior, and disability in osteoarthritis patients: The role of catastrophizing. *Pain* 87: 325–334.

Larson BS (1991). Somatic complaints and their relationship to depressive symptoms in Swedish adolescents. *J Child Psychol Psychiatry* 32(5): 821–832.

Lester N, Lefebvre JC, and Keefe FJ (1994). Pain in young adults: I. Relationship to gender and family pain history. *Clin J Pain* 10(4): 282–289.

Lester P, Stein JA, and Bursch B (2003). Developmental predictors of somatic symptoms in adolescents of parents with HIV: A 12-month follow-up. *J Dev Behav Pediatr* 24(4): 242–250.

Livingston R (1993). Children of people with somatization disorder. *J Am Acad Child Adolesc Psychiatry* 32(3): 536–544.

Livingston R, Witt A, and Smith GR (1995). Families who somatize. *J Dev Behav Pediatr* 16: 42–46.

Ljungman G, Gordh T, Sorensen S, Sörensen S, and Kreuger A (1999). Pain in paediatric oncology: Interviews with children, adolescents and their parents. *Acta Paediatrica* 88: 623–630.

Logan DE and Scharff L (2005). Relationships between family and parent characteristics and functional abilities in children with recurrent pain syndromes: An investigation of moderating effects on the pathway from pain to disability. *J Pediatr Psychol* 30(8): 698–707.

Lovell D and Walco GA (1989). Pain associated with juvenile rheumatoid arthritis. *Pediatr Clin North Am* 36: 1015–1027.

Manassis K, Bradley S, Goldberg S, Hood J, and Swinson RP (1995). Behavioural inhibition, attachment and anxiety in children of mothers with anxiety disorders. *Can J Psychiatry* 40: 87–92.

McCaig LF and Nawar E (2006). National Hospital Ambulatory Medical Care Survey: 2004 emergency department summary. *Adv Data* (372): 1–29.

McEwen BS and Seeman T (1999). Protective and damaging effects of mediators of stress: Elaborating and testing the concepts of allostasis and allostatic load. *Ann N Y Acad Sci* 896: 30–47.

McGrath PJ, Johnson G, Goodman JT, Schillinger J, Dunn J, and Chapman J (1985). CHEOPS: A behavioral scale for rating postoperative pain in children. In: *Advances in Pain Research and Therapy*, HL Fields, R Dubner, and F Cervero (eds.). New York: New York Raven Press, 395–401

McLendon D, Check J, Carteaux P, Michael L, Moehring J, Secrest JW, Clark SE, Cohen H, Klein SA, Boyle D, George JA, Okuno-Jones S, Buchanan DS, McKinley P, and Whitfield JM (2003). Implementation of potentially better practices for the prevention of brain hemorrhage and ischemic brain injury in very low birth weight infants. *Pediatrics* 111(4 Pt 2): e497–e503.

Merkel SI, Voepel-Lewis T, Shayevitz JR, and Malviya S (1997). The FLACC: A behavioral scale for scoring postoperative pain in young children. *Pediatr Nurs* 23: 293–297.

Merskey H, Albe-Fessard DG, Bonica JJ, Carmon A, Dubner R, Kerr FWL, Lindblom U, Mumford JM, Nathan PW, Noordenbos W, Pagni CA, Sternbach RA, and Sunderland SS. (1979). Pain terms: A list with definitions and notes on usage. *Pain* 6: 249–252.

Mitchell A and Boss B (2002). Adverse effects of pain on the nervous systems of newborns and young children: A review of the literature. *J Neurosci Nurs* 34: 228–236.

Pagé MG, Fuss S, Martin AL, Escobar EM, and Katz J (2010). Development and preliminary validation of the Child Pain Anxiety Symptoms Scale in a community sample. *J Pediatr Psychol* 35(10): 1071–1082.

Petty RE, Southwood TR, Manners P, Baum J, Glass DN, Goldenberg J, He X, Maldonado-Cocco J, Orozco-Alcala J, Prieur AM, Suarez-Almazor ME, and Woo P (2004). International League of Associations for Rheumatology classification of juvenile idiopathic arthritis, 2nd rev., Edmonton, 2001. *J Rheumatol* 31: 390–392.

Piira T, Taplin JE, Goodenough B, and von Baeyer CL (2002). Cognitive-behavioral predictors of children's tolerance of laboratory-induced pain: Implications for clinical assessment and future directions. *Behav Res Ther* 40: 571–584.

Rossi AF, Seiden HS, Sadeghi AM, Nguyen KH, Quintana CS, Gross RP, and Griepp RB (1998). The outcome of cardiac operations in infants weighing two kilograms or less. *J Thorac Cardiovasc Surg* 116: 28–35.

Schanberg LE, Anthony KK, Gil KM, and Maurin EC (2003). Daily pain and symptoms in children with polyarticular arthritis. *Arthritis Rheum* 48: 1390–1397.

Schanberg LE, Keefe FJ, Lefebvre JC, Kredich DW, and Gil KM (1998). Social context of pain in children with Juvenile Primary Fibromyalgia Syndrome: Parental pain history and family environment. *Clin J Pain* 14(2): 107–115.

Sherry DD, Bohnsack J, Salmonson K, Wallace CA, and Mellins E (1990). Painless juvenile rheumatoid arthritis. *J Pediatr* 116: 921–923.

Spierings C, Pocls PJ, Sijben N, Gabreëls FJ, and Renier WO (1990). Conversion disorders in childhood: A retrospective follow-up study of 84 inpatients. *Dev Med Child Neurol* 32: 865–871.

Steinhausen HC, von Aster M, Pfeiffer E, and Göbel D (1989). Comparative studies of conversion disorders in childhood and adolescence. *J Child Psychol Psychiatry* 30(4): 615–621.

Stickler GB and Murphy DB (1979). Recurrent abdominal pain. *Am J Dis Child* 133: 486–489.

Stinson J, Yamada J, Dickson A, Lamba J, and Stevens B (2008). Review of systematic reviews on acute procedural pain in children in the hospital setting. *Pain Res Manag* 13(1): 51–57.

Stuart S and Noyes R (1999). Attachment and interpersonal communication in somatization. *Psychosomatics* 40: 34–43.

Sullivan MJ, Thorn B, Haythornthwaite JA, Keefe F, Martin M, Bradley LA, and Lefebvre JC (2001). Theoretical perspectives on the relation between catastrophizing and pain. *Clin J Pain* 17: 52–64.

Taddio A, Shah V, Gilbert-MacLeod C, and Katz J (2002). Conditioning and hyperalgesia in newborns exposed to repeated heel lances. *JAMA* 288: 857–861.

Tamminen TM, Bredenberg P, Escartin T, Kaukonen P, Puura K, Rutanen M, Suominen I, Leijala H, and Salmelin R (1991). Psychosomatic symptoms in preadolescent children. *Psychother Psychosom* 56(1–2): 70–77.

Taylor S (1999). Anxiety sensitivity: Theory, research and treatment of the fear of anxiety. London: Lawrence Erlbaum Associates.

Thastum M, Zachariae R, and Herlin T (2001). Pain experience and pain coping strategies in children with juvenile idiopathic arthritis. *J Rheumatol* 28: 1091–1098.

Thastum M, Zachariae R, Scholer M, Bjerring P, and Herlin T (1997). Cold pressor pain: Comparing responses of juvenile arthritis patients and their parents. *Scand J Rheumatol* 26: 272–279.

Thomsen AH, Compas BE, Colletti RB, Stanger C, Boyer MC, and Konik BS (2002). Parent reports of coping and stress responses in children with recurrent abdominal pain. *J Pediatr Psychol* 27(3): 215–226.

Tobiansky R, Lui K, Roberts S, and Veddovi M (1995). Neurodevelopmental outcome in very low birthweight infants with necrotizing enterocolitis requiring surgery. *J Paediatr Child Health* 31: 233–236.

Tsao JC, Meldrum M, Kim SC, and Zeltzer LK (2007). Anxiety sensitivity and health-related quality of life in children with chronic pain. *J Pain* 8(10): 814–823.

von Baeyer CL and Spagrud LJ (2007). Systematic review of observational (behavioral) measures of pain for children and adolescents aged 3 to 18 years. *Pain* 127(1–2): 140–150.

Walker LS, Garber J, and Greene JW (1991). Somatization symptoms in pediatric abdominal pain patients: Relation to chronicity of abdominal pain and parent somatization. *J Abnorm Child Psychol* 19(4): 379–394.

Walker LS, Garber J, and Greene JW (1993). Psychosocial correlates of recurrent childhood pain: A comparison of pediatric patients with recurrent abdominal pain, organic illness, and psychiatric disorders. *J Abnorm Psychol* 102: 248–258.

Walker LS, Garber J, Smith CA, Van Slyke DA, and Claar RL (2001). The relation of daily stressors to somatic and emotional symptoms in children with and without recurrent abdominal pain. *J Consult Clin Psychol* 69(1): 85–91.

Walker LS, Smith CA, Garber J, and Van Slyke DA (1997). Development and validation of the Pain Response Inventory for children. *Psychological Assessment* 9: 392–405.

Walker LS and Zeman JL (1992). Parental response to child illness behavior. *J Pediatr Psychol* 17: 49–71.

Wasserman AL, Whitington PF, and Rivara FP (1988). Psychogenic basis for abdominal pain in children and adolescents. *J Am Acad Child Adolesc Psychiatry* 27(2): 179–184.

Whitfield MF and Grunau RE (2000). Behavior, pain perception, and the extremely low-birth weight survivor. *Clin Perinatol* 27(2):363–379.

Zuckerman B, Stevenson J, and Bailey V (1987). Stomachaches and headaches in a community sample of preschool children. *Pediatrics* 79: 677–682.

Pediatric Iatrogenic Trauma Symptoms

Psychological distress in response to serious pediatric illness is common, but surprisingly not universal. A review of research studies of pediatric heart transplant recipients found that only 20%–24% of these children experienced significant psychological distress (Todaro et al. 2000). However, even in children undergoing a simple tonsillectomy, 17% of 89 children followed prospectively had temporary symptoms consistent with a depressive episode (Papakostas et al. 2003).

An area of increasing clinical focus is illness- or treatment-related trauma symptoms (iatrogenic trauma). This type of trauma is caused by frightening experiences in a health-care facility, with medical personnel, and/or with medical procedures. Children with serious illness are often exposed to many potentially traumatizing situations. Examples of potentially traumatizing events include receiving a frightening diagnosis, experiencing painful procedures, coping with unfamiliar and complex medical technologies without the support of a parent, and watching one's body change and abilities decrease. For example, Kean et al. (2006) found that adolescents with asthma, especially those who have experienced a life-threatening event, have high levels of posttraumatic stress symptoms, with 20% meeting diagnostic criteria for posttraumatic stress disorder (PTSD). In a review of research published on children who survived a hospital admission in a pediatric intensive care unit (PICU) (Knoester et al. 2007), trauma symptoms were found in 11 of the 74 evaluated children. Colville, Kerry, and Pierce (2008) found that 33 of 102 (32%) children interviewed three months after discharge from a PICU reported delusional memories and distressing hallucinations. The delusional memories were associated with the duration of time the children were taking opiates and/or benzodiazepines, and with an increased risk of developing posttraumatic stress symptoms.

Rennick et al. (2002, 2004) reported that children who were younger, more severely ill, and who experienced more invasive procedures had significantly more medical fears, a lower sense of control over their own health, and chronic posttraumatic stress symptoms for six months after hospital discharge. Exposure to more medical procedures was the strongest predictor of posttraumatic stress symptoms at six weeks after hospital discharge.

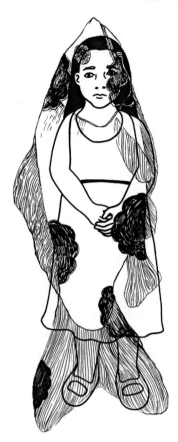

This chapter provides the reader with information on the impact of iatrogenic trauma on the child, developmental considerations, and interviewing techniques for use with traumatized children.

IMPACT OF IATROGENIC TRAUMA ON CHILDREN

The symptoms assessed in most of the pediatric trauma research do not meet criteria for a DSM-IV (American Psychiatric Association 1994) PTSD diagnosis, possibly because nearly half of the diagnostic criteria of this disorder require the child to give verbal descriptions of his/her experiences and internal states. As described in chapter 2 on the developmental guidelines, young children have little ability for introspection, do not spontaneously provide information on their experiences without developmentally oriented questions, and are not always cognizant of their emotions and mood states (see chapters 3–4). Nevertheless, posttraumatic stress symptoms are a significant problem for traumatized children as they are associated with a decrease in normal functioning (Winston et al. 2003). In the following example, a child who does not meet DSM-IV (1994) criteria for PTSD is clearly very debilitated by her trauma symptoms.

Disabling Trauma Symptoms

Six-year-old Sally experienced a very traumatic event six weeks ago when she was emergently prepared for surgery after a bowel perforation. She has severe, recurrent, intrusive petrifying memories of the event. She is afraid to eat because she believes it will happen again. She is extremely distressed psychologically and physically when she thinks of the event, demonstrated by the fact that she vomits several times a day and has lost 6 pounds. She refuses to say the name of the hospital and will not get in the car for her follow-up medical appointment. She denies decreased interest, difficulty remembering important details about the event, restricted range of affect, or foreshortened future. However, she endorses extreme difficulty sleeping and cannot sleep for more than an hour at a time. She also jumps when she hears the slightest sound.

Young children may be especially vulnerable to traumatic experiences and they may be more likely to suffer adverse outcomes because of their (1) limited coping skills; (2) dependence on their primary caregiver to protect them, who, in turn, may also be traumatized and/or impaired (see Knoester et al. 2007); and (3) vulnerable brain, which organizes and develops in response to sensory and emotional experiences during childhood (Perry 2001). In addition to PTSD, research suggests that young traumatized children also appear to be at greater risk for anxiety, depression, attention deficit/hyperactivity (ADHD), and oppositional defiant disorders (ODD) (Scheeringa and Zeanah 2008; Scheeringa et al. 2003). However, since internalizing symptoms (e.g., depression, anxiety, fears) can be difficult to assess in a young child, it could be that the more easily observable symptoms in children with high emotionality and deregulated behavior may cause them to mistakenly receive diagnoses such as ADHD and ODD instead of PTSD (Scheeringa and Zeanah 2008). (See chapters 3–6 covering mood, anxiety, fears, attention, and aggression for additional information on misdiagnosis and mislabeling of young children's behavior.)

It is reasonable to surmise (based mostly on clinical observations) that trauma might also interrupt key developmental tasks, such as emotion regulation, secure attachments, autonomy, and socialization skills (Gaensbauer and Siegel 1995). Supporting these clinical observations, it does appear that children do not simply "grow out of" PTSD (Cohen and Scheeringa 2009). If left untreated, trauma during early childhood can lead to a chronic and unremitting course (Laor et al. 1996, 1997, 2001; Meiser-Stedman et al. 2008; Scheeringa et al. 2005). Research suggests that a secure attachment to a caregiver, healthy parental psychological functioning, effective parenting skills, and cohesive family functioning may protect children from the negative effects of trauma (Laor et al. 1996).

Developmental Considerations

The perceptual, affective, behavioral, and social developmental capacities needed to manifest PTSD symptoms emerge around approximately 7 months of age (Scheeringa and Gaensbauer 2000). The ability to develop autobiographical memories of traumatic events, verbally express trauma narratives, and describe internalizing symptoms evolves after 18 months of age. Therefore, young children can retain memories of traumatic events and exhibit emotional and behavioral trauma symptoms. However, they are limited in their verbal abilities when it comes to describing symptoms. Consequently, the clinical interview of a young traumatized patient can be particularly challenging.

The most commonly reported trauma symptoms among young children include repeatedly talking about the event, distress upon reminders of the trauma, nightmares, new separation anxiety or clinginess, new fears, crying, sleep disturbance, increased motor activity, and more irritability or tantrums (Graham-Bermann et al. 2008; Klein et al. 2009; Levendosky et al. 2002; Saylor et al. 1992; Scheeringa et al. 2001, 2003; Zerk et al. 2009). As illustrated in the example of Sally presented earlier in this chapter, studies with preschoolers using diagnostic interviews have shown that the DSM–IV (1994) PTSD criteria under-identify children with clinically significant and debilitating PTSD symptoms. In fact, the subjective interpretation of a traumatic event, not the objective nature of the event, has been associated with more emotional difficulties (De Young et al. 2011a; Taylor and Weems 2009).

Research has revealed that reexperiencing and hyperarousal symptoms are common among traumatized children, particularly in the first month following the trauma. Yet it is rare for young children to describe or exhibit enough avoidance/numbing symptoms to meet the DSM–IV (1994) or proposed DSM–5 thresholds for PTSD diagnosis (De Young et al. 2011a). Therefore, diagnostic algorithms with developmentally consistent accommodations appear to be more appropriate for young children (De Young et al. 2011b).

It is also important to remember that many preschool children associate pain with punishment and may believe they did something wrong when they are in pain, or that they somehow caused their illness or the injury. For example, they may think back to times when they did not wear a sweater outside, or when they ate too much candy, because these are both transgressions that they were told could lead to illness. It may not occur to a child to share this thought with an adult. Consequently, unless discussed, the child may feel excessive guilt about his/her condition.

Not always able to understand the intentions of others, young children can also get angry or frustrated with the medical provider who is administering a painful procedure. Thus, such a child might feel medical providers are mean and do not care about the child's distress. The child might also become angry at a parent who is perceived as not adequately protecting the child from pain.

Finally, preschool children generally do not understand that some losses are permanent, such as a physical disability. Although this perception might initially be protective, the permanency of certain losses will only become evident to some children over time. Consequently, it is possible that an appreciation for the severity of his or her medical condition may evolve over time as the child matures and develops an awareness of loss permanency.

CLINICAL INTERVIEW

This section describes the assessment of specific symptom constellations, including reexperiencing the trauma, avoidance/numbing, and hyperarousal. It also reviews other features and risk factors that should be evaluated in a child suspected of suffering from iatrogenic trauma.

Reexperiencing

Symptoms associated with reexperiencing the trauma are the most common in young children and may be observed in the young child's play (Gaensbauer 1995). Play suggestive of trauma reexperiencing includes the rigid, repetitive, and anxious reenactment of trauma-related themes (Lieberman and Knorr 2007). The young child may also experience distressing nightmares, with or without trauma-related themes (Scheeringa et al. 2003). Flashbacks and dissociative episodes are much less common, but may be reported by caregivers.

Trauma reminders/triggers can cause intense emotional or physical reactions, such as a child who starts to scream "You're hurting me!" as soon as a clinician wearing a white coat enters the patient room. Such severe reaction to health-care professionals can make a clinical interview itself potentially quite distressing to the child. Avoiding triggers (such as a white coat) and informing the child you do not plan to touch them can be helpful when you interview a child about iatrogenic trauma symptoms.

While symptoms related to re-experiencing are largely behavioral, some children can talk about it. This is illustrated in the following dialogue:

Trauma Reexperiencing
INTERVIEWER: *How are you feeling today, Brooke?*
CHILD: *Tired*
INTERVIEWER: *Did you sleep okay last night?*
CHILD: *Kind of.*
INTERVIEWER: *Does that mean kind of okay and kind of not okay?*
CHILD: *Yeah.*
INTERVIEWER: *I see. What makes it hard to sleep?*
CHILD: *Scary dreams.*
INTERVIEWER: *Oh, I see. Do you remember what happens in your scary dreams?*
CHILD: *I keep dreaming my house is burning down, but I can't find my mom.*
INTERVIEWER: *Wow. That does sound scary. Has that ever happened to you in real life?*
CHILD: *I don't think so.*
INTERVIEWER: *I am glad about that. It is still a scary dream though, isn't it?*
CHILD: *Yes.*
INTERVIEWER: *Have you told your mom about your bad dreams?*
CHILD: *No, she hasn't been spending the night at the hospital.*
INTERVIEWER: *I see. What is it like for you when your mom doesn't spend the night?*
CHILD: *I don't like it.*
INTERVIEWER: *What don't you like about it?*
CHILD: *They hurt me and she isn't there to help me.*
INTERVIEWER: *They hurt you when your mother is not there?*
CHILD: *Yes.*
INTERVIEWER: *Oh my. What happened?*
CHILD: *Well, they might hurt me.*

Some children have difficulty recognizing and/or directly discussing trauma symptoms, but they can readily discuss these topics within the context of play. This is illustrated in the following dialogue:

Using Play to Communicate

INTERVIEWER: *Hi, Brooke. I see you are playing with your doll. Does your doll have an IV?*

CHILD: *Yes. She is sick, in the hospital. Her name is Amy.*

INTERVIEWER: *Are you Amy's mother or her doctor?*

CHILD: *I am her nurse.*

INTERVIEWER: *I see. Can I play with you?*

CHILD: *Yeah; you can hold her down while I change her bandages.*

INTERVIEWER: *Okay. Why do I need to hold her down?*

CHILD: *Because she screams like a little baby.*

INTERVIEWER: *Oh my. What makes her scream?*

CHILD: *It hurts to change bandages. I know.*

INTERVIEWER: *I see. That must be very hard for Amy. Does it hurt when you have your bandages changed?*

CHILD: *No. I am not a baby—I am not allowed to scream.*

INTERVIEWER: *What helps you when you have your bandages changed?*

CHILD: *Watching cartoons.*

INTERVIEWER: *What a good idea. Shall we put cartoons on for Amy?*

CHILD: *It's not time for cartoons.*

INTERVIEWER: *Oh. That is a problem, isn't it? What do you do when you have your bandages changed and it's not time for cartoons?*

CHILD: *Sometimes I scream.*

INTERVIEWER: *I see. Hmm. Have you ever tried playing a game when you have your bandages changed?*

CHILD: *What kind of game?*

INTERVIEWER: *Have you ever seen the one where you try to find as many animals in the picture as you can?*

CHILD: *No.*

INTERVIEWER: *Do you want to try it next time you have your bandages changed and it's not time for cartoons?*

CHILD: *Okay.*

Avoidance/Numbing

Young children may exhibit trauma-related avoidance of discussions of the trauma as well as of people, places, things or situations that remind them of the trauma. They may refuse to get in the car to go to dialysis, avoid taking needed immuno-suppressant medication, or close their eyes and pretend to sleep when clinicians enter their hospital room. Young children may display emotional numbing by withdrawing from family members and from play (Pynoos et al. 2009; Scheeringa et al. 2003). In an extreme state, the child might curl up in a ball and completely refuse to engage. Withdrawal behaviors are unusual in most children and should alert the clinician that trauma (of any kind) could be a factor.

The use of drawing and storytelling can be very effective when assessing trauma in a young child. As illustrated the in the dialogue that follows, it can become derailed if it becomes too personal. It is recommended that the interviewer take the lead from the child when making a sensitive transition from the story to talking about real life.

Use of Drawings to Communicate

INTERVIEWER: *How are you feeling today, Maria?*

Maria doesn't answer.

INTERVIEWER: *Are you feeling like you don't want to talk today?*

Maria doesn't answer.

INTERVIEWER: *Can you tell me what is making it hard to talk today?*

Maria doesn't answer.

INTERVIEWER: *Hmm. Sometimes kids don't want to talk because they are mad, or they are sad, or they don't feel good. Are you feeling one of those things today?*

Maria doesn't answer, but looks interested.

INTERVIEWER: *I have an idea. Instead of talking, let's draw and tell a story about what we draw.*

CHILD: *Okay.*

– –

INTERVIEWER: *Wow, Maria, what a good drawing of the fish. Can you tell me about the fish?*

CHILD: *He's mad.*

INTERVIEWER: *He's mad. What is making him mad?*

CHILD: *They keep taking pieces of him.*

INTERVIEWER: *They keep taking pieces of him. Can you tell me more about that?*

CHILD: *All the time, biopsies, biopsies, biopsies.*

INTERVIEWER: *The fish is mad because he has to have biopsies all the time?*

CHILD: *The poor fish is full of holes—he doesn't want anyone to touch him anymore.*

INTERVIEWER: *That makes sense. I think I would feel that way if I were the fish. What about you?*

CHILD: *Let's draw flowers now.*

In the dialogue above, the interviewer made a helpful choice, to suggest Maria draw and talk about her drawing. This format of communication engaged Maria, who was then able to talk about her drawing and the trauma the fish in her drawing experienced. This successful approach continued until the interviewer prematurely asked Maria a personal question about how she would feel if she were the fish. Maria, unable to tolerate this question, then changed topics and stopped talking about her drawing. This barrier to communication could have been avoided had the interviewer waited for Maria to make a personal statement before asking a personal question.

Hyperarousal

Disturbed sleep, increased irritability, fussiness, temper tantrums, hypervigilance, exaggerated startle response, impaired concentration, and/or increased activity levels are signs of hyperarousal that may be seen in the young traumatized child (Lieberman and Knorr 2007; Pynoos et al. 2009; Scheeringa et al. 2003). Caregivers may be better able than the child to describe these changes in the child. As revealed in the following dialogue between a pediatrician and a young child, hyperarousal might be directly observed in the traumatized child.

A night nurses' tool box
by Aaron Watson

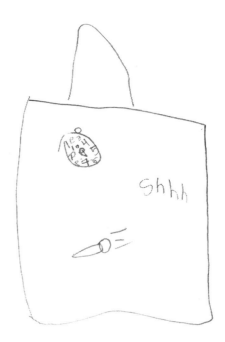

Shhh

Hyperarousal

INTERVIEWER: *How are you feeling today Jimmy?*

CHILD: *Okay. What's that?*

INTERVIEWER: *You mean my stethoscope?*

Jimmy doesn't answer, looks wary.

INTERVIEWER: *You've seen this before. It let's me hear your heart and your breathing.*

CHILD: *What else do you have?*

Jimmy looks around.

INTERVIEWER: *Nothing else. You look worried. Is there something you are worried about?*

CHILD: *You're not going to give me a shot, are you?*

Jimmy looks around.

INTERVIEWER: *Oh. I am sorry if I scared you. I do not plan to give you a shot or touch you at all. I am just here to talk.*

Nurse walks into the room.

CHILD (looking at nurse): *What do you have?*

Other Features

Traumatized young children may also exhibit increases in separation anxiety, clinginess, or physical aggression; developmental regression; and/or new fears with or without obvious links to the trauma (Scheeringa et al. 2003; Zero to Three 2005). In the following example, the child demonstrates aggression as she is using medical play to cope with her own trauma of experiencing multiple needle sticks.

Aggression
INTERVIEWER: *Hi, Brooke. I see you are playing with your doll Amy. Are you giving her a shot?*
CHILD: *No, I am giving her an IV.*
INTERVIEWER: *It looks like you are having to poke her over and over again.*
CHILD: *Yes. She is a hard stick and she is a baby.*
INTERVIEWER: *I see. What is a hard stick?*
CHILD: *I don't know.*
INTERVIEWER: *How long do you have to keeping poking her?*
CHILD: *Until she stops screaming. Amy, be a big girl and hold still.*
INTERVIEWER: *Amy must be very upset. Do you think you are hurting her?*
CHILD: *The sooner she calms down, the sooner it will be over.*
INTERVIEWER: *I see. Do you think it would help if we helped Amy calm down before you poked her again?*
CHILD: *I do not have time to baby her. I have other kids waiting to get IVs. Amy needs to be a big girl and not waste my time.*

General Risk Factors

Additional risk factors that a young child might be able to discuss include prior traumatic experiences, prior posttraumatic stress symptoms, current additional stressors, a history of anxiety, and lack of strong social support.

Prior Traumatic Experiences and Support
INTERVIEWER: *Keenan, we've been talking a lot about what's been happening to you. I know it has been hard and scary.*
CHILD: *Yeah.*
INTERVIEWER: *Before this happened, had you ever been to a hospital?*
CHILD: *Just to see my grandpa.*
INTERVIEWER: *Was that scary?*
CHILD: *No. He was sick, but he got better.*
INTERVIEWER: *Have you ever had anything really bad or really scary happen to you before?*
Keenan doesn't answer, looks away.
INTERVIEWER: *Is it hard to talk about it?*
CHILD: *Yeah.*
INTERVIEWER: *Would you rather make a drawing of it?*
CHILD: *No. I don't like to think about it. I'll tell you, real quick. I saw my dog get hit by a truck.*

INTERVIEWER: *Oh my. What happened?*

CHILD: *He ran into the street and a big truck smashed him. He was dead and squished.*

INTERVIEWER: *And, you don't like to think about it?*

CHILD: *No. Because, then I can't stop.*

INTERVIEWER: *I see. How can you stop?*

CHILD: *If I think about something happy instead.*

INTERVIEWER: *Do you ever talk to your dads about it?*

CHILD: *No. They get mad if I talk about it.*

INTERVIEWER: *I see. So you just try to think of something happy?*

CHILD: *Yeah.*

INTERVIEWER: *Can you do that now?*

CHILD: *Okay. Will you play a game with me?*

INTERVIEWER: *Sure.*

In the dialogue above, the interviewer took the cue from Keenan that he would not be able to tolerate much discussion about seeing his dog hit by a truck. Nevertheless, even in this short conversation, the interviewer was able to discern that this event was very distressing to him, that his fathers do not talk to him about it, and that he avoids thinking about it. The interviewer does not leave the interview until he supports Keenan in his efforts to cope by switching topics and playing a game. Based on this exchange, the interviewer learned that Keenan has a history of a prior traumatic event and limited social support from his parents, both issues worthy of treatment recommendations.

Potentially difficult for a young child to communicate, the following questions can be asked of family members and/or a medical record review might provide information about these potential risk factors:

Information to Collect from Parents
- Did the trauma happen suddenly or was there a gradual onset?
- Is the condition life threatening or life limiting?
- What was the intensity and the length of exposure to traumatic event(s)?
- What is the likelihood of subsequent or ongoing medical/health complications?
- Are the health effects obvious or visible to others?
- What is the degree to which other family members were directly affected?
- What is the degree to which the family had to reorganize their lives and relationships?
- Was the trauma caused by another person? If so, was it intentional or unintentional?
- Is there a history of past trauma, abuse, neglect?

SUMMARY
- Psychological distress in response to serious pediatric illness is common, but surprisingly not universal.
- Iatrogenic trauma is caused by medical personnel or procedures or develops through exposure to the environment of a health-care facility.
- Young children may be especially vulnerable to traumatic experiences and they may be more likely to suffer adverse outcomes because of their limited

> coping skills; their dependence on their primary caregiver to protect them; and their vulnerable brain, which organizes and develops in response to sensory and emotional experiences during childhood.

- Young traumatized children appear to be at greater risk for anxiety, depression, ADHD, and oppositional defiant disorders.
- A secure attachment to a caregiver, healthy parental psychological functioning, effective parenting skills, and cohesive family functioning may protect children from the negative effects of trauma.
- Reexperiencing and hyperarousal symptoms, rather than avoidance or numbing symptoms, are common among traumatized children, particularly in the first month following the trauma. The most commonly reported trauma symptoms among young children include talking about the event, distress upon reminders of the trauma, nightmares, new separation anxiety or clinginess, new fears, crying, sleep disturbance, increased motor activity, and increased irritability or tantrums.
- The use of play, drawing and storytelling can be very effective when assessing trauma in a young child.

REFERENCES

American Psychiatric Association. (1994). *Diagnostic and statistical manual of mental disorders* (4th ed., DSM-IV). Washington, DC: American Psychiatric Association.

Cohen JA and Scheeringa MS (2009). Post-traumatic stress disorder diagnosis in children: Challenges and promises. *Dialogues Clin Neurosci* 11(1): 91–99.

Colville G, Kerry S, and Pierce C (2008). Children's factual and delusional memories of intensive care. *Am J Respir Crit Care Med* 177(9): 976–982.

De Young AC, Kenardy JA, and Cobham VE (2011a). Diagnosis of posttraumatic stress disorder in preschool children. *J Clin Child Adolesc Psychol* 40(3): 375–384.

De Young AC, Kenardy JA, and Cobham VE (2011b). Trauma in early childhood: A neglected population. *Clin Child Fam Psychol Rev* 14(3): 231–250.

Gaensbauer T J (1995). Trauma in the preverbal period: Symptoms, memories, and developmental impact. *Psychoanal Study Child* 50: 122–149.

Gaensbauer TJ and Siegel CH (1995). Therapeutic approaches to posttraumatic stress disorder in infants and toddlers. *Infant Mental Health Journal* 16(4): 292–305.

Graham-Bermann SA, Howell K, Habarth J, Krishnan S, Loree A, and Bermann EA (2008). Toward assessing traumatic events and stress symptoms in preschool children from low-income families. *Am J Orthopsychiatry* 78(2): 220–228.

Kean EM, Kelsay K, Wamboldt F, and Wamboldt MZ (2006). Posttraumatic stress in adolescents with asthma and their parents. *J Am Acad Child Adolesc Psychiatry* 45(1): 78–86.

Klein TP, Devoe ER, Miranda-Julian C, and Linas K (2009). Young children's responses to September 11th: The New York City experience. *Infant Mental Health Journal* 30(1): 1–22.

Knoester H, Grootenhuis MA, and Bos AP (2007). Outcome of paediatric intensive care survivors. *Eur J Pediatr* 166(11): 1119–1128.

Laor N, Wolmer L, and Cohen DJ (2001). Mothers' functioning and children's symptoms 5 years after a SCUD missile attack. *Am J Psychiatry* 158(7): 1020–1026.

Laor N, Wolmer L, Mayes LC, and Gershon A (1997). Israeli preschool children under scuds: A 30-month follow-up. *J Am Acad Child Adolesc Psychiatry* 36(3): 349–356.

Laor N, Wolmer L, Mayes LC, Golomb A, Silverberg D, and Weizman R (1996). Israeli preschoolers under scud missile attacks: A developmental perspective on risk-modifying factors. *Arch Gen Psychiatry* 53(5): 416–423.

Levendosky AA, Huth-Bocks AC, Semel MA, and Shapiro DL (2002). Trauma symptoms in pre-school-age children exposed to domestic violence. *J Interpers Violence* 17(2): 150–164.

Lieberman AF and Knorr K (2007). The impact of trauma: A development framework for infancy and early childhood. *Pediatr Ann* 36(4): 209–215.

Meiser-Stedman R, Smith P, Glucksman E, Yule W, and Dalgleish T (2008). The posttraumatic stress disorder diagnosis in preschool- and elementary school-age children exposed to motor vehicle accidents. *Am J Psychiatry* 165(10): 1326–1337.

Papakostas K, Moraitis D, Lancaster J, and McCormick MS (2003). Depressive symptoms in chil-dren after tonsillectomy. *Int J Pediatr Otorhinolaryngol* 67(2): 127–132.

Perry BD (2001). The neurodevelopmental impact of violence in childhood. In: *Textbook of child and adolescent forensic psychiatry*, D Schetky and E Benedek (eds.). Washington, D.C.: American Psychiatric Press, Inc., 221–238.

Pynoos RS, Steinberg AM, Layne CM, Briggs EC, Ostrowski SA, and Fairbank JA (2009). DSM-V PTSD diagnostic criteria for children and adolescents: A developmental perspective and rec-ommendations. *J Trauma Stress* 22(5): 391–398.

Rennick JE, Johnston CC, Dougherty G, Platt R, and Ritchie JA (2002). Children's psychological responses after critical illness and exposure to invasive technology. *J Dev Behav Pediatr* 23(3): 133–144.

Rennick JE, Morin I, Kim D, Johnston CC, Dougherty G, and Platt R (2004). Identifying chil-dren at high risk for psychological sequelae after pediatric intensive care unit hospitalization. *Pediatr Crit Care Med* 5(4): 358–363.

Saylor CF, Swenson CC, and Powell P (1992). Hurricane Hugo blows down the broccoli: Preschoolers' post-disaster play and adjustment. *Child Psychiatry Hum Dev* 22(3): 139–149.

Scheeringa MS and Gaensbauer TJ (2000). Posttraumatic stress disorder. In: Handbook of infant mental health, 2nd ed., CH Zeanah Jr (ed.). New York, NY: Guilford Press, 369–381.

Scheeringa MS, Peebles CD, Cook CA, and Zeanah CH (2001). Toward establishing procedural, criterion, and discriminant validity for PTSD in early childhood. *J Am Acad Child Adolesc Psychiatry* 40(1): 52–60.

Scheeringa MS and Zeanah CH (2008). Reconsideration of harm's way: Onsets and comorbidity patterns of disorders in preschool children and their caregivers following Hurricane Katrina. *J Clin Child Adolesc Psychol* 37(3): 508–518.

Scheeringa MS, Zeanah CH, Myers L, and Putnam FW (2003). New findings on alternative crite-ria for PTSD in preschool children. *J Am Acad Child Adolesc Psychiatry* 42(5): 561–570.

Scheeringa MS, Zeanah CH, Myers L, and Putnam FW (2005). Predictive validity in a prospective follow-up of PTSD in preschool children. *J Am Acad Child Adolesc Psychiatry* 44(9): 899–906.

Taylor LK and Weems CF (2009). What do youth report as a traumatic event? Toward a develop-mentally informed classification of traumatic stressors. *Psychol Trauma* 1(2): 91–106.

Todaro JF, Fennell EB, Sears SF, Rodrigue JR, and Roche AK (2000). Review: Cognitive and psy-chological outcomes in pediatric heart transplantation. *J Pediatr Psychol* 25(8): 567–576.

Winston FK, Kassam-Adams N, Garcia-España F, Ittenbach R, and Cnaan A (2003). Screening for risk of persistent posttraumatic stress in injured children and their parents. *JAMA* 290: 643–649.

Zerk DM, Mertin PG, and Proeve M (2009). Domestic violence and maternal reports of young children's functioning. *Journal of Family Violence* 24(7): 423–432.

Zero to Three (2005). *Diagnostic classification of mental health and developmental disorders of infancy and early childhood* (DC: 0–3R), rev. ed. Washington, DC.

Pediatric Terminal Illness

Among family members and clinicians alike, one of the most difficult events to cope with is a terminal illness and death of a child. In this chapter, the reader will be provided information about how physical, emotional, environmental, and family factors impact the terminally ill child; how children understand and cope with a terminal illness; and interviewing techniques to help the child communicate about their symptoms and experience.

The majority of the example dialogues in this chapter are between a mental health clinician and a 9-year-old girl with leukemia named Reece. Although children with leukemia are typically successfully treated, Reece and her family have to cope with treatment resistant disease. The example dialogues will illustrate some of the common concerns of terminally ill children and helpful interviewing techniques for these children.

FAMILY AND MEDICAL SETTING CONTEXT

Family Context

The response of a family to the death of a child depends on a number of factors and greatly impacts the experience of the child. For example, parental feelings of guilt (related to earlier medical decision making or to a spiritual belief that they must have done something deserving of such harsh punishment) can impact future medical decision making as well as their communication with the child. Prior experience with death may also impact parental expectations about the process of death for their child. They may feel conflicted in some situations, such as wanting to interact with their dying child but also wanting sufficient pain control, which may be sedating. Another common dilemma is whether or not to spend the last days of the child's life in the hospital or with the dying child at home, which may require the parent to provide a degree of medical care and may expose siblings to the death (Brown et al. 1990). Parents may find that their preferences and/or coping styles are not aligned with each other. For example, one parent may wish to talk about the expected death of the child and the other may wish to hold out hope or concentrate on the day-to-day tasks (Koocher and MacDonald 1992).

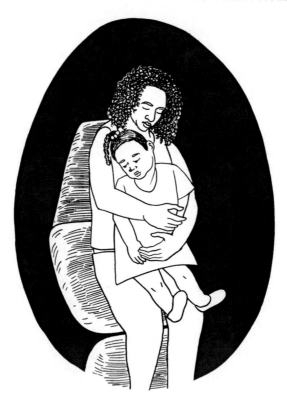

Likewise, parents may experience differing trauma symptoms. Some may be flooded with memories or reminded of the impending death by seemingly innocent objects or events, causing them distress. Others may feel numbed or blunted (Kazak, et al. 1997; Stuber et al. 1996). Preexisting family or marital conflict, or psychopathology in a parent, can exacerbate all of these problems (Davies et al. 1994). The dying child may also be aware that his/her parents are under additional stress due to the needs of other family members, job requirements, the loss of time for enjoyable activities, and the financial strain associated with lost work and medical expenses.

Medical Setting Context

Many factors related to the medical setting can complicate communication with a terminally ill child. For example, disagreements may occur within the medical team or between the medical team and the child and/or family about whether the death of the child is inevitable or not. Cultural or philosophical differences may influence beliefs and, therefore, communication. Physicians responding to the parents' hope to cure their child may conflict with nurses who believe that the child's quality of life is being adversely impacted by futile medical interventions. Medical teams sometimes view deeply religious families, who remain hopeful for a miracle, as being in "denial." Family members may request that clinicians withhold potentially upsetting information from the child to protect the child from distress. The dying child and family members might have different treatment goals, such as the level of pain control desired.

CHILDREN'S DEVELOPMENTAL UNDERSTANDING OF DEATH

Until relatively recently it was believed that children did not comprehend death and that it would be harmful to attempt to discuss it with them (Kastenbaum and Costa 1977). This led to the practice of hiding poor prognostic information from children (Evans 1968). In the mid-1960s, it was discovered that children sensed the concern and anxiety of their doctors and parents, despite these caretakers attempts to be cheerful (Vernick and Karon 1965). It appeared that it was parental discomfort that inhibited seriously ill children from discussing death (Kubler-Ross 1969). Research then revealed that children as young as six years old understand the life-threatening nature of their leukemia (Spinetta 1973).

Despite individual differences, research has revealed that a child's understanding of the meaning of death normally correlates with the age of the child (Christ 2000). In a qualitative study related to grief, 157 children (3 to 17 years old) who lost a parent to cancer demonstrated these developmental differences. The 3 to 5-year-old group exhibited regressive behaviors and irritability. They were initially confused by the absence of the parent and exhibited separation anxiety, only understanding the permanence of the separation over time. The 6-to-8 year old children immediately understood the permanence of the death. In addition to their common grief symptoms including sadness and anger, they also had worries about their potential role in the death. For example, they were prone to worrying that their bad behaviors or wishes had brought about the death. Sometimes confusing to adults, they were also able to joyfully reminisce about the deceased parent. By contrast, the 9 to 11-year olds were most likely to request detailed factual information about the death, but were typically avoidant of strong emotions.

ASSESSMENT: GENERAL APPROACH

Facilitating communication about the topic of death can significantly improve the quality of life for the child and family. To determine the level of understanding of the child and the types of communication transpiring between child and parent, assessment should include discussions with both the child and parents. Parent education may be warranted for those parents who are being unrealistically withholding of information and for those who are overwhelming their child with too much or overly complex information. Likewise, the level of involvement of the child in medical decision making should be assessed and modified if it is inappropriate to the developmental level and medical status of the child. Parents often have questions about how to communicate with their child about death and are grateful to discuss this topic.

Family

Although parents may ask clinicians to withhold a poor prognosis from a child, qualitative studies suggest that children often have awareness that they may soon die (Sourkes 1996). Available evidence also suggests that parents may regret not discussing death with their child. One study (Kreicbergs et al. 2004) demonstrated that none of the 147 parents (of 429 parents whose children had died of cancer) who talked with their child about death regretted having had the discussion. On the other hand, 69 of the 258 parents who did not discuss death with their child regretted not having done so.

Open family communication about death allows concerns to be shared and appropriate actions to be taken. For example, supportive interventions might include increased emotional support for the child, reassurance about unwarranted worries, and practical assistance with problems perceived by the child (Share 1972). Open communication about death has been found to help prevent depression and reduce isolation for the child (Kellerman et al. 1977; Vernick and Karon 1965). While not forcing the children to deal with more than they are ready to handle, parents and caregivers are encouraged to bring up the topic rather than wait for the child to initiate questions (Koocher 1974; Spinetta 1980).

Medical Team

Open and sensitive communication about death by physicians with pediatric patients and their parents is also correlated with parents' ratings of high quality end-of-life care. Mack and colleagues (2005) telephone surveyed 144 parents of children who received cancer treatment. Parents rated care higher when physicians clearly told them what to expect at the end of life, communicated in a sensitive and caring manner, and appropriately communicated with the child.

Child

Effective communication with a child requires an assessment of his or her developmental level and understanding of the situation (such as of the medical diagnosis and concept of death). Communication should then be based on the child's ability to comprehend the information, using words and concepts the child understands. Some children use words they have heard from staff or parents without an appreciation of their meaning, making it important to ask the child to provide detailed explanations in order to fully assess his/her understanding. It is also important to avoid causing secondary fears in an attempt to provide explanations. For example, equating death with unending sleep can cause a fear of going to sleep (Stuber and Mesrkhani 2001). Interviewers should remember that a neutral stance, together with positive reinforcement for communicating, and the use of "What" questions typically yield the best information.

ASSESSMENT: ASSESSING DEVELOPMENTAL LEVEL AND UNDERSTANDING

The interviewer can assess the child's developmental level and understanding of their situation with the following techniques and questions.

1. Asking the Child to Explain His or Her Medical Condition

Explaining Medical Condition

INTERVIEWER: *What are you doing in the hospital, Reece?*

CHILD: *I am getting chemo.*

INTERVIEWER: *That is interesting. What is the chemo for?*

CHILD: *For my leukemia.*

INTERVIEWER: *Leukemia. What is leukemia?*

CHILD: *I think it is cancer.*

INTERVIEWER: *What makes you think that?*

CHILD: *Because one of the nurses said that.*

INTERVIEWER: *Oh. And what do your parents say?*

CHILD: *They say I have leukemia.*

INTERVIEWER: *Okay. Can you help me understand? What is leukemia?*

CHILD: *My parents said it means my blood is sick and the chemo will fix it.*

INTERVIEWER: *Well, that is interesting. Is that the same thing or different than cancer?*

CHILD: *I don't know. I think you die when you have cancer.*

INTERVIEWER: *Hmm. Do you think you might die?*

CHILD: *Maybe.*

INTERVIEWER: *Is that something you would like to ask your parents about?*

CHILD: *Maybe.*

INTERVIEWER: *Some kids worry about asking that question. Are you worried about asking it?*

CHILD: *Maybe.*

INTERVIEWER: *Can you help me understand—what are your worries about asking your parents if you might die?*

CHILD: *They might get mad or maybe they will cry.*

INTERVIEWER: *I see. Does that sometimes happen?*

CHILD: *Yes. My mom cries a lot.*

In the dialogue above, the interviewer was careful to use "What" rather than "Why" questions and did not assume that the child knew the meaning of the words she used to explain why she was in the hospital. This approach revealed that the young girl was somewhat confused about both her diagnosis and her prognosis. It further revealed that she was uncomfortable about asking her parents for additional explanation due to her concerns about upsetting them. It is important that the interviewer refrain from giving his/her own definition or clinical information to the child, recognizing that it would be more helpful to everyone if efforts were made to improve the communication among the family members.

2. Asking the Child about His or Her Beliefs about Death

Beliefs About Death

INTERVIEWER: *Earlier you told me that you thought you might die. Do you remember?*

CHILD: *Yes.*

INTERVIEWER: *Can you help me understand—what happens when you die?*

CHILD: *You go in a box and they bury you and have a party.*

INTERVIEWER: *Hmm. Do you know someone who died?*

CHILD: *Yes. My grandma died and she went into a box. They buried her in the ground and then there was a party.*

INTERVIEWER: *What did you think about that?*

CHILD: *I don't know.*

INTERVIEWER: *What else happened when your grandma died?*

CHILD: *Hmm. Let me think. Lots of people cried, but not everyone. We don't go to her house anymore. Her cat lives with us now.*

INTERVIEWER: *What do you think would happen if you died?*

CHILD: *I don't know. Maybe I would go in the box with my grandma?*

INTERVIEWER: *That is a good question. Is that something you would like to ask your parents about?*

CHILD: *Maybe.*

In the dialogue above, the interviewer was again respectful of the family belief system by refraining from giving opinions about what happens when someone dies. The interviewer was careful to encourage continued discussion by remaining neutral and asking questions, rather than attempting to reassure the child that she is unlikely to die. While it is sometimes tempting to provide such reassurances, the child may interpret this as a message that it is not appropriate to discuss fears or thoughts about death. This dialogue revealed that, commensurate with her developmental level, the child's thoughts about what happens when you die are concrete in nature. She was not thinking about the spiritual aspects of this question as an older child might. Instead, she was literally thinking about where her body would be placed. Because this might not be what her parents would be expecting her to be thinking about, the interviewer identified another potentially important opportunity to improve family communication.

3. Assessing the Child's Concerns Related to Death or Dying

Concerns Related to Dying

INTERVIEWER: *Remember yesterday when we had the meeting with your doctor and your parents?*

CHILD: *Yes.*

INTERVIEWER: *Do you remember what they said?*

CHILD: *Yes.*

INTERVIEWER: *Can you remind me—what did they say?*

CHILD: *They said that my chemo isn't fixing my leukemia.*

INTERVIEWER: *That's right. What else did they say?*

CHILD: *They said that maybe I will have stronger chemo or maybe I will die.*

INTERVIEWER: *That's right. What do you think about that?*

CHILD: *I don't know.*

INTERVIEWER: *Sometimes kids get confused or mad or sad. What about you?*

CHILD: *No.*

INTERVIEWER: *Sometimes kids get worried. Can you tell me if you have any worries?*

CHILD: *Maybe it will hurt.*

INTERVIEWER: *You think it might hurt?*

CHILD: *Yes.*

INTERVIEWER: *I see. That is important. Thank you for telling me. What other worries do you have?*

CHILD: *I have to feed my grandma's cat.*

INTERVIEWER: *Oh. Hmm. Are you worried that you won't be able to feed the cat if you die?*

CHILD: *Yes.*

INTERVIEWER: *I see. That is important, too. Thank you for telling me. What other worries do you have?*

CHILD: *Nothing.*

INTERVIEWER: *No more worries?*

CHILD: *No.*

INTERVIEWER: *Okay. Well, maybe I will ask you again tomorrow to see if you thought of more. Is that okay?*

CHILD: *Okay.*

INTERVIEWER: *So, earlier you said that you are worried it might hurt. Is that right?*

CHILD: *Yes.*

INTERVIEWER: *Can you tell me more about that?*

CHILD: *When I had chemo before, I got sores in my mouth and I couldn't eat.*

INTERVIEWER: *Oh, I see. And are you worried that might happen again?*

CHILD: *Yes.*

INTERVIEWER: *What do you think we could do about that?*

CHILD: *Nothing.*

INTERVIEWER: *Maybe we could think of some things. Shall we try?*

CHILD: *Okay.*

In the dialogue above, by asking the child to recount what had been communicated to her, the interviewer was careful not to assume that the child remembered or understood what was conveyed to her during the meeting with her doctor and parents. The interviewer normalized having an emotional reaction to this information by informing the child that other children sometimes have fears or worries. The interviewer encouraged further communication by thanking the child for sharing the information and by letting her know that the interviewer would ask her about her worries again tomorrow. While her parents are likely to be feeling extremely distraught and helpless as a result of the new information that the chemo is not working, it might be possible to successfully address the patient's concerns to improve her emotional state and quality of life.

ASSESSMENT: ASSESSING SYMPTOMS

Common Symptoms in the Terminally Ill Child

A study designed to inventory physical, psychological, and social symptoms of children with terminal cancer queried 32 parents of children who had died 1 to 3 years earlier (Theunissen et al. 2007). Near the end of life, the children had an average of

6.3 (SD 2.7) physical symptoms and 3.2 (SD 2.2) psychological symptoms. The most common physical symptoms were pain, poor appetite, fatigue, lack of mobility, and vomiting. The most common psychological symptoms were sadness, difficulty talking to their parents about their illness and death, and fear of being alone. Goldman and associates (2006) also studied symptoms in 185 children (4 months to 19 years old) who had died from cancer, finding that anxiety was one factor that was significantly associated with the presence of pain.

ANXIETY

Factors that may contribute to symptoms of anxiety in a dying child include alarming physical symptoms (such as difficulty breathing or pain), the hospital environment, separation from family members (including pets), distressing and/or painful procedures, upsetting emotional responses of others, fear of death, and/or lack of accurate, age-appropriate, and consistent information. Signs/symptoms of anxiety might include an increase in clinginess, crying, or tantrums; physical symptoms, including pain, nausea, or other symptoms; withdrawal from friends, family, or peers; seemingly oppositional behavior; and intense fear or guilt. Sometimes children simply quietly worry without any observable sign of anxiety. As illustrated below, it is important to take a careful assessment to discern the source of a child's anxiety.

Anxiety

INTERVIEWER: *How are you feeling today Reece?*
CHILD: *Okay.*
INTERVIEWER: *What is happening today?*
CHILD: *A bone marrow.*
INTERVIEWER: *Oh. Is that easy or hard for you?*
CHILD: *It depends.*
INTERVIEWER: *What does it depend on?*
CHILD: *If I am awake or asleep.*
INTERVIEWER: *I see. What do you like better?*
CHILD: *I like to be awake as long as they do not give me the medicine that makes me feel funny.*
INTERVIEWER: *What is better about being awake?*
CHILD: *I won't end up on the breathing tube.*
INTERVIEWER: *What makes you think that could happen?*
CHILD: *When I was sick, they put me asleep and I woke up on the breathing tube.*
INTERVIEWER: *I see. Is that something you have been thinking about?*
CHILD: *Yeah. I don't want to do that again.*
INTERVIEWER: *Have you told anyone that you have been thinking about that?*
CHILD: *No.*
INTERVIEWER: *What if you found out that you would be awake for your bone marrow today?*
CHILD: *Happy!* (pauses) *But, I don't want that medicine that makes me feel funny.*
INTERVIEWER: *What medication is that?*
CHILD: *My mom knows.*

INTERVIEWER: *Okay. How about if I find out the name of the medication from your mom and then we ask your doctor to come in to your room so we can ask about the bone marrow and the medicine?*

CHILD: *Okay.*

Medical staff and parents often assume that a child would prefer to be sedated for a procedure or provided with an antianxiety medication. However, the dialogue above demonstrates the anxiety that can accompany such well-meaning interventions. It is not uncommon for young children to dislike antianxiety medications because it can make them feel out of control and/or strange. Likewise, because young children might not realize that some procedures are less complicated, shorter in duration, or conducted when the child is less medically vulnerable, they might believe that all procedures carry the same risk (such as waking up on a ventilator). Again, in the above example, the interviewer encouraged communication by not prematurely attempting to reassure the child and sought to improve communication with the medical team by suggesting they speak with the team together.

DEPRESSION/SUICIDALITY

While terminally ill children may sometimes feel sad or depressed as they grieve multiple losses, few suffer from a major depressive disorder (Kersun and Shemesh 2007). As described in chapter 3 on Mood, Anger, and Irritability, the most difficult task may be in determining if depressive symptoms are explained by the medical condition. This raises the question about whether or not to include somatic symptoms of depression (such as changes in appetite or weight, poor sleep, and lack of energy) in the assessment. However, because existing evidence suggests that depression in children is often either unrecognized or undertreated, it is recommended that somatic symptoms be considered symptoms of depression even if they could be medically explained (Ortiz-Aguayo and Campo 2009). Because medically ill children normally maintain an interest in engaging in pleasurable activities, a lack of interest in such activities is a particularly notable symptom in a child who would otherwise be considered well enough to play (Kersun and Shemesh 2007).

Little data exists to suggest that terminally ill children are at greater risk to be suicidal. One study of suicide in childhood cancer patients failed to find any evidence that children are likely to commit suicide as a means to control the dying process (Kunin et al. 1995). Although completed suicides are uncommon among young children, it is important to ask about suicidal thoughts. Assessment of suicidality includes specifically asking about suicidal thoughts and plans, differentiating between fantasy and intention to act, assessing incidents of past self-injurious behaviors, discerning what the child thinks would happen if suicide were attempted/achieved, concepts and experiences of death, depression and other affects, family situations, and environmental situations (Pfeffer 1986). As is evident in the following dialogue, it is important not to assume the child has suicidal ideation simply because she talks about death or wanting to be dead.

Suicidality vs. Talking about Death and Dying

INTERVIEWER: *Hi, Reece. How are you doing?*

CHILD: *Fine.*

INTERVIEWER: *Your nurse asked me to come see you because she said you mentioned to her that you wish you were dead. Did you say that to her?*

CHILD: *Yeah.*

INTERVIEWER: *I see. Can you tell me more about how you are feeling?*

CHILD: *I don't know.*

INTERVIEWER: *Do you still wish you were dead?*

CHILD: *I don't like taking my pills.*

INTERVIEWER: *I see. So, you wish you were dead so you don't have to take your pills?*

CHILD: *Yeah.*

INTERVIEWER: *What about at other times? Do you wish you were dead when you are not taking your pills?*

CHILD: *Of course not!*

INTERVIEWER: *So, you only wish you were dead when you have to take your pills?*

CHILD: *Right.*

INTERVIEWER: *When you have to take your pills and you wish you were dead, do you ever think about doing something to hurt yourself or to kill yourself?*

CHILD: *Like what?*

INTERVIEWER: *I don't know. I want to know what you think during those times.*

CHILD: *I just think I have to take my pills fast so I can play.*

INTERVIEWER: *What a good idea.*

Insomnia

Causes of insomnia in children with terminal illness are multiple and might be difficult to determine. Nevertheless, the assessment of insomnia in young children should include possible contributing factors including physical symptoms (such as pain or itching), anxiety (often mild), depression, sleeping during the day instead of at night, bladder or bowel distention, frequent urination, night sweats, or withdrawal from barbiturates or benzodiazepines (Doyle 1984; Levy and Catalano 1985). Environmental factors that might contribute to insomnia include position of the bed, noise, lighting, and room temperature.

Pain

Pain can be the result of the child's terminal illness, medical treatments and procedures, as well as injuries or disorders that are independent of the terminal illness. As described in chapter 14, pain can be classified by location on the body, duration (acute, recurrent, chronic), intensity (mild, moderate, severe), cause (malignant vs. nonmalignant disease), and presumed physiological mechanism. A biopsychosocial model can be used for the evaluation and treatment of all types of pain (see Chapter 14).

It is important to remember that children may not exhibit the "pain behaviors" that one would expect to see in adults. Children experiencing pain are very good at distracting themselves with play or withdrawing into sleep. Children who lack verbal skills may be unable to express that they are in pain and appear irritable or oppositional. Some children may not complain of pain because they assume their pain is being managed as well as possible, they may not want to admit they have pain for fear that will lead to medical procedures, or they may not have the skills of assertion to report pain to their clinicians. Family member's experience with or fear of addiction to pain medications can also result in a child's reluctance to admit they are in pain.

ASSESSMENT: ALTERNATE TECHNIQUES

It can be particularly challenging to assess a child who is nonverbal, a child with parents who do not wish open communication to transpire, and/or a child with an unclear prognosis. Nevertheless, there are a variety of assessment techniques that can allow the child to indirectly communicate beliefs, concerns, and symptoms. In addition to using art, music, games, or storytelling to communicate, it is important for the interviewer to be aware that even children sometimes speak in simple metaphor, as illustrated in this clinical example.

Terminal Illness and Metaphor
INTERVIEWER: *How are you feeling today, Reece?*
CHILD: *Good.*
INTERVIEWER: *Remember the other day when we were talking about worries?*
CHILD: *Yeah.*
INTERVIEWER: *I thought I would check in with you to see if you thought of any more worries. What other worries have you been thinking about?*
CHILD: *Nothing.*
INTERVIEWER: *Oh, I see. What have you been thinking about?*
CHILD: *I am going on a trip soon.*
INTERVIEWER: *That is interesting. Where are you going?*
CHILD: *I am going on a boat.*
INTERVIEWER: *I see. I am very interested in hearing about your trip. Will you tell me about it?*
CHILD: *I haven't told anybody.*
INTERVIEWER: *Oh? And why haven't you told anybody?*
CHILD: *Because my parents will miss me if I go.*
INTERVIEWER: *I see. Do you think you would want to say good-bye to them?*
CHILD: *Yes. They don't like saying good-bye.*
INTERVIEWER: *Hmm. How do you know that?*
CHILD: *They just like talking about happy things.*
INTERVIEWER: *I see. Do you think you'd like to draw them a picture or write them a letter? If you want, maybe you could say good-bye in it.*
CHILD: *Okay.*

A common challenge when interviewing a young child about death and dying is that the child may ask the interviewer questions. In many circumstances, it may not be appropriate to directly answer questions posed by the child. Examples might be questions with answers that depend upon family belief systems, such as what happens after death, or questions with answers that best come from someone else, such as how much longer the hospitalization will be. It is important that the interviewer not feel the need to answer all questions posed by a child during an interview as in the next clinical example.

Managing Rather Than Answering Questions
INTERVIEWER: *Hi, Reece. What are you doing?*
CHILD: *Drawing a picture of my grandma.*
INTERVIEWER: *Oh. Is that the grandma who died?*

CHILD: *Yes.*

INTERVIEWER: *Have you been thinking about her?*

CHILD: *Yes.*

INTERVIEWER: *Hmm. What have you been thinking about?*

CHILD: *Do you think she can hear me?*

INTERVIEWER: *What an interesting question. What do you think?*

CHILD: *I don't know.*

INTERVIEWER: *Would you like to talk to her?*

CHILD: *Yes.*

INTERVIEWER: *What would you like to say to her?*

CHILD: *I don't know.*

INTERVIEWER: *Would you like to ask your parents if they think she can hear you?*

CHILD: *My mom said my grandma can hear me.*

INTERVIEWER: *I see. And, what have you been thinking?*

CHILD: *I can't see her and I can't hear her.*

INTERVIEWER: *Oh, I see. That is confusing, isn't it? Do you think maybe she can hear you even though you can't hear her?*

CHILD: *I don't know.*

INTERVIEWER: *Sometimes kids wonder what it will be like if they were to die. What about you—do you wonder about that kind of thing?*

CHILD: *No. My mom said not to talk about it.*

INTERVIEWER: *I see. Why doesn't she want you to talk about it?*

CHILD: *It makes her cry.*

INTERVIEWER: *What would you want to ask your mom if you could?*

CHILD: *Do you have to go to school in heaven?*

INTERVIEWER: *That is an excellent question. Could you ask your dad that question?*

CHILD: *Maybe.*

INTERVIEWER: *Do you want to pretend with me? We can practice asking and then maybe I can help you ask your dad. What do you think?*

CHILD: *That sounds good.*

In the dialogue above, the interviewer was careful not to impose any beliefs upon the child but instead encouraged the child to talk about her questions and helped her problem-solve how to communicate with her family about her questions. When asked directly by the child if her grandmother could hear her, the interviewer responded that the child asked a good question and then asked her what she thought. This exchange reveals the child's confusion about the information she has from her mother (that her grandmother can hear her even though the child cannot see or hear the grandmother). Additionally, it becomes apparent that the child does not feel she can discuss what happens after death with her mother.

SUMMARY

- Young children can understand the life-threatening nature of a serious illness.
- Facilitating communication about the topic of death can prevent depression and reduce isolation for the child, and improve the quality of life of the child and family.

- The most common physical symptoms among terminally ill children are pain, poor appetite, fatigue, lack of mobility, and vomiting.
- The most common psychological symptoms are sadness, difficulty in talking to their parents about their illness and death, and fear of being alone.
- It can be particularly challenging to assess a child who is nonverbal, a child whose parents do not wish open communication to transpire, and/or a child with a prognosis that is unclear or might be terminal. Art, music, games, or storytelling can assist a young child in communicating.
- It is important that the interviewer not feel the need to answer all questions posed by a terminally ill child, especially if the question relates to a cultural family belief or to a topic better answered by another member of the medical team.

REFERENCES

Brown P, Davies B, and Martens N (1990). Families in supportive care: II. Palliative care at home: A viable care setting. *J Palliat Care* 6(2): 8–16.

Christ GH (2000). Impact of development on children's mourning. *Cancer Pract* 8: 72–81.

Davies B, Reimer JC, and Martens N (1994). Family functioning and its implications for palliative care. *J Palliat Care* 10(1): 29–36.

Doyle D (1984). Palliative symptom control. In: *Palliative Care: The Management of Far-Advanced Illness*, D Doyle (ed.). Philadelphia, PA: The Charles Press, 95–116.

Evans AE (1968). If a child must die. *N Engl J Med* 278: 138–142.

Goldman A, Hewitt M, Collins GS, Childs M, and Hain R (2006). United Kingdom Children's Cancer Study Group/Paediatric Oncology Nurses' Forum Palliative Care Working Group. Symptoms in children/young people with progressive malignant disease: United Kingdom Children's Cancer Study Group/Paediatric Oncology Nurses Forum survey. *Pediatrics* 117(6): e1179–e1186.

Kastenbaum R and Costa PT (1977). Psychological perspectives on death. *Ann Rev Psychol* 28: 225–249.

Kazak AE, Barakat LP, Meeske K, Christakis D, Meadows AT, Casey R, Penati B, and Stuber ML (1997). Post traumatic stress symptoms, family functioning, and social support in survivors of childhood leukemia and their mothers and fathers. *J Consult Clin Psychol* 65(1): 120–129.

Kellerman J, Rigler D, and Siegal SE (1977). Psychological effects of isolation in protected environments. *Am J Psychiatry* 134: 563–565.

Kersun LS and Shemesh E (2007). Depression and anxiety in children at the end of life. *Pediatr Clin N Am* 54(5): 691–708, xi.

Koocher GP (1974). Talking with children about death. *Am J Orthopsychiatry* 44: 404–411.

Koocher GP and MacDonald BL (1992). Preventive intervention and family coping with a child's life-threatening or terminal illness. In: *Family Health Psychology. Series in Applied Psychology: Social Issues and Questions*, TJ Akamatsu, MA Parris Stephens, SE Hobfoll, and JH Crowther (eds.). Washington, DC: Hemisphere Publishing Corp., 67–86.

Kreicbergs U, Valdimarsdottir U, Onelov E, Henter JI, and Steineck G (2004). Talking about death with children who have severe malignant disease. *N Engl J Med* 351(12): 1175–1186.

Kubler-Ross E (1969). *On Death and Dying.* New York: Macmillan Publishing Co.

Kunin HM, Patenaude AF, and Grier HE (1995). Suicide risk in pediatric cancer patients: An exploratory study. *Psycho-oncology* 4: 149–155.

Levy MH and Catalano RB (1985). Control of common physical symptoms other than pain in patients with terminal disease. *Semin Oncol* 12(4): 411–430.

Mack JW, Hilden JM, Watterson J, Moore C, Turner B, Grier HE, Weeks JC, and Wolfe J (2005). Parent and physician perspectives on quality of care at the end of life in children with cancer. *J Clin Oncol* 23(36): 9155–9161.

Ortiz-Aguayo R and Campo JV (2009). Treating depression in children and adolescents with chronic physical illness. In: *Treating Child and Adolescent Depression*, JM Rey and B Birmaher (eds.). Baltimore, MD: Lippincott, Williams and Wilkins, 295–309.

Pfeffer CR (1986). *The Suicidal Child.* New York: Guiliford Press.

Share L (1972). Family communication in the crisis of a child's fatal illness: A literature review and analysis. *Omega* 3: 187–201.

Sourkes BM (1996). The broken heart: Anticipatory grief in the child facing death. *J Palliat Care* 12: 56–59.

Spinetta JJ (1973). Anxiety in the dying child. *Pediatrics* 52: 841–845.

Spinetta JJ (1980). Disease-related communication: How to tell. In: *Psychological Aspects of Childhood Cancer*, J Kellerman (ed.). Springfield, IL: Charles C Thomas, 190–224.

Stuber ML, Christakis D, Houskamp BM, and Kazak AE (1996). Post trauma symptoms in childhood leukemia survivors and their parents. *Psychosomatics* 37: 254–261.

Stuber ML and Mesrkhani VH (2001). "What do we tell the children?" Understanding childhood grief. *West J Med* 174(3): 187–191.

Theunissen JM, Hoogerbrugge PM, van Achterberg T, Prins JB, Vernooij-Dassen MJ, and van den Ende CH (2007). Symptoms in the palliative phase of children with cancer. *Pediatr Blood Cancer* 49(2): 160–165.

Vernick J and Karon M (1965). Who's afraid of death on a leukemia ward? *Am J Dis Child* 109: 393–397.

PART V

Brief Review and Next Steps

"Guess What? We Are Done. You Are Such a Good Talker and Did Such a Great Job!"

"GUESS WHAT?"

Both knowledge and skill acquisition increase competence and facilitate the transition from being a novice to an expert clinical interviewer. The reader is now equipped with developmental guidelines to better understand how young children understand and respond to questions about their illness, emotions, difficulties, problems, and worries, and how they use language to formulate and communicate their thoughts and feelings to the listener. By demonstrating how to use developmentally sensitive interview tools, the clinical examples have provided the reader with techniques for interviewing young children about difficult and complex topics.

However, knowledge and skill acquisition is only the first step. The reader should next practice the interview techniques in order to become a competent interviewer. In this concluding chapter, we briefly review the developmental guidelines and recommended interview techniques. The chapter concludes with practical suggestions to accelerate the transition to expert interviewer.

REVIEW OF DEVELOPMENTAL GUIDELINES

Children Are Not Little Adults

- The language and communication skills of young children differ from those of adults in both quality and quantity.
- The developmental guidelines address the main features of these qualitative and quantitative differences.

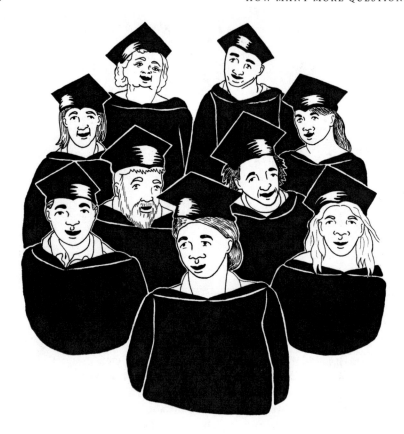

Young Children Do Not Initiate Speech with Strangers

- Young children rarely engage in spontaneous speech with professionals.
- The responsibility is, therefore, on the professional to encourage the child to talk and provide the information needed.
- This can be done using developmentally sensitive interview techniques.

Young Children Do Not Elaborate on the Topic of Conversation

- Children speak in mini-paragraphs of one to two sentences (nondiscursive speech).
- If a child's response yields insufficient detail, the interviewer should help the child elaborate by using "What" and "How" questions, expressing empathy, repeating a statement the child made followed by a pause, making an open-ended statement, asking an open-ended question, and praising the child for answering questions.

Young Children Are Concrete Thinkers

- Concrete thinking refers to thoughts about actions, objects, events, and people rather than thoughts about ideas and concepts.

- Children with concrete thinking understand and use the literal rather than the figurative meaning of words, phrases, sentences, and idioms.
- Young children express their thoughts and ideas concretely.
- Adults are often unaware of the abstract nature of how they speak, as well as of young children's limited abstract thinking and understanding of abstract language.
- The interviewer should use concrete language and reformulate abstract concepts into action-based language by using verbs.

Young Children Have Poor Perception of Chronology and Time

- Children are poor historians regarding the onset, duration, frequency, and recurrence of their symptoms.
- Interviewers should refrain from asking children to tell them "When," "How long," and "How often" they have symptoms.
- Parents are usually better informants on the chronology, evolution, and duration of physical and externalizing behavior symptoms but not of internalizing symptoms.

Young Children Try to Please Adults

- Young children typically want to make a good impression on adults. During an interview they achieve this by answering questions.
- Interviewers should structure their questions so that young children can successfully provide them with the needed information.
- Young children do not volunteer that they are having difficulty understanding adults or that they do not know the answer to a question an adult asks.
- Signs suggesting a child has difficulty answering questions include repeated "Yes/No," "Maybe," "I'm not sure," "I guess," "A little," and "Because" answers, and repeatedly confirming the last option in a series that the interviewer presents in a question.
- When young children appear to be "uncooperative" or "resistant" to answering questions in an interview, the interviewer should determine what has made the child feel she/he cannot answer the questions.
- Children are happy to help adults understand what they are trying to communicate as they usually are in the reverse role and need adults to help them.
- Some children fear that sharing their painful feelings, such as sadness, anger, and fear, might make their parents angry. Therefore, whenever possible, young children should be interviewed separately from their parents in order to obtain valid information on their emotions and behavior.

Young Children Figure Out What the Interviewer Wants to Hear

- Children respond to leading questions that either maximize or minimize pathology with the information the interviewer seems to want to hear.
- Interviewers should ask neutral questions to avoid leading the child to answer in the way the child thinks she/he is supposed to answer.

Young Children Talk If They Feel Comfortable

- Establishing good rapport during an interview helps an interviewer obtain optimal information from young children.
- The interviewer should refrain from telling the child that the interviewer will ask the child questions. Rather, the interviewer might tell the child he wants to chat with the child in order to get to know the child and understand what brought the child to the professional today.
- Children do not feel good about their negative behaviors. Hearing from the interviewer that the parent is talking about their negative behaviors is not conducive to making the child feel comfortable and willing to talk about them.
- The interviewer should only approach "sensitive" topics such as the parents' main complaint once the child appears comfortable enough to talk about it.
- The interviewer should let the child continue with activities during the interview unless they distract her so that she cannot speak.
- Providing the child with positive feedback about being a good talker and expressing empathy for the information obtained from the child encourage the child to talk more.
- Interviewers should not repeat questions the child does not answer (or answers inadequately) because this indirectly communicates the interviewer's dissatisfaction with the child.
- The interviewer should reformulate the question, change the topic, or offer some concrete response options if the child does not understand or has trouble answering the question because the topic is emotionally laden. Alternatively, the interviewer can revisit the question when the child appears to be feeling more comfortable and talkative.
- An interview of a young child should last no longer than 60 minutes.
- The interviewer should "normalize" behaviors such as sadness, anger, and fears that might make the child embarrassed.

Young Children Do Not Like "Why" Questions

- "Why" questions require children to tap into their analytical skills and come up with a logical answer.
- Rather than posing "Why" questions, interviewers can obtain information on causality by asking young children "What" questions or by providing response options.
- "How" questions can be useful as long as they do not require the child's reasoning.
- "What" and "How" questions also help children elaborate on the topic of conversation.

"Yes/No" Questions Yield Minimal Information

- When adults are presented with a "Yes/No" question during an interview, they usually elaborate on their answer. However, young children do not spontaneously elaborate.

- "Yes/No" questions can be cumbersome and prolong the interview because of the need to validate the child's answers through additional "What" and "How" questions.

Use Simple Sentences to Ask Short Focused Questions

- Young children respond well to questions made up of short simple sentences.
- When an interviewer uses complex sentences to ask a question, a child's response might address only part of the question.
- Follow-up validation questions of answers to complex sentences are necessary to determine to which part of the question the child responded and to prevent the interviewer from reaching erroneous conclusions.

Work on Understanding

- The interviewer is the child's communication assistant.
- The interviewer should listen and pay attention to every word the child says during the interview.
- The interviewer should get a sense of a child's cognitive and linguistic developmental level and communicate with the child at that level.
- If the interviewer has some difficulty comprehending what the child is saying, she should explain to the child that, to best help the child, everything he tells her is important.
- The interviewer should thank and compliment the child for this help.
- The interviewer should have no preconception of what the child should be saying in answer to a question.
- When faced with what appears to be derailment of conversation, the interviewer should always determine if the child is trying to provide the interviewer with information that the child deems important, is avoiding the topic, or has not understood the question.
- The interviewer should consider that a child might have linguistic, cognitive, or both linguistic and cognitive problems if he appears to struggle to understand her questions.

NEXT STEPS: HOW TO BECOME AN EXPERT INTERVIEWER

Interviewers interested in achieving an expert level of competence now require targeted and sustained interviewing experience. Expert interviewers possess a consistent and proficient ability to apply the knowledge presented in this book in a flexible manner to complex real world cases. As the reader practices the guidelines and associated techniques presented in this book, the nuances of expert interviewing will be learned and refined over time. Those who master the ability to expertly interview and correctly interpret the communication of young, medically ill children will also be well equipped to apply these skills to other challenging interviews, such as with older individuals with cognitive limitations.

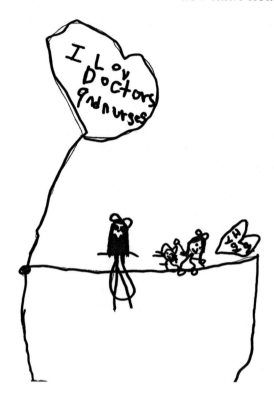

Interviewer Checklist

✓ Interview child separately from the parent if possible.

✓ Use literal concrete language.

✓ Speak in simple sentences without clauses to ask short focused questions.

✓ Word questions at the appropriate developmental level and using words the child understands.

✓ Use "What" and "How" questions.

✓ Avoid "Yes/No," "When," "How long," "How often," and "Why" questions.

✓ Leave sensitive topics to later in the interview when rapport is strengthened.

✓ Allow the child to continue to engage in an activity that does not demand the child's full attention.

✓ Carefully listen to the child and ask for the child's help if you do not understand.

✓ Let the child know that he is doing a good job or is a good talker periodically during the interview if the child is, in fact, talking.

✓ When the child's does not answer a question, reformulate the question or provide a choice of response options.

✓ Express empathy for the child's difficulties and problems.

✓ When possible "normalize" negative feelings to encourage the child to talk about them.

✓ Direct "When" and frequency questions to parents.

There are a number of additional things the reader can do to accelerate the transition to expert interviewer. First, interviewing practice that includes detailed feedback and expert mentorship contributes to the development of complex knowledge structures that can be generalized to other situations. Second, review of videotaped recordings conducted by the interviewer help sensitize him/her to the technical strengths and weaknesses of the interview. Third, a deliberate progression from more basic interviews to more complex and challenging interviews will enable a helpful progression of mastery. Fourth, adaptation of the suggested techniques to the specific learning and practice style of the reader will allow for better integration and adoption of effective methods. Finally, as expertise develops, the reader will become less consciously dependent on the specific techniques presented in this book, will be increasingly intuitive when conducting a challenging interview, and will surely develop additional effective interview techniques.

CPSIA information can be obtained at www.ICGtesting.com
Printed in the USA
BVOW042054060912

299479BV00003B/5/P

9 780199 843824